Magnetic Resonance Angiography
Techniques, Indications and Practical Applications

G. Schneider • M.R. Prince • J.F.M. Meaney • V.B. Ho (Eds)

Magnetic Resonance Angiography

Techniques, Indications and Practical Applications

Foreword by
E. J. Potchen

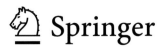
Springer

Günther Schneider
Department of Diagnostic and
Interventional Radiology
Saarland University Hospital
Homburg/Saar, Germany

Martin R. Prince
Departments of Radiology
Weill Medical College
of Cornell University and
Columbia College
of Physicians and Surgeons
New York, USA

James F. M. Meaney
MRI Department
St. James's Hospital
Dublin, Ireland

Vincent B. Ho
Department of Radiology
and Radiological Sciences
Uniformed Services
University of the Health Sciences
Bethesda, USA

Anatomical drawings by **Nadia Simeoni** (Turin, Italy)

ISBN 88-470-0266-4 Springer Milan Berlin Heidelberg New York

Library of Congress Control Number: 2004116342

Springer is a part of Springer Science+Business Media
springeronline.com
© Springer-Verlag Italia 2005
Printed in Italy

Cover design: Simona Colombo, Milan
Typesetting: Compostudio, Cernusco s/N (Milan)
Printing and binding: Arti Grafiche Nidasio, Assago (Milan)

Foreword

Those of us involved in the development of magnetic resonance angiography (MRA) in the late 1980's could hardly envision the routine application of MRA in every MR facility everyday. In those years there was spectacular development of many new MR clinical applications. Many pioneering researchers investigated various strategies exploiting the effects of blood flow on the MR signal to optimize clinical MRA. Remarkable successes were demonstrated in rapid succession. It is very alluring to attempt to catalogue the significant contributions in the founding of clinical MRA here, but that comprehensive effort is best relegated to the careful authors of history chapters in MRA books. The following are a few milestones from the early years of MRA development.

The first research meeting devoted to Magnetic Resonance Angiography was hosted by Roberto Passariello in L'Aquila, Italy in 1989. This meeting gave rise to formation of the MR Angio Club, which then held its first meeting at Michigan State University in 1990. Those were the days when three-dimensional phase contrast MRA would take some 19 hours from the time the patient entered the magnet until images could be seen: one hour to acquire the image and 18 hours of overnight image post processing. Seeing vasculature for the first time in 3D display is when we all realized the future potential clinical utility of MRA. Computational capabilities of modern equipment have reduced the delay to a few seconds. Post processing now has taken a more central role in the communication of enormous amounts of data with less cumbersome two- or three-dimensional projections. Many variations on the MRA theme have been presented over the ensuing 15 years. For example, Dennis Parker developed the 3D multi-slab time-of-flight MRA technique which remains in routine clinical use to this day. Pulse sequence design plays a major role in the continuing advancements in the field, most notably as a consequence of more sophisticated and novel k-space filling strategies.

The work of Kent Yucel and Martin Prince at the Massachusetts General Hospital in 1992 brought gadolinium-enhanced MR angiography to clinical utility. The first-pass dynamic contrast-enhanced MRA method provides robust and reproducible imaging results that have propelled the adoption of MRA into wider clinical use. This advance reliably produced images of sufficient quality to replace invasive catheter-based x-ray contrast angiography for most diagnostic purposes. Now it is possible to acquire a high quality MR angiography study in seconds.

The advent of very high field clinical scanners operating at 3.0 Tesla is now reinvigorating earlier non-contrast methods. 3.0 T MRA benefits from two key phenomena: (1) the signal to noise of 3.0 T is twice that of the 1.5 T, offering the opportunity to either increase the spatial resolution or to shorten scan times by up to a factor of four, and, (2) the longer T1's of tissues at 3.0 T, ~20-40% higher than 1.5T, provides better background suppression, additional inflow enhancement, and improved contrast-to-noise. Magnetization transfer would normally be considered SAR prohibitive at 3.0 T, but novel pulse sequence design has overcome this challenge. The appropriate choice of imaging parameters can minimize artifacts and exploit T1 prolongation at higher fields for better quality MRA. The availability of scanners capable of parallel imaging along with growing availability of multi-channel coils is coincident with the arrival of these very high field scanners. The future potential is bright. Early results using these combined advancements for intracranial MRA yield spatial resolution exceeding invasive DSA and provide breathtaking visualization of small arteries such as the lenticulostriate vasculature. The efficiency of the parallel imaging approach will also compliment the quality of time resolved MR techniques.

Where are we going from here? Highest on the cardiovascular unresolved diagnostic problem list is the localization and assessment of unstable plaques. Specifically designed contrast agent(s) targeted to a characteristic within the unstable plaque will comprise a Molecular MRA procedure. Clearly, the domain of MRA is embracing this pursuit. It is remarkable that, after 15 years, we are still searching for the MRA technique to completely assess atherosclerotic disease in the carotid artery. Insights into bifurcation disease drive the quest for ever higher spatial resolution and SNR to assess plaque structure and stability. In this regard, carotid MRA will require integrating the newly available technologies to achieve the necessary spatial resolution.

Fusion MRA can refer to integrated multidimensional presentations of the MRA anatomy merged with other anatomical and functional modalities. We are now beginning to see presentations of MR and CT coronary angiography fused with PET myocardial perfusion images, or short-axis MR cardiac function images, or MR perfusion reserve images. Fusing MRA images to MRI, MR CSI, PET, nuclear medicine, and CT will be a direction that this field will take.

How do we optimize the present value of this potential? The persistent need for comprehensive outcome studies for MRA endures. A persistent challenge, however, is that by the time these studies are completed, the best methods may well have changed. We, who are students of changing technologies and best practices, need to further develop methodologies to measure the merits of alternative diagnostic procedures. MRA has the probability of becoming the standard for future non-invasive technologies.

This book presents an up-to-date treatise, a much needed presentation of the current practice of clinical MRA fully exploiting the benefits of dynamic contrast-enhanced MRA. I compliment Drs. Schneider, Prince, Meaney, and Ho on producing a definitive work on a rapidly moving target. This book provides the benchmark against which future MRA developments will be measured.

E. James Potchen, M.D.
Department of Radiology
Michigan State University, USA

Contents

SECTION VI – Abdomen

SECTION VII – Peripheral Arteries

SECTION VIII – MR Angiography in Pediatrics

SECTION IX – MR Venography

SECTION X – Clinical Implications

Contributors

Nicoletta Anzalone
Department of Neuroradiology
Scientific Institute and University
H. S. Raffaele
Milan, Italy

Martin Backens
Centre for Radiology
Work Group
Magnetic Resonance Imaging
Saarland University Hospital
Homburg/Saar, Germany

Baocheng Chu
Department of Radiology
University of Washington
Seattle, USA

William R. Corse
Department of Radiology
Doylestown Hospital
Doylestown, USA

Milind Y. Desai
Departments of Medicine
and Radiology
Johns Hopkins University
Baltimore, USA

Philippe C. Douek
Department of Radiology
CREATIS, CNRS Research Unit
(UMR 5515) affiliated to INSERM
Lyon, France

Peter Fries
Department of Diagnostic and
Interventional Radiology
Saarland University Hospital
Homburg/Saar, Germany

Jeffrey P. Goldman
Mount Sinai School of Medicine
Dept. of Radiology
New York, USA

Mathias Goyen
University Medical Center
Hamburg-Eppendorf
Hamburg, Germany

Marcela Hernández-Hoyos
Department of Radiology
CREATIS, CNRS Research Unit
(UMR 5515) affiliated to INSERM
Lyon, France

Vincent B. Ho
Department of Radiology
and Radiological Sciences
Uniformed Services
University of the Health Sciences
Bethesda, USA

Robert A. Lookstein
Division of Interventional Radiology
Mount Sinai Medical Center
New York, USA

Miles A. Kirchin
Worldwide Medical Affairs
Bracco Imaging SpA
Milan, Italy

Michael V. Knopp
Ohio State University Hospital
Columbus, USA

Jeffrey H. Maki
Department of Radiology
University of Washington
Seattle, USA

Kenneth R. Maravilla
Department of Radiology
University of Washington
Seattle, USA

James F. M. Meaney
MRI Department
St. James's Hospital
Dublin, Ireland

Maciej Orkisz
Department of Radiology
CREATIS, CNRS Research Unit
(UMR 5515) affiliated to INSERM
Lyon, France

F. Scott Pereles
Department of Radiology
Feinberg School of Medicine
Northwestern University
Chicago, USA

Martin R. Prince
Departments of Radiology
Weill Medical College
of Cornell University and
Columbia College
of Physicians and Surgeons
New York, USA

Stefan G. Ruehm
David Geffen School
of Medicine at UCLA
Los Angeles, USA

Bernd Schmitz
Department of Radiology
University Hospitals Ulm
Ulm, Germany

Günther Schneider
Department of Diagnostic and
Interventional Radiology
Saarland University Hospital
Homburg/Saar, Germany

Stefan Schoenberg
Institute of Clinical Radiology
University Hospitals
Grosshadern
Munich, Germany

Roland Seidel
Department of Diagnostic and
Interventional Radiology
Saarland University Hospital
Homburg/Saar, Germany

Matthias Stuber
Departments of Medicine,
Radiology and Electrical Engineering
Johns Hopkins University
Baltimore, USA

Armando Tartaro
Department of Clinical Sciences and
Bioimaging
Section of Radiological Sciences
G. D'Annunzio Foundation
University of Chieti (Pescara), Italy

Martin N. Wasser
Department of Radiology
Leiden University Medical Center
Leiden, The Netherlands

Honglei Zhang
Department of Radiology
Weill Medical College
of Cornell University
New York, USA

SECTION I

Technical Background

I.1

Unenhanced MR Angiography

Martin Backens and Bernd Schmitz

Introduction

In conventional x-ray digital subtraction angiography (DSA), administration of contrast agent is necessary in order to depict blood vessels. After arterial catheterization and injection of an iodinated contrast agent, two-dimensional projection images of the lumen of the vessel are acquired from chosen angles. For every new projection this procedure has to be repeated. The availability of 3D rotational angiography and CT angiography may help to overcome this problem but at the expense of high radiation doses.

Unenhanced MR angiography (MRA) differs from DSA and other angiographic techniques in that blood vessels are depicted non-invasively in the absence of contrast agent injection. Unenhanced MR techniques allow the acquisition of 3D datasets or stacks of 2D images that contain all vessels in the volume of interest. The acquired images included in the 3D data set are called "source images". Projectional angiographic displays of the vessel are subsequently reconstructed from the data using the maximum intensity projection (MIP) postprocessing algorithm, which generates angiogram-like images from the entire dataset or a subset from any desired viewing angle without the need for further measurement. Another advantage of MRA versus x-ray angiography derives from the fact that extravascular tissue is depicted together with the vessels, thereby permitting the correlation of blood flow abnormalities with associated soft tissue pathologies (Table 1).

Contrast in MR images depends principally on static tissue parameters: longitudinal relaxation time T1, transverse relaxation time T2, and proton density. In addition, the MR signal is sensitive to flow and movement which frequently leads to artifacts in MR imaging. MR angiographic sequences, however, use flow-induced signal variations to depict blood vessels or even to obtain quantitative information about blood flow in terms of velocity and direction.

Unenhanced MRA comprises those MR techniques that rely solely on flow effects. Unlike contrast-enhanced MRA (CE MRA) and x-ray angiography, which depict the vessel lumen filled with contrast agent, it is just the **movement** of blood that is seen in the unenhanced MR-angiogram.

Flow effects can be grouped into two fundamentally different categories:

- **Amplitude effects (time-of-flight)** Blood flowing into or out of a chosen slice has a different **longitudinal** magnetization compared to stationary spins, depending on the duration of stay (time-of-flight) in the slice.
- **Phase effects** Blood flowing along the direction of a magnetic field gradient is subject to changes of its **transverse** magnetization compared to stationary spins.

In principle, both flow phenomena are effective simultaneously leading either to a decrease or an increase of the MR signal depending on the type of sequence used. Appropriate sequence techniques have been developed which emphasize one of the flow effects and suppress the other. Typically, MR angiography techniques are designed in such a way that flowing blood produces **hyper**intense signal while the background signal from stationary tissue remains largely suppressed ("bright-blood" angiography). Alternatively, flowing spins can be

Table 1. Advantages of MR angiography

Advantages of MR angiography
No ionizing radiation
Non-invasive
Any projection can be reconstructed from 3D datasets
Depiction of extravascular tissue
Flow quantification in terms of velocity and direction

Table 2. Techniques of unenhanced MR angiography

Time-of-Flight (TOF) angiography:
Flow changes longitudinal magnetization
Phase-contrast (PC) angiography:
Flow changes transverse magnetization

made to appear **hypo**intense compared to the stationary background ("black-blood" angiography). In the clinical setting "bright-blood" MRA is the more widely accepted of the two techniques. There are two approaches to performing "bright-blood" MRA: time-of-flight (TOF) and phase-contrast (PC) angiography (Table 2).

Although intravenous contrast administration is not required in TOF and PC MRA, it can be applied in certain situations to improve vessel contrast.

Since unenhanced MRA is based on complex flow phenomena, physiological conditions of flow in the vascular territory of interest are of major importance for the applicability of the method. Advantageous conditions are found especially in the vessels of the brain because of the nearly laminar flow in this territory. Moreover, flow is largely constant during the heart cycle (Fig. 1), making ECG triggering unnecessary for imaging of brain vessels. The high velocity of arterial flow (50–100 cm/sec) provides good vessel-background contrast and moderate acquisition times. In clinical routine, unenhanced MRA has proven to be a robust and versatile method for non-invasively imaging of brain vessels (circle of wilis, sagittal sinus). In addition, this technique is also suitable for depicting extracranial carotid arteries and short segments of peripheral vessels (e.g. lower leg).

A major limitation of unenhanced MRA, however, is a susceptibility to signal loss in areas of turbulent or very slow flow. In severe cases, this may lead to a misdiagnosis of the pathologic condition (stenosis, aneurysm). Additionally, TOF and PC angiography are highly sensitive to motion artifacts. Although motion artifacts often arise due to patient movement because of the need for relatively long acquisition times, they may also occur in areas of very pulsatile flow such as that occurring in the carotids, aorta, and especially, in the peripheral arteries, and in the thoracic and abdominal regions due to breathing and heart actions. Whereas ECG triggering may reduce or eliminate those artifacts associated with pulsatile flow, the availability of contrast-enhanced MR angiography (CE MRA) has largely made unenhanced MRA redundant for most vascular territories outside of the brain. However if unenhanced MRA techniques are performed, a thorough understanding of the underlying physical and technical mechanisms is prerequisite to performing imaging and to correctly interpreting the acquired angiograms.

Understanding Flow Effects

Outflow-related Signal Loss (washout effect, T2 flow void)

When images are obtained with a spin-echo (SE) pulse sequence, blood flowing at a high velocity perpendicular to the imaging plane produces a weaker signal than the surrounding stationary tissue. This phenomenon is caused by the washout of flowing spins from the slice during the imaging process.

Spin-echo techniques are characterized by a sequence of slice-selective 90° and 180° radio frequency (RF) pulses. Only those tissue components that are affected by both pulses can provide an MR signal. Moving material, such as blood in the vessels, flowing through the excited slice at a suffi-

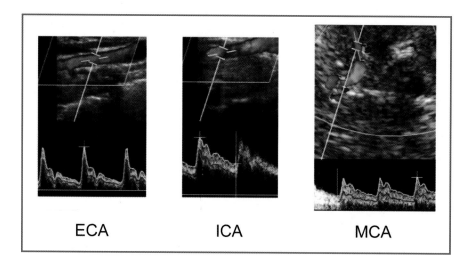

ECA   ICA   MCA

Fig. 1. Comparison of flow profiles in the external carotid artery (ECA), the internal carotid artery (ICA) and the middle cerebral artery (MCA). There is very pulsatile flow in the ECA. However, in the intracranial vessels, the variation of flow during heart cycle is much less pronounced [Courtesy of Steffi Behnke, MD, Dept. of Neurology, Saarland University Hospitals]

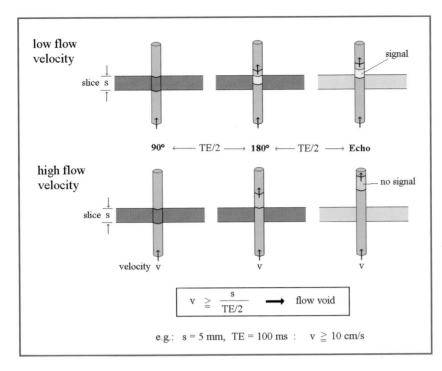

Fig. 2. In spin-echo sequences, blood flowing out of the measured slice in the time between 90°- and 180°-radiofrequency pulses leads to signal loss

ciently high velocity, is affected by only one of these pulses, and therefore does not contribute to the MR signal. This is the so-called flow void (Fig. 2).

The intensity of the vascular signal declines with

- decreasing slice thickness, s,
- increasing echo time, TE,
- increasing flow velocity, v.

If the blood flow velocity is so high that all spins leave the slice between the 90°- and 180°-pulses ($v \geq s/(TE/2)$), there will be no signal at all and the vessel will appear dark.

Spins flowing within the imaging plane are not affected by this phenomenon.

The washout effect is observed only for SE sequences and is most pronounced on T2- weighted imaging because of the long echo times used. With gradient-echo (GRE) techniques, the echo is refocused without a 180° pulse simply by reversing the imaging gradients. Since only one RF pulse is needed to form an echo, the washout effect does not occur.

With standard SE sequences the washout effect provides valuable and reliable information about blood flow. The absence of a flow void on T2-weighted imaging should be considered as indicative of very slow flow or even occlusion of the vessel (Fig. 3). On the other hand, occlusion of the vessel can be excluded if a flow void is present.

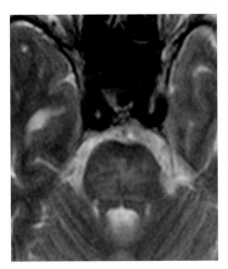 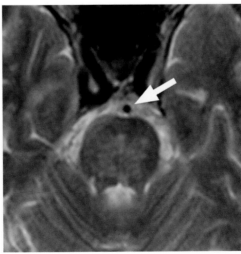

Fig. 3. Axial T2-weighted spin-echo image of the pons region. *Left:* Missing flow void in the basilar artery indicates thrombosis of the vessel. *Right:* After thrombolysis, the vessel (*arrow*) appears dark due to restored flow

Inflow-related Signal Enhancement (Inflow Effect)

Although the signal of blood flowing quickly **out** of the measured slice is reduced with SE sequences, under certain circumstances the opposite effect may occur: spins flowing **into** the slice may generate a higher signal than the surrounding tissue. This effect is referred to as inflow enhancement.

On T1-weighted imaging, contrast is generated by repeated RF pulses that are applied with a time interval (repetition time, TR) that is shorter than the T1 relaxation time of the tissue (typically TR < 700 msec). As a result, the tissue components are saturated unequally, depending on their individual T1 times. This is the basis of T1-weighted image contrast (Fig. 4). Irrespective of flow effects, blood in the vessels would appear hypointense on a normal T1-weighted image due to its relatively long T1 time.

The signal emitted by the tissue diminishes when the TR is reduced. With GRE sequences, repetition times shorter than 50 msec can be achieved. This allows the majority of non-moving spins to become saturated, thus minimizing the background signal.

Spins outside the excited slice (or volume) are not influenced by the RF pulses. Consequently, blood entering into the slice being imaged is fully relaxed, experiencing not more than a few excitations on its way through the slice. As a result, flowing blood gives rise to considerably higher signal intensity relative to that of the saturated spins in the stationary tissue. This effect is called "inflow enhancement" or "flow-related enhancement" (Fig. 5).

The signal intensity of flowing blood increases with:
- decreasing slice thickness s,
- increasing flow velocity v.

If the blood flow velocity is so high that all vessel spins are replaced by unsaturated spins in the time interval TR (i.e. v > s/TR), flow enhancement is maximal and the vessel appears bright on a gray or black background (Fig. 6).

Although the inflow effect occurs both with SE and GRE sequences, SE sequences are not practical for the TOF method because the competing washout effect (see above) tends to overbalance the inflow effect at higher flow velocities, leading to decreased flow signal.

Consequently, flow-related enhancement using GRE sequences to produce bright-blood images is the basis of time-of-flight angiography.

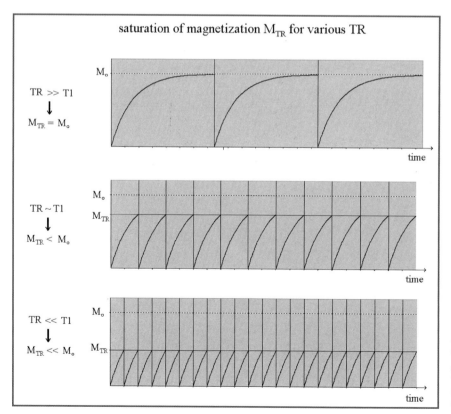

Fig. 4. With a very long repetition time TR, the magnetization fully relaxes yielding maximum signal strength M_o. Shortening of the TR leads to partially saturated magnetization and therefore decreased signal

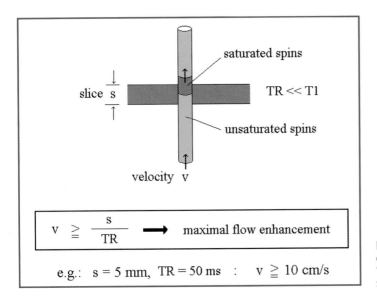

$$v \geqq \frac{s}{TR} \quad \longrightarrow \quad \text{maximal flow enhancement}$$

e.g.: $s = 5$ mm, $TR = 50$ ms : $v \geqq 10$ cm/s

Fig. 5. Inflow effect: In the interval between two RF excitations, the blood in the vessel is replaced by "fresh", unsaturated blood, while the stationary tissue in the slice is saturated due to the short TR

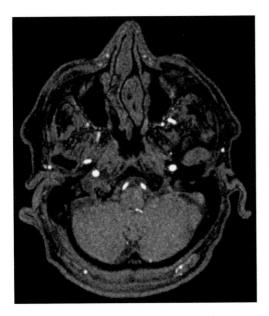

Fig. 6. Brain vessels, axial slice. Due to the inflow effect, there is high contrast between the vessels and the surrounding tissue

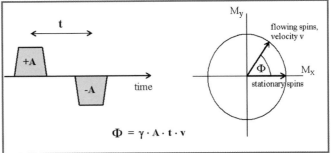

$$\Phi = \gamma \cdot A \cdot t \cdot v$$

Fig. 7. Spins moving along bipolar magnetic field gradients experience a phase shift Φ of their transverse magnetization proportional to the gradient A, the time interval t between the pulses, and the velocity v of the spins along the gradient direction. In contrast, the phase shift for stationary spins is zero

Phase Effects

Phase effects concern the transverse component of the magnetization. They occur whenever spins are moving in the presence of magnetic field gradients, as are applied for spatial encoding of the MR signal.

Magnetic field gradients provoke a change in the Larmor frequency depending on gradient strength and spin position. A gradient pulse of certain length and amplitude therefore induces a phase shift of the transverse magnetization, which can be compensated by a second gradient pulse with identical strength and duration but opposite sign. Thus, for stationary spins the net phase shift is zero. In contrast, the same gradients applied on a flowing spin generate a non-zero phase shift. Since the spins change their position during the bipolar gradient application, the second gradient pulse is no longer able to completely compensate for the phase shifts induced by the first gradient. The remaining phase shift Φ is proportional to the velocity component v of the spins along the gradient direction (Fig. 7).

On standard MR imaging, this flow-induced phase shift causes a spatial misencoding of the sig-

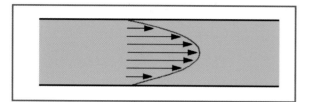

Fig. 8. Blood vessel exhibiting laminar flow with a parabolic flow profile. The flow velocity is indicated by the length of the arrows showing an increase from the border towards the center

nal leading to ghost artifacts that are typically found in the phase-encoding direction.

Spins in a blood vessel are moving with different velocities. Often, a parabolic flow profile is found (Fig. 8). Spins moving faster experience a larger phase shift than those moving more slowly. If there is a velocity distribution inside a voxel, phase dispersion (intra-voxel dephasing) occurs resulting in decreased signal in the blood vessel (Fig. 9). The extent of spin-dephasing depends on the strength and time interval of the gradient pulses, as well as the distribution of spin velocities. When complex flow patterns are encountered, for example in vessels with turbulent flow, there may be a very broad spectrum of velocities within a voxel, leading to total signal loss in the vessel (Fig. 9 c).

Using additional gradient pulses of appropriate amplitude and duration, flow-induced phase shifts can be compensated, thus eliminating any signal loss. This technique is called "gradient motion rephasing (GMR)" or just "flow compensation" [1]. However, GMR is normally restricted to first-order movements, i.e. spins that move at a constant velocity. Turbulent flow and effects of acceleration cannot be completely compensated by GMR.

Optimal reduction of flow-induced phase effects can be achieved by combining GMR with as short a TE as possible, in order to reduce the time available for spin dephasing. Short echo times also diminish the impact of pulsatile blood flow and turbulence.

Time-of-Flight (TOF) Angiography

Techniques

The contrast mechanism of TOF MRA is based on the inflow effect. Fully relaxed blood entering the measured volume behaves as an endogenous contrast agent, by producing a bright signal. The bright depiction of flowing blood, however, requires the use of flow rephasing techniques (GMR) in order to overcome the effects of spin dephasing due to transverse magnetization. TOF MRA using GRE sequences has several advantages: Firstly, GRE sequences are not affected by the wash-out phenomenon that diminishes the signal of fast flowing blood when using SE techniques. Secondly, GRE techniques permit the use of short repetition times (TR < 40 msec), which are needed to efficiently saturate stationary tissue. Thirdly, echo times can be kept short (TE < 5 msec), thus further reducing spin dephasing. Generally, it is advisable to apply in-phase echo times in order to avoid opposed-phase effects at the vessel walls that would impair the depiction of small vessels. Finally, GRE techniques are characterized by short acquisition times which are important when acquiring volume (3D) datasets.

TOF techniques can be divided into three groups (Fig. 10):

- sequential 2D multi-slice method,
- 3D single-slab method,
- 3D multi-slab method.

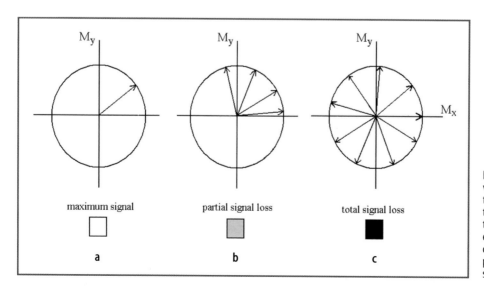

Fig. 9a-c. a If all spins in a voxel have the same velocity the signal is maximal. **b** If there is velocity distribution, loss of phase coherence occurs resulting in decreased signal intensity. **c** If phase dispersion is total, the signal intensity is zero

maximum signal

partial signal loss

total signal loss

a

b

c

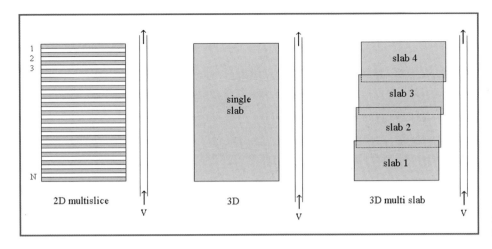

Fig. 10. TOF-techniques: 2D multi-slice, 3D single-slab, 3D multi-slab

With **2D techniques,** the vessel is imaged by sequentially scanning multiple thin slices. This method has two advantages in comparison to the interleaved multi-slice technique: Firstly, very short TR times can be used which boost the inflow effect, and secondly, partially saturated blood is hindered from flowing from one slice to another. The method guarantees sufficient inflow enhancement even in vessels with a very slow flow and produces constant vessel-background contrast in the covered region, because each slice is an entry slice [2].

Problems arise with 2D TOF MRA if the vessels to be imaged do not flow in a perpendicular direction to the imaging plane. If the vessels run partly inside the slice (i.e. in-plane) or return to the slice in a looped form, then signal loss may occur due to the partial saturation of flow.

In order to achieve a sufficient signal-to-noise ratio, a slice thickness of at least 2-3 mm is necessary. However, this results in reduced spatial resolution and increased spin dephasing due to the larger voxel size required. 2D slices do not have rectangular RF profiles and therefore exhibit signal variations at the edges that can lead to step-like artifacts in maximum intensity projection (MIP) reconstructions. However, this effect can be largely overcome by overlapping the slices.

In vessels exhibiting very pulsatile flow, the extent of inflow enhancement varies during the heart cycle. The periodic change of inflow enhancement generates ghost images of the vessels. Saturation of blood spins can occur due to slow flow in the diastolic phase. The use of ECG triggered 2D TOF sequences may overcome many of these problems by confining data acquisition to the phase of maximum inflow. Thus, blood signal is enhanced and ghost artifacts are eliminated. By synchronizing data acquisition with the heart cycle, the vessel is mapped in each slice with equal intensity. Unfortunately, a drawback of this approach is the prolonged acquisition time.

In **3D** TOF MRA, the entire imaging volume, usually 30 – 60 mm thick, is excited simultaneously and then partitioned into thin slices by an additional phase encoding gradient along the slice-select direction [3]. 3D TOF MRA has the advantage of high spatial resolution together with high signal-to-noise ratio, thereby facilitating the improved depiction of particularly small vessel structures. The technique allows slices of less than 1 mm thickness and isotropic voxels to be acquired easily.

One major problem of the 3D technique, however, is the progressive saturation that occurs when blood flowing through the volume is subjected to repeated RF pulses. As a result, the signal intensity decreases continuously in the direction of flow. The extent of saturation depends on the length of time in which the blood stays inside the volume. In slow flow vessels, signal begins to diminish when only a short distance has been covered. Conversely, in faster flowing blood the signal remains visible for a greater distance. Consequently, the maximum volume thickness should be kept as small as possible, matched to the size of the vessel region of interest. A reduction of saturation can also be achieved by increasing the TR (see Fig. 5).

Larger vessel sections can be investigated by subdividing the volume of interest into several thin 3D slabs that are acquired sequentially [4]. One such **multi-slab** technique, which retains the advantages of 3D TOF yet has reduced saturation effects like 2D TOF, is called multiple overlapping thin slab acquisition (MOTSA). Generally, the chosen slab thickness has to be small enough to avoid saturation within the slabs. However, adjacent slabs must overlap by about 20 – 30% in order to compensate for signal attenuations arising at the slab edges due to non-rectangular excitation profiles. This results in compromised time efficiency and longer overall acquisition times.

The advantages and disadvantages of 2D and 3D TOF MRA are summarized in Table 3.

Table 3. Comparison of 2D TOF and 3D TOF angiography

2D TOF	3D TOF
Strong inflow effect, minimal saturation	
• sensitive even to slow flow (veins)	More saturation effects
• sensitive to rather fast flow (arteries)	
Relatively poor signal-to-noise ratio	High signal-to-noise ratio
Short scan times	Poor background suppression
Relatively thick slices	
• suitable for large vessels	Thin slices, allows isotropic voxels
• suitable for small vessels	
Poor in-plane flow sensitivity	
• for straight, unidirectional flow	Better than 2D TOF for tortuous vessels
Long echo times	Short echo times, less dephasing
Step artifacts at the vessel wall	Smoother vessel walls

Table 4. Options to improve TOF angiography

Orientation of slices or volume perpendicular to flow direction
2D for slow flow, 3D for fast flow
3D multi-slab for larger vessel sections
Spatial presaturation to isolate arteries and veins
Use of minimum TE reduces signal loss due to spin dephasing
TONE pulse reduces saturation effects in 3D TOF
Magnetization transfer (MTC) and fat suppression improve vessel contrast

Frequently, 2D TOF MRA is favored for imaging veins because of the high sensitivity to slow flow. 3D TOF MRA, on the other hand, is more appropriate for fast arterial flow and for those cases in which high spatial resolution is required.

Optimization (Table 4)

In TOF MRA, arteries and veins are often displayed simultaneously, since the inflow enhancement is equally effective for directly opposed flow directions. As a result, there may be an interfering overlap of arterial and venous vessels in the MIP reconstruction which hampers the detection or assessment of vessel lesions. This drawback can be overcome by applying additional presaturation slabs that saturate and dephase spins before they enter the image slice. A selective arteriograph is generated if the presaturated area is placed distal to the imaging volume, i.e. at the entry side of the veins. In this case, inflowing venous spins are saturated in a manner similar to stationary spins and therefore do not produce a bright signal. Conversely, presaturation of arterial inflow permits the selective depiction of veins. In order to achieve sufficient suppression even of fast flowing blood, presaturation slabs of several centimeters thickness must be positioned close to the imaging volume. In case of 2D TOF sequences traveling presaturation slabs may be employed that move along with the imaged slice but at a constant distance from the actually imaged slice.

For all TOF techniques, it is important to position the imaging volume (slices or slabs) perpendicular to the vessel to minimize the length of the vessel section in the slice or slab and to reduce the saturation effects. As intracranial vessels run in different directions, it is not possible to simultaneously orientate the imaging volume perpendicular to all vessels. Consequently, the 3D multi-slab technique has proven to be the best method for investigating brain arteries. In order to guarantee optimal coverage of the arterial vessel tree with minimal slab thickness it is advisable to tilt the slabs slightly from the axial to the coronal orientation (Fig. 11). The resulting MIP reconstruction gives excellent visualization of the brain arteries (Fig. 12).

The depiction of venous brain vessels using the TOF technique can be optimized by choosing a sagittal slice orientation tilted slightly towards coronal and axial directions (Fig. 13). As a result of this spatial orientation, saturation of blood in the sagittal sinus that could occur due to long-range flow within one single slice is prevented. Inflow enhancement is sufficient for all veins, regardless of their flow direction (Fig. 14).

The flip angle of a GRE sequence considerably

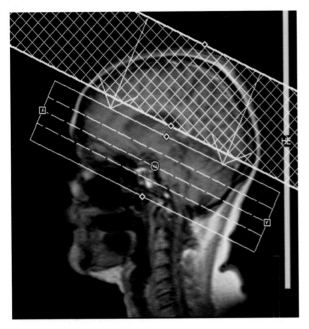

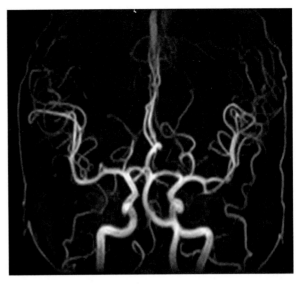

Fig. 11. Typical position of a 3D TOF multi-slab. The presaturation slab above the imaging volume suppresses the signal of venous flow

Fig. 12. MIP reconstruction from a 3D multi-slab TOF MRA dataset of the brain arteries

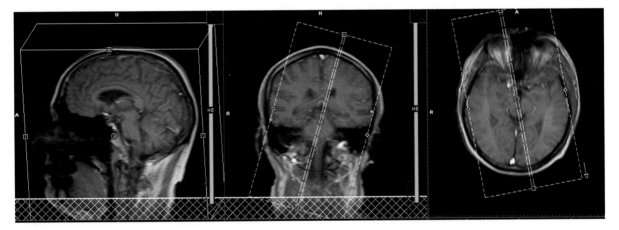

Fig. 13. Imaging volume of a 2D TOF MRA of the brain veins. By tilting the sagittal slices in an axial and coronal orientation, saturation of venous blood in the sinus sagittalis is avoided. The saturation slab located beneath the imaging volume suppresses the arterial flow signal

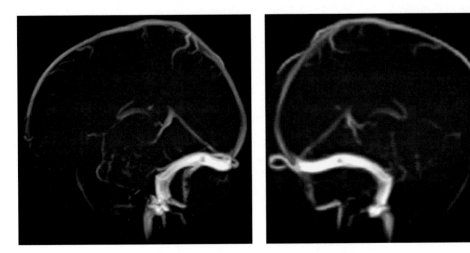

Fig. 14. MIP reconstruction of a 3D TOF MRA dataset of the venous brain vessels

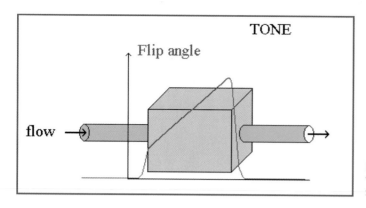

Fig. 15. By linearly varying the flip angle across the volume (TONE), the progressive saturation of the flow signal occurring with 3D TOF MRA can be reduced

influences the vessel-background contrast. Large flip angles generate a high signal at the entry side of the blood, but also provoke rapid signal decrease along the course of the vessel due to saturation. Small flip angles produce a lower vessel-background contrast but less saturation. 2D TOF typically uses flip angles in the range of 30° - 70°, whereas 3D TOF employs lower angles between 15° and 20° to reduce saturation. In the technique referred to as TONE (Tilted, Optimized, None-Saturating Excitation) [5], the flip angle is varied linearly in the slice direction, beginning with small values at the entry side and ending with high values at the exit side of the volume (Fig. 15). In this way, saturation across 3D slabs can partially be compensated to achieve a more uniform signal distribution along the course of the vessel. The extent of the flip angle variation depends on flow direction, flow velocity (slow, medium, fast) and slab thickness. Therefore, sequence protocols that utilize TONE are optimized for specific vessel regions.

Further suppression of background signal can be achieved using magnetization transfer contrast (MTC) [6, 7]. By applying a radio pulse at a much different frequency from that of water resonance, protons of motionally restricted macromolecules are saturated. In contrast mobile water protons that generate the MR signal in vessels and tissues are not affected by this off-resonance pulse. By cross-relaxation and chemical exchange, the saturation is transferred to the neighboring free protons, thus significantly reducing the measured MR signal. This effect can be seen in the gray and white brain matter (reduction of signal by 15-40%) but not in blood. Consequently, the contrast between the vessel and the surrounding tissue is enhanced. This is particularly useful for depiction of small vessels and slow flowing blood which are made appreciably more visible.

Unfortunately, fat does not exhibit magnetization transfer. Therefore, to avoid enhanced fat contrast, MTC should be used in combination with fat suppression techniques. Effective suppression of the signal of fat may be achieved either by direct frequency-selective saturation of the fat signal or by selective excitation of water (Fig. 16). The dis-

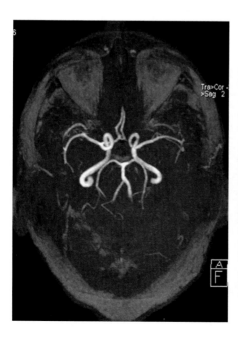
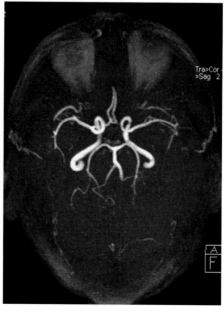

Fig. 16. *Left*: non-selective excitation. *Right*: fat suppression using selective water excitation

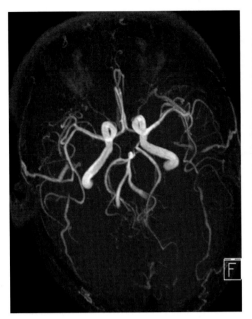 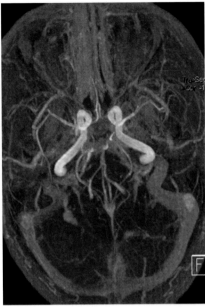

Fig. 17. TOF MRA pre (*left*) and post (*right*) administration of gadolinium contrast agent. After contrast injection, the suppression of veins is no longer effective

advantage of fat saturation in comparison with water excitation is that water protons instead of fat protons could be accidentally affected by the pre-saturation pulse in regions outside the shim volume (i.e. in the less homogeneous magnetic field) resulting in unwanted reduction of inflow effect.

Unlike unenhanced MRA, contrast-enhanced MRA (CE MRA) is usually achieved through the application of an exogenous gadolinium-based MR contrast agent which shortens the T1 relaxation time of proton spins in its immediate vicinity. After intravenous administration, the T1 of blood is strongly reduced, thereby counteracting problems associated with the saturation of spins flowing across the volume. As a consequence, the contrast between blood vessels and surrounding tissues is improved, primarily for small vessels and those with slow flow. There are, however, two major disadvantages arising from contrast agent administration: First, if soft tissue in the imaging

area shows considerable contrast enhancement, the background signal will also be enhanced. Second, due to the fast T1 relaxation of blood protons, suppression of either the signal from the arteries or veins using presaturation pulses will malfunction (Fig. 17). In such cases, evaluation of source images or multiplanar reconstructions may yield more information than MIP reconstructions.

Pitfalls (Table 5)

Tissues with very short T1 relaxation times, such as fat, methemoglobin after intracranial hemorrhage or in fresh thrombi, and contrast enhancing structures, pose a problem for TOF MRA. As a result of inefficient saturation, these tissues often produce a very bright signal which may render them undistinguishable from flowing blood. For example, methemoglobin in a hemorrhage (Fig.

Table 5. Pitfalls with TOF MRA

Methemoglobin in thrombosed vessels (cavernous: sinus thrombosis) may mimic blood flow (i.e., vessel patency)
Workaround: compare MIP with pre-contrast T1 images or use phase contrast MRA
Short T1 tissues (fat, bleeding, tissue that take up contrast) may simulate vessels
Pulsation artifacts in CSF may simulate vessel lesions
Signal loss occurring with turbulent or very slow flow causes overestimation of stenosis and artifacts in the depiction of aneurysms
Signal loss due to susceptibility artifacts (coils, clips)
Signal loss in case of in-plane flow (2D) or slow flow (3D)
Overlap of arteries and veins after contrast administration, particularly in intracranial MRA

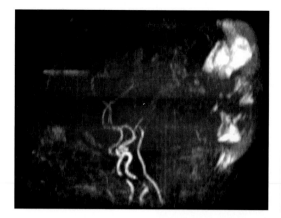
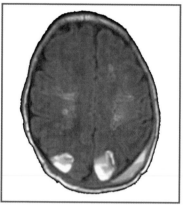

Fig. 18. Methemoglobin in an intracranial hemorrhage. *Left*: MIP reconstruction. *Right*: T1-weighted image

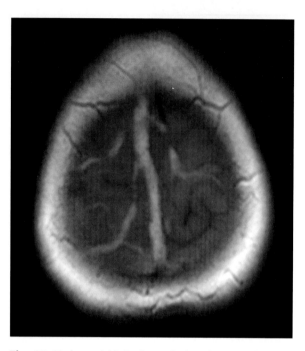

Fig. 19. Methemoglobin in sinus vein thrombosis. Bright depiction of the occluded veins in the unenhanced T1-weighted image

18) may be mistaken for an aneurysm while occluded vessels, such as sinus thrombosis (Fig. 19), may be misinterpreted as perfused. Confusions of this kind can be avoided by comparing the TOF data with precontrast T1-weighted acquisitions.

As shown in Fig. 20, pulsating cerebrospinal fluid (CSF) may cause artifacts on TOF MRA. In this case the 3D TOF multi-slab technique provokes strong inflow enhancement at the entrance of the upper slab, generating a bright signal of the CSF in the cerebral aqueduct of Sylvius on the sagittal reconstruction of the source images (Fig. 20 c). In the projection reconstructions obtained by MIP postprocessing (Fig. 20 a, b), this structure may be misinterpreted as a vessel lesion.

Distal to a stenosis or near arteriosclerotic alterations of the vessel wall, turbulent and accelerating flow may lead to signal loss due to spin de-

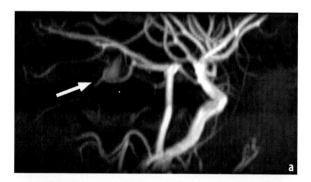
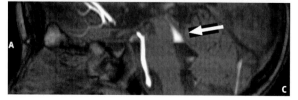

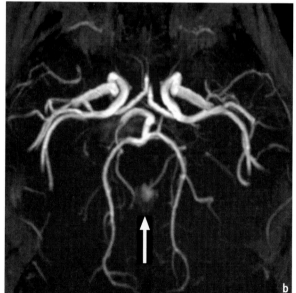

Fig. 20a-c. Artifact (*arrows*) in the sagittal (**a**) and axial (**b**) MIP reconstructions, caused by pulsating cerebrospinal fluid (**c**, *arrow*) in the cerebral aqueduct as shown in a reconstructed sagittal slice

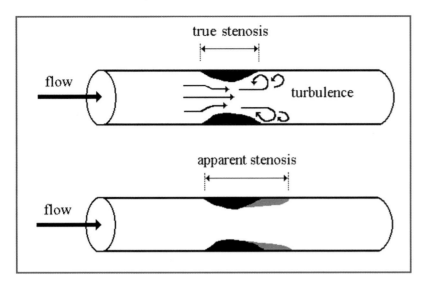

Fig. 21. Overestimation of the length of a stenosis due to turbulence

phasing. The degree of stenosis may therefore be overestimated (Fig. 21). The problem can be reduced, if not entirely eliminated, by the use of very short TE values. In addition, the low flow velocities that may exist in severely stenotic vessels may lead to increased saturation effects and hence reduced flow contrast.

Similarly, the evaluation of aneurysms is susceptible to artifacts caused by turbulence or very slow flow.

Further pitfalls associated with TOF MRA derive from the fact that GRE sequences in general are sensitive to distortions of the magnetic field originating from metallic implants (clips, coils, etc.). Likewise, signal loss due to magnetic susceptibility artifacts may simulate an interrupted vessel, while signal decrease resulting from saturation effects is always a major problem with TOF MRA.

In 2D TOF MRA, signal loss should be considered if vessels are running within the imaging plane. It is therefore essential to place the slices perpendicular to the vessel. In 3D TOF MRA, saturation occurs if thick slabs are applied to vessels with slow flow.

Phase Contrast Angiography

Whereas phase effects are suppressed as fully as possible in TOF MRA, it is the flow-induced phase shift of the transverse magnetization that is employed to image blood vessels with phase contrast techniques. There are two ways of using phase effects to selectively depict blood flow:
- magnitude contrast (rephased-dephased) method
- phase contrast method

Today, magnitude contrast is only rarely used. Conversely, techniques that in a stricter sense are referred to as "phase contrast", have gained greater importance both as an imaging method and as an accurate approach to measuring blood flow velocity and direction.

Magnitude Contrast Technique

The concept of magnitude contrast angiography is analogous to x-ray digital subtraction angiography (DSA). The basic idea is to acquire two datasets: one flow-**re**phased and one flow-**de**phased [8]. First a flow-compensated measurement is performed using GMR in order to image flowing blood with high signal intensity. In the second acquisition, flow-sensitizing bipolar gradient pulses are applied specifically to induce velocity-dependent phase shifts of moving spins. If the flow-sensitizing gradient is strong enough, the spins within a voxel possessing different velocities may totally dephase resulting in dark vessel signal (Fig. 22). Since stationary tissue appears the same in both acquisitions, subtraction of one dataset from the other results in the signal of the stationary tissue being cancelled leaving only the moving blood as visible (Fig. 23). Interleaving the acquisition of both datasets can diminish the impact of motion artifacts on the subtraction process.

The signal intensity in the subtracted image depends only on the velocity component along the flow-sensitizing gradient which is normally applied in the frequency-encoding direction. Therefore, the imaging volume should be oriented in such a way that the main flow direction in the vessel of interest is parallel to the read-out direction.

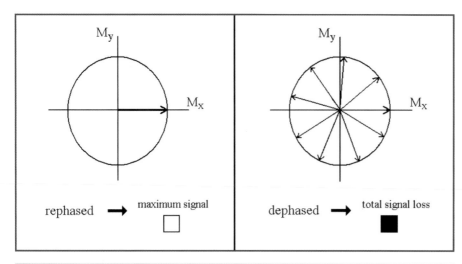

Fig. 22. *Left*: Using flow compensation (GMR), the phases of all spins regardless of their velocity are aligned. Thus, the signal is maximal, the vessel appears bright. *Right*: Using strong flow-sensitizing gradients, complete dephasing of the spins occurs due to their different velocities. In this case, the signal is nulled, the vessel appears black

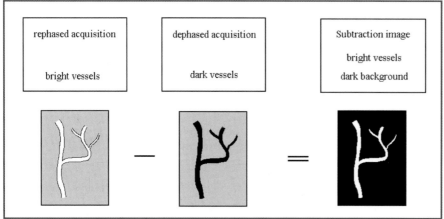

Fig. 23. Principle of magnitude contrast angiography. First a flow-**re**phased dataset is acquired followed by a flow-**de**phased acquisition. After pixel by pixel subtraction (similar to x-ray digital subtraction angiography (DSA)) only the signal of flowing blood remains, while background signal is nulled

Information about all three orthogonal flow directions can be obtained by repeating the flow-encoded acquisition with altered gradient orientations. As a result, a total of four acquisitions has to be performed (one rephased, three dephased), which impacts on the overall acquisition time.

Although not in widespread use, magnitude contrast MRA can be considered applicable for imaging of peripheral vessels (arm, leg) since it allows larger sections of arteries to be visualized. If flow is unidirectional, a single pair of rephased and dephased acquisitions is sufficient, thereby reducing the overall acquisition time.

Magnitude contrast MRA requires a spectrum of flow velocities within a voxel. Laminar flow with its parabolic flow profile is therefore readily detected. The signal acquired is a direct result of the velocity distribution in each voxel, ensuring complete background suppression. The method is well adapted for depicting slow flow with good spatial resolution, covering larger sections of vessels. One disadvantage arises from the fact that this technique does not provide any information on flow direction or flow velocity.

Phase Contrast Technique

Similar to magnitude contrast, phase contrast angiography is based on the acquisition of two datasets that differ in the phase of moving spins [9, 10]. At first, a flow-rephased sequence (S_1) is applied which defines the phase of transverse magnetization under conditions of total flow compensation. The second measurement (S_2) is flow-sensitive, utilizing special flow-encoding gradients to provoke a measurable phase shift. Contrary to the magnitude contrast technique, the chosen gradient is weak enough to avoid complete phase dispersion arising from the velocity distribution of the spins. Complex subtraction of the two datasets S_1 and S_2 yields the phase difference Φ as well as the difference vector ΔS, both of which depend on the velocity component of the spins along the flow-encoding gradient (Fig. 24).

There are two different approaches to utilizing flow-induced phase shifts to generate angiographic images. In the so-called **phase map** images, it is the phase difference Φ that is depicted as signal intensity. The sign of the phase shift encodes the

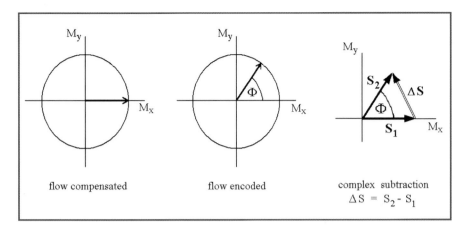

Fig. 24. Principle of phase contrast angiography: A flow-compensated (S_1) and a flow-sensitive (S_2) dataset are acquired. Complex subtraction yields the phase difference Φ and the difference vector ΔS. Both quantities depend on the local flow velocity and can be used for generating flow images

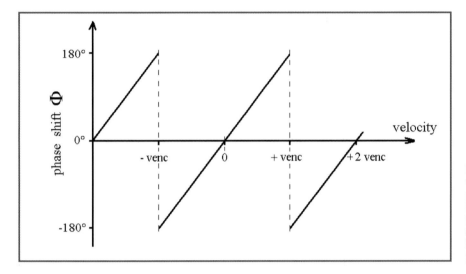

Fig. 25. In the phase image, the value of the phase shift Φ is depicted as signal intensity. In the range from −venc to +venc, the phase shift is directly proportional to the flow velocity. Flow that is faster leads to a turnover of the phase (aliasing)

flow direction. Non-moving tissue appears as a medium shade of gray while flowing blood is either brighter or darker, according to the direction of flow. As the intensity of each pixel is linearly proportional to flow velocity, phase images are particularly well suited for flow quantification and for identifying flow direction.

In the second approach **Magnitude** images, which reveal the length of the difference vector ΔS, are applied to anatomically image the vessels. However, while the brightness in each pixel is a measure of the local flow velocity, there is no information about the flow direction.

The difference vector ΔS increases with rising spin velocity, reaching a maximum at $\Phi=180°$. The corresponding critical velocity is called flow sensitivity or velocity encoding (venc) and is determined by the strength of the bipolar flow-encoding gradients. The manufacturers of MR scanners provide a set of sequences adapted to different velocity ranges. In clinical practice, it is important to estimate the maximum flow velocity expected to occur in the vessel in advance in order to choose the phase contrast sequence with an adequate venc value.

With phase contrast, only those velocities ranging between −venc and +venc, corresponding to phase shifts between −180° and +180°, can be uniquely detected. If the flow velocity exceeds the venc value, there is an abrupt change of signal intensity in the phase image from bright to dark or vice versa (Fig. 25). Blood flow that provokes a phase shift of 190° cannot be distinguished from oppositely directed flow that generates a phase shift of −170°. This ambiguity is called aliasing.

In the magnitude image, maximum intensity is reached when the flow velocity equals the venc value (Fig. 26). At higher velocities, the signal intensity begins to decrease again. If the flow velocity in a voxel is exactly twice the venc value, no signal emanates from the voxel, and the vessel appears to be interrupted.

As an example, for a venc value of 40 cm/sec spins flowing at a rate of 40 cm/sec provoke a phase shift of 180° yielding maximum signal intensity. Spins that flow at 60 cm/sec possess a phase shift higher than 180°. Therefore, on the magnitude image they appear less bright than the spins flowing at 40 cm/sec, but equally as bright as spins flowing at a rate of 20 cm/sec. Likewise, if there are spins flow-

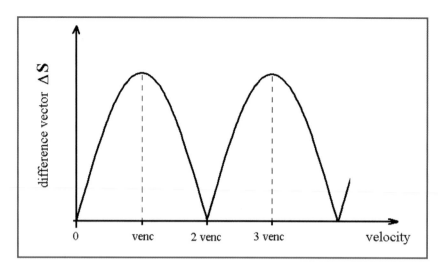

Fig. 26. In the magnitude image, the length of the difference vector DS is depicted as signal intensity. Brightness is maximal at the venc value and decreases at higher flow rates. If the velocity is twice the venc value, the signal intensity is zero

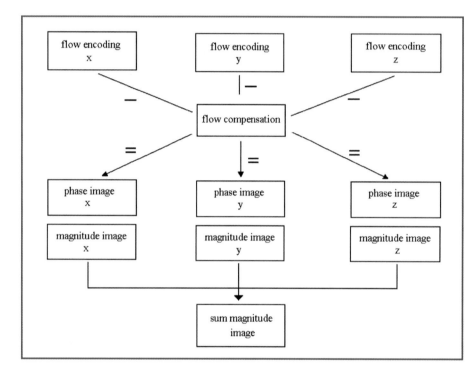

Fig. 27. Complex subtraction of the flow-encoded and flow-compensated datasets yields phase- and magnitude images for the three directions in space. By combining the magnitude images, a sum magnitude image can be obtained that gives a vessel image that is independent of flow direction

ing at a rate of 80 cm/sec, they will provide zero signal and appear as stationary spins.

The phase contrast method is sensitive only for the velocity component along the flow-encoding gradient. In order to obtain information on all flow directions, one dedicated flow-encoding gradient for each orthogonal direction of space is required. Thus, a phase contrast sequence comprises a total of four acquisitions: one flow-compensated measurement and three flow-encoded acquisitions in the x-,

y-, and z-directions. Interleaving the four datasets can reduce artifacts caused by patient motion.

Phase and magnitude images of the flow components in the three orthogonal directions are obtained by complex subtraction of flow-encoded and flow-compensated datasets (Fig. 27). The three magnitude subtraction images can be added to obtain a sum magnitude image that depicts blood flow with bright signal regardless of flow direction (Figs. 27, 28).

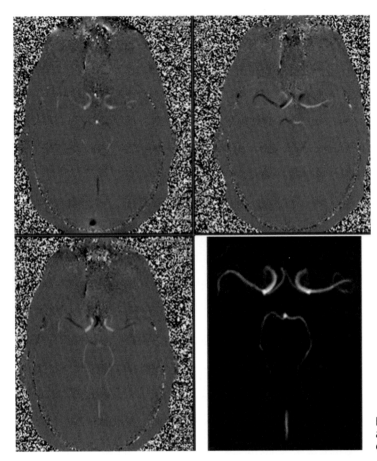

Fig. 28. 2D phase contrast angiography: phase images encoded for the x, y, and z-directions and the corresponding sum magnitude image

Optimization (Table 6)

The correct choice of the flow sensitivity of a phase contrast sequence is critical to the quality of vessel depiction. If the chosen venc value is too high, the acquired signal-to-noise ratio is poor due to the small difference between signals. Conversely, venc values that are two low lead to aliasing artifacts and flow voids which may be misconstrued as stenosis. Typical flow velocities in some larger vessels, which may indicate the appropriate venc values to use, are given in Table 7.

Blood flow in arteries and veins is rarely constant during the heart cycle. Therefore, given that phase contrast sequences require several minutes of acquisition time, it is not the maximum but the mean flow velocity averaged over the heart cycle that is relevant. In the brain the vessels are highly tortuous and thus blood flow is hardly ever directed along one single phase encoding direction. Hence, in practice, the maximum signal intensity is obtained when the chosen venc value is about half the maximum flow velocity, as demonstrated in Fig. 29.

Due to the irregular course and position of vessels in the brain, it is reasonable to encode one single flow sensitivity in all three orthogonal directions. Conversely, in the peripheral arteries, there is one main flow direction, but a great variation of flow velocities. Consequently, in the peripheral arteries a "multi-venc" measurement can be performed in which three flow velocities (e.g. 30, 60,

Table 6. Options for improving phase contrast MRA

Adapting flow sensitivity (venc) to maximum flow velocity
Encoding different flow velocities (multivenc) or different flow directions
Contrast agent improves flow signal
2D acquisition provides one *single* projection within a short acquisition time,
3D acquisition permits MIP postprocessing
ECG triggering can be applied in cases of pulsatile flow
Presaturation pulses can separate arteries and veins

Table 7. Flow velocities in some large vessels
(according to Siemens application manual Magnetom Vision)

Vessel	Flow velocity (cm/s)
Ascending aorta	50 – 100
Descending aorta	100
Aortic stenosis	150 – 500
Aortic valve insufficiency	150 – 200
Common carotid artery	60 – 80
Carotid artery stenosis	100 – 500
Middle cerebral artery	60
Basilar artery	40 – 50
Femoral artery	60 – 80
Popliteal artery	35 – 40
Vena cava	5 – 40
Portal vein	5 – 10

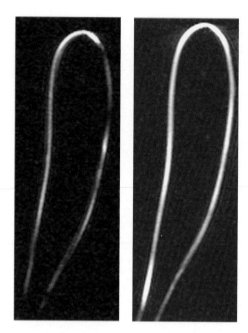

Fig. 29. Phase contrast study on a flow phantom with pulsating flow. *Left*: venc = v_{max} ; *Right*: venc = $v_{max}/2$.
Due to vessel tortuosity and the time varying flow velocity, the signal intensity is higher when the flow sensitivity (venc) of the sequence is half the maximum flow velocity

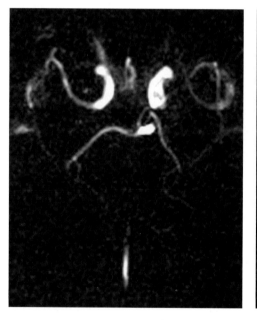
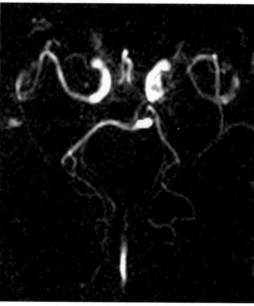

Fig. 30. Phase contrast angiography before (*left*) and after (*right*) administration of a gadolinium contrast agent. Due to T1 shortening, the signal-to-noise ratio increases, thereby improving the detection of small vessels

and 90 cm/sec) are encoded simultaneously but in only one encoding direction. All three acquired images are then combined to form a sum image.

In CE MRA, the signal-to-noise ratio of the blood increases after contrast agent administration because the greater T1 shortening of the spins leads to more signal. Phase contrast angiography, unlike TOF angiography, can benefit from this ef-fect without the penalty of increased background signal. The additional signal afforded by the application of a contrast agent (already at a dose of 4 ml) is particularly beneficial for the visualization of small vessels with low flow velocity when working at lower field strength (Fig. 30).

As with TOF MRA, both 2D and 3D phase contrast MRA techniques are available. However, un-

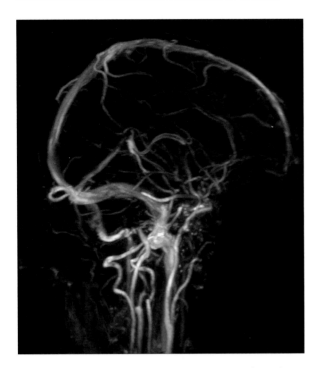

Fig. 31. Phase contrast angiogram of the intracranial vessels

contrast sequence is significantly greater than that of a 3D TOF sequence, because four data volumes need to be acquired rather than just one.

The possibility to combine ECG- or peripheral pulse triggering with the 2D phase contrast sequence may allow the acquisition of time-resolved images of pulsating blood flow in vessels. A series of cine velocity images can be obtained that spans the cardiac cycle. If an optimal depiction of pulsating blood flow is required rather than time resolution, it is advantageous to confine the acquisition to the cardiac interval of maximum flow velocity.

As with TOF MRA, phase contrast techniques can be combined with presaturation pulses in order to eliminate unwanted vessels from the reconstruction. However, because phase contrast sequences are independent of inflow effects, the separation of arteries and veins is not as successful as in TOF-MRA.

Due to the flow encoding gradients, TE values are prolonged compared with those employed in TOF sequences, because the bipolar gradient pulses have to be applied within the TE interval. As a result, phase contrast sequences are sensitive to phase errors caused by, for example, susceptibility effects or turbulent flow.

The sensitivity for flow is proportional to the flow encoding gradient area (gradient amplitude * gradient length). Therefore, the encoding of low flow velocities requires longer TE values. Shortening of TE values can be achieved with stronger gradients, by keeping the gradient area constant. In this way, phase contrast MRA benefits from stronger gradient systems.

like TOF MRA, phase contrast MRA does not impose any restrictions on image orientation, because the method is not dependent on inflow effects.

2D phase contrast sequences are well suited for imaging vessels in a large volume. Because only moving spins contribute to the measured signal, the background signal is very effectively suppressed. Even thick single slices of about 100 mm can be imaged and the overall acquisition times are relatively short (about 1-2 min). The result is a projection image in which all the vessels in the excited slice volume are depicted (Fig. 31). A drawback, however, is that it is not possible to reconstruct projections from another perspective.

With 3D phase contrast MRA datasets, as well as with stacks of 2D phase contrast acquisitions, MIP reconstructions can be acquired in any projection, in a manner similar to that performed in 3D TOF MRA. However, depending on the number of partitions, the acquisition time for a 3D phase

Summary

In clinical practice, unenhanced MRA techniques are mainly employed for imaging of the intracranial vasculature. Although they are also applicable to imaging of blood vessels in the neck, arm and leg, CE MRA is now firmly established as the dominating approach in the extracranial and peripheral regions. A summary of the different areas of application for the different MRA techniques is given in Table 8.

Table 8. Application areas of MRA techniques

	3D-TOF	2D-TOF	3D-PC	2D-PC	Magnitude contrast	CE MRA
Intracranial:						
- Arteries	***		*			*
- Veins	*	***	**	*		*
Carotids	**	**				***
Peripheral vessels		**			*	***

*** method of choice; ** second-best alternative or for additional information; * working technique, but with sub-optimal results
TOF MRA: Time-of-Flight MRA; PC MRA: Phase Contrast MRA; CE MRA: Contrast Enhanced MRA

Table 9. Benefits and limitations of TOF and phase contrast MRA

	TOF-MRA	Phase contrast MRA
Advantages	Simple to implement, robust	No saturation effects
	High spatial resolution	Excellent background suppression
	Shorter acquisition time (in 3D)	Enables quantitative flow measurement
Disadvantages	Reduced sensitivity to slow flow	Prior knowledge about flow rates required
	Restrictions to size and orientation of the imaging volume	Very long acquisition times for 3D techniques
	Short T1 tissue may be mistaken for flowing blood	Susceptible to phase errors

TOF and phase contrast MRA are based on very different physical and technical mechanisms. As a result, there are advantages and limitations to both methods, which have to be taken into account when deciding on the appropriate method for a given vasculature territory (Table 9).

The TOF technique is robust and easy to implement. In the intracranial territory, it is established as a screening method that allows good-quality visualization of the vascular anatomy. 3D TOF acquisitions are particularly appropriate for imaging of arterial flow. 3D TOF MRA provides high spatial resolution with a significantly shorter acquisition time than that required for 3D phase contrast MRA. Problems due to saturation effects can partly be avoided with the use of multi-slab and TONE techniques. 2D TOF MRA is advantageous when imaging veins, because of its higher sensitivity to slow flow. On the other hand, it should be noted that the quality of TOF MRA is strongly influenced by flow velocity, the course of the vessels, and the size and orientation of the imaging volume. The use of very short TE values minimizes phase effects while poor background suppression can be improved by applying magnetization transfer. However, stationary tissue with short T1 may sometimes be mistaken for flowing blood.

Unlike TOF MRA, phase contrast MRA is not dependent on inflow effects. Therefore, the size and orientation of the imaging volume can be chosen arbitrarily. The method allows large sections of vessels to be depicted almost without saturation effects. 2D phase contrast MRA requires only a short acquisition time to generate a projection image of one single thick slice while 3D phase contrast acquisitions require a long time, since four datasets have to be acquired to obtain full flow information in all three orthogonal directions. Phase contrast MRA is sensitive to slow flow rates and is applicable mainly for imaging veins. Background suppression is excellent and short T1 tissues do not appear in the reconstructed angiograms. Because the signal intensity is directly proportional to the velocity of local blood flow, phase contrast MRA permits quantitative evaluations, such as flow quantification or determination of flow direction. Problems with phase contrast MRA may arise because prior knowledge about blood flow rates is required in order to avoid aliasing artifacts and flow voids.

References

1. Lenz G, Haacke E, Masaryk T, Laub GA (1988) In-plane vascular imaging: pulse sequence design and strategy. Radiology 166:875-882
2. Keller PJ, Drayer BP, Fram EK, Williams KD et al (1989) MR angiography with two-dimensional acquisition and three-dimensional display. Radiology 173:527-532
3. Laub GA, Kaiser WA (1988) MR angiography with gradient motion refocusing. J Comput Assist Tomogr 12:377-382
4. Parker GL, Yuan C, Blatter DD (1991) MR angiography by multiple thin-slab 3D acquisitions. Magn Res Med 17:434-451
5. Tkach J, Masaryk T, Ruggieri P et al (1992) Use of Tilted Optimized Nonsaturating Excitation. SMRM abstract 2:3905
6. Atkinson D, Brant-Zawadzki M, Gillan G et al (1994) Improved MR angiography: Magnetization transfer suppression with variable flip angles excitation and increased resolution. Radiology 190:890-894
7. Edelman RR, Ahn SS, Chien D et al (1992) Improved time-of-flight MR angiography of the brain with magnetization transfer contrast. Radiology 184:395-399
8. Axel L, Morton D (1987) MR flow imaging by velocity-compensated/uncompensated difference images. J. Comp Assist Tomogr 11:31-34
9. Dumoulin CL, Hart HR (1986) Magnetic Resonance Angiography. Radiology 161:717-720
10. Dumoulin CL, Souza SP, Walker MF, Wagle W (1989) Three-dimensional phase contrast angiography. Magn Res Med 9:139-149

I.2

Contrast-Enhanced MR Angiography: Theory and Technical Optimization

Vincent B. Ho, William R. Corse and Jeffrey H. Maki

Introduction

Contrast-enhanced magnetic resonance angiography (CE MRA) has emerged as a technique of choice for vascular imaging [1-3]. Technical improvements in CE MRA over the past decade have significantly improved not only image quality but also its speed, reliability and ease of use. Performed using traditional extracellular gadolinium(Gd)-chelate contrast media, CE MRA yields angiographic data that are comparable to–and in some instances, superior to–those of conventional catheter angiography. CE MRA, moreover, is non-invasive and has inherent clinical benefits compared to catheter x-ray angiography and CT angiography in that there is no exposure to ionizing radiation or nephrotoxic iodinated contrast media. The latter issue of nephrotoxicity is a major consideration in patients with vascular disease as many also have diabetes mellitus and/or renal insufficiency, making the use of iodinated contrast agents undesirable. CE MRA relies on the T1 shortening effect of Gd-chelate contrast agents in blood [4-8]. This is different from the flow-based time-of-flight (TOF) and phase-contrast (PC) MRA techniques which exploit the inherent motion of blood flow to generate vascular signal. By relying on the presence of Gd within vessels, the vascular signal on CE MRA is not hampered by the numerous flow-related artifacts such as signal loss from spin saturation or slow flow that can degrade flow-based MRA techniques, often resulting in the overestimation of stenoses or the mimicking of a vascular occlusion [9].

With CE MRA, arteries will be visualized if image acquisition is performed during the arterial phase of the bolus. If, on the other hand, imaging is performed later during the venous or delayed phase of the bolus, veins will be visualized. As in conventional angiography, imaging a contrast agent during its vascular transit enables the generation of a "luminogram". Since vascular enhancement is a transient and dynamic process, the critical element for CE MRA, as with catheter-based x-ray angiography, is timing of the imaging. Data from CE MRA can be post-processed to yield projections very similar to those of conventional catheter angiography. CE MRA, generally performed using three-dimensional (3D) MRA pulse sequences, has the added benefit of yielding volumetric data sets which can also be post-processed using multiplanar reformation and various 3D visualization techniques, notably maximum intensity projection (MIP) and volume rendered (VR) display (see Chapter 2). These tools often enable a greater appreciation of vascular segments that would otherwise be obscured by overlying structures on planar projections from conventional catheter angiography (Fig. 1).

Over the past decade, CE MRA has benefited from numerous improvements in scanner hardware and from the development of specialized CE MRA software. As a result, it has progressively evolved into the technique of choice for many – if not most – common clinical vascular indications, such as the carotid arteries [10-14], the aorta [15-19], the renal arteries [19-25], and the peripheral vasculature [25-39]. These applications will be described more extensively in the chapters to follow. In this chapter, the basic principles of CE MRA will be reviewed, and the practical issues related to patient preparation and set up, timing,

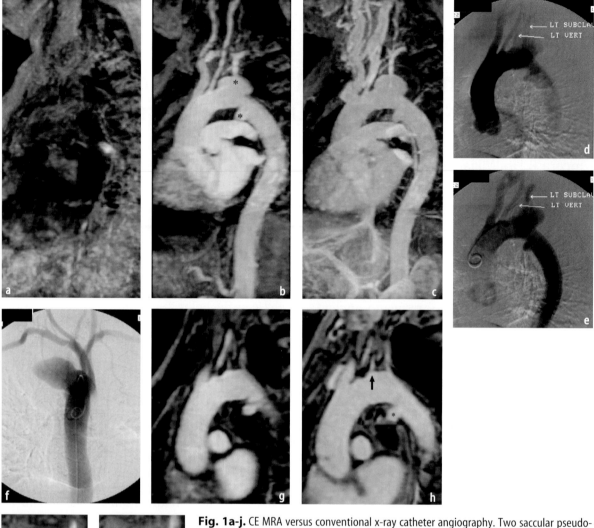

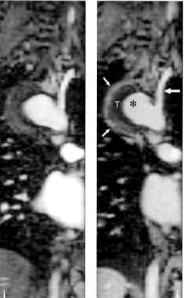

Fig. 1a-j. CE MRA versus conventional x-ray catheter angiography. Two saccular pseudo-aneurysms of the thoracic aorta in this patient with a remote history of a severe motor vehicle accident are well visualized on 3D CE MRA. The MR exam included pre-contrast 3D MRA (**a**, sagittal MIP) to assure that artifacts (e.g. phase wrap, etc) are minimal and that adequate anatomic coverage is achieved. The pre-contrast MRA also serves as a useful practice scan for both the patient and the operator prior to contrast administration. The visualization of the two saccular aneurysms (∗) on dual phase 3D CE MRA, consisting of arterial-phase (**b**, sagittal MIP) and delayed-phase (**c**, sagittal MIP) 3D MRA, compares favorably with that of conventional x-ray angiography (**d** and **e**, left anterior oblique projections; **f**, frontal projections). While traditional MIP projections (**b** and **c**) give a good large view of the thoracic aorta, 3D CE MRA benefits from its ability to provide improved illustration of the actual neck of the saccular aneurysms as well as their relationship with adjacent arch vessels using multi-planar reformation (MPR) of the volumetric data sets. Oblique sagittal MPR images (**g**, arterial phase; **h**, delayed phase) show the neck of the smaller saccular aneurysm (∗) and aberrant origin of the left vertebral artery (*arrow*) from the aortic arch. The left vertebral artery is better visualized on the delayed phase image (**h**) because of its small size and relatively slower flow that hampered adequate Gd concentration during the arterial phase. This highlights the benefit of dual phase imaging when performing CE MRA (especially when using ultra fast 3D MRA acquisitions) as slow filling structures may not be seen as they have yet to accumulate sufficient Gd concentration. 3D CE MRA has the advantages of MPR for improved visualization of individual vascular segments and their relationships. In this case, the aberrant left vertebral artery origin is better seen on MPR of the 3D CE MRA than on corresponding planar projections of conventional x-ray angiography (**d** and **e**), in which filling of the large superior saccular aneurysm quickly obscures the left vertebral and left subclavian artery origins. On coronal MPR (**i**, arterial phase; **j**, delayed phase), the neck of the larger superior saccular aneurysm (∗) and its relationship to the origin of the left subclavian artery (large arrow) can be evaluated *en face* (compare to conventional x-ray angiogram image, **f**). On delayed phase images (**j**), peri-aneurysmal enhancement (*small arrows*) aids in the identification of thrombus (T) within the larger superior saccular aneurysm (Reprinted and adapted with permission from [17])

imaging parameters and contrast agent administration will be discussed. In each section, potential artifacts and pitfalls, as well as strategies for their minimization or avoidance, will be highlighted.

CE MRA: Theory

Vascular visualization on CE MRA relies on the concentration of Gd-chelate contrast agent within the vascular bed during image acquisition [4-8]. Ideally, imaging is performed during peak enhancement of the target vessel when overlapping structures and background tissue are not enhanced. For arterial depiction, this means synchronizing imaging for the period of preferential arterial enhancement when arterial Gd concentration is high and no significant venous or background enhancement has occurred (Fig. 2).

For CE MRA at 1.5 Tesla, the T1 shortening effects of Gd-chelate contrast agents can be estimated by the equation [5, 40]:

$$1/\mathbf{T1} = 1/1200 + \mathbf{R}_1\,[\mathbf{Gd}]$$

where $T1$ is the T1 value of contrast-enhanced blood, R_1 is the field-dependent T1 relaxivity of the gadolinium chelate, and $[Gd]$ is the concentration of gadolinium chelate. In this equation 1200 (msec) represents the T1 of blood at 1.5 Tesla in the absence of Gd contrast agent. Thus, increases in Gd concentration will result in shorter T1. It is the shortening of blood T1 by the arrival of Gd that results in preferential vascular visualization (i.e. vascular image contrast) on CE MRA (Fig. 3).

Patient Preparation

As with any MR scan, proper patient preparation will minimize exam duration and improve clinical

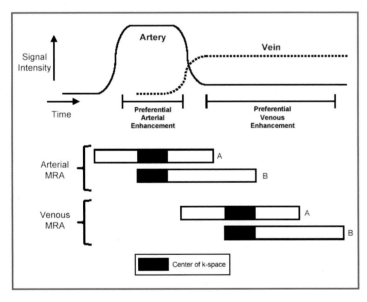

Fig. 2. Contrast bolus timing for 3D CE MRA. At the top of this figure, representative contrast enhancement curves for arteries and veins are shown. Arteries are best visualized if the critical center of k-space data is acquired during the peak and preferential arterial enhancement period. This will minimize possible venous contamination of the data set that may hamper proper separation of arterial structures. There are several methods for acquiring central k-space data. With the traditional sequential or linear method, the center of k-space is sampled during the middle of the acquisition ("**A**"). With centric phase ordered k-space acquisition "schemes" ("**B**"), which include elliptical centric and reverse sequential partial Fourier acquisitions (see Fig. 8), the center of k-space is sampled earlier during the beginning of the imaging period. Thus, proper timing of CE MRA depends not only on the arrival time of contrast in the target vessels but also on knowledge of the type of k-space sampling that is being used for the 3D imaging sequence (Reprinted and adapted with permission from [18])

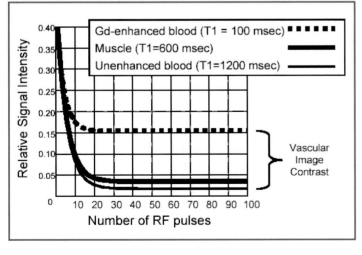

Fig. 3. Vascular Image Contrast on CE MRA. On CE MRA, the repetitive application of radiofrequency pulses generates the necessary image contrast to distinguish Gd-enhanced blood from unenhanced structures. Proper timing of imaging to occur during the phase of preferential arterial enhancement will thus result in the selective visualization of Gd-enhanced arteries over adjacent un-enhanced veins and background tissue (e.g. muscle)

efficiency. In addition to screening for the usual contraindications for MR scanning (e.g. pacemakers) and for the use of Gd-chelate contrast agents (e.g. pregnancy), patients scheduled for a CE MRA examination should also be asked about underlying pulmonary disease and their ability to hold their breath. Intra-abdominal and thoracic CE MRA image quality is markedly improved when performed during a breath hold. Even patients with diminished breath-hold capacity, however, can typically hold their breath for 20-25 seconds if proper coaching is performed in advance and breath holding is optimized by the use of supplemental oxygen and hyperventilation [41]. For multi-station CE MRA examinations (i.e. bolus chase CE MRA) it is also important to know if the patient has any underlying condition that may prevent them from staying still for even short periods of time (e.g. history of Huntington disease or severe back pain), as image subtraction is usually necessary for these exams [42]. Patient motion between pre- and post-contrast data sets can result in spatial mis-registration leading to degraded image subtraction. Patients should also be asked about prior interventions, especially vascular or endovascular procedures. Knowledge of extra-anatomic bypass grafts or stent grafts will ensure proper scan prescription and planning.

During the physical examination, patients should also be assessed for venous access. Ideally, for CE MRA, the intravenous catheter is placed in the antecubital fossa and should be sufficiently large (i.e. at least 22 gauge) to support a bolus rate of at least 2 mL/sec. When imaging the aortic arch and great vessel origins, it is preferable to place the intravenous catheter in the right arm, as left sided venous contrast administration can cause T_2* artifacts due to the high concentration of Gd within the left bracheocephalic vein en route to the right heart. This can often be mistaken for a proximal great vessel stenosis (Fig. 4) [43]. For multi-station bolus chase exams, care must be taken to ensure that the intravenous catheter is stabilized and that the tubing is sufficiently long to allow free movement of the patient and table during the bolus chase table translation. It is frequently advisable to firmly tape the tubing to the patient and to cover potential areas that may snare the tubing. Snaring of the tubing during table translation may not only pull the intravenous catheter out, but also stop table translation as some scanners will automatically stop if any resistance or hindrance to table translation is detected.

For most CE MRA examinations, patients are positioned feet first in the supine position in the bore of the magnet. The one exception is neurovascular imaging which requires the use of a head or neurovascular head and neck coil and thus requires patients to be placed head first into the scanner. Vascular signal-to-noise (SNR) can be improved by the use of phased array coils and, additionally, by the proper centering of the coil elements about the region(s) of interest. For this reason it is well worth the time to ensure proper coil

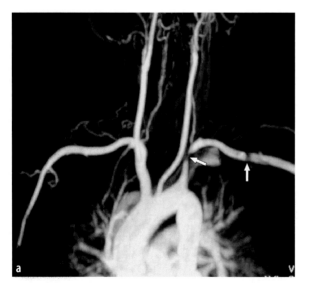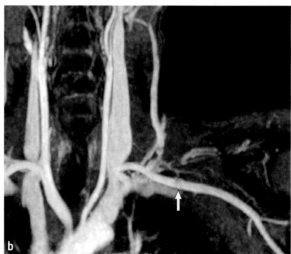

Fig. 4a, b. T2* artifact from left antecubital injection. **a** On the initial arterial-phase, 3D CE MRA of the aortic arch vessels (coronal MIP), there is suggestion of two stenoses (*arrows*) of the left subclavian artery. **b** On delayed-phase images (sub-volume MIP), however, both regions are noted to have a normal caliber (proximal left subclavian artery not shown). The apparent narrowing of the arch vessels on arterial-phase images results from T2* susceptibility artifact resulting from the high concentration of Gd within adjacent veins and is more commonly seen following a left upper extremity injection. As shown in this case in which a left antecubital vein was used for contrast administration, this T2* artifact can occur in any arterial segment close to the left subclavian vein and left bracheocephalic vein. As a practice, dual phase acquisitions will greatly assist in the recognition of this artifact, as delayed phase images will invariably demonstrate normal arterial caliber (Reprinted and adapted with permission from [18])

positioning. A growing number of third party vendors now offer dedicated coils for vascular imaging, primarily for peripheral and neurovascular imaging. With the advent of new scanners with increased numbers of reception channels, coverage of the entire body of the patient with multiple coils is now possible allowing whole body imaging without moving the patient. The use of phased array coils provides the additional benefit of markedly shortening image acquisition times or, with the use of parallel imaging schemes (see below), of acquiring higher spatial resolution image sets in the same time period.

Timing

The adage that "timing is everything" is certainly true for CE MRA. Since CE MRA depends substantially on Gd concentration, and contrast enhancement is a dynamic process, it is not surprising that vascular visualization relies heavily on timing–i.e. the moment in which imaging is actually performed [4-8]. With traditional extracellular Gd-chelate contrast agents, much of an intravenously administered dose will diffuse rapidly out of the vascular space into adjacent tissues within 5 minutes, thereby increasing background signal and reducing the vascular contrast-to-noise ratio (CNR).

In most instances, CE MRA is performed for arterial evaluation. As previously mentioned, arteries are best imaged if imaging data are acquired during peak arterial enhancement (i.e. when the concentration of Gd is greatest, see Fig. 2). The arrival time for the contrast bolus in the region of interest depends on the patient's cardiac output and the status of the intervening vascular anatomy. For example, the arrival of contrast agent into the iliac arteries might be significantly delayed in patients with congestive heart failure. Individual contrast arrival times can vary significantly. Peak contrast enhancement of the abdominal aorta, for example, has been shown to range from 10 seconds to as long as 60 seconds, with the longest delay occurring in a patient with inherently slow flow due to the presence of a large thoracoabdominal aneurysm [44].

Fundamental to the proper synchronization of arterial CE MRA is the acquisition of imaging data (specifically central k-space data, see below) during the period of preferential arterial enhancement prior to the occurrence of significant venous enhancement. This period varies with each vascular territory and can be quite short. For example in the carotid-jugular circulation it can be a mere 5 seconds [14, 45] (Figs. 5, 6). Similarly, accurate timing is exceedingly important for CE MRA of the renal arteries due to the comparatively rapid enhancement of the renal veins.

Accurate determination of the appropriate delay time between contrast administration and image acquisition can therefore be challenging. Prior to the availability of MR compatible injectors and fast imaging methods, an empiric estimation of the bolus arrival time was used. This technique, also called "best guess" or "educated guess," used pre-determined times (e.g. a 10 second delay for CE MRA of the thoracic aorta and a 12 second delay for renal CE MRA) but generally required higher doses of Gd-chelate (e.g. 40 to 60 mL or 0.2 to 0.3 mmol/kg) to ensure sufficiently long arterial phase duration of an adequate Gd concentration [4,5]. As mentioned above, peak arterial enhancement is highly variable between individual patients and is rarely estimated reliably on the basis of physiologic parameters alone [46]. Whereas CE MRA techniques based on fixed timing delays are frequently successful, these methods typically require higher doses of contrast agent – thereby, increasing study costs – and have an increased rate of failure. This is particularly evident for CE MRA of the carotid arteries [47] and renal arteries because the windows of preferential arterial enhancement are brief.

Tailoring CE MRA for individual variations in contrast arrival times by using a timing method,

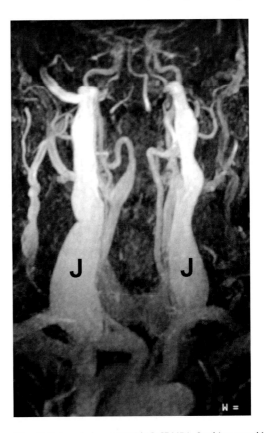

Fig. 5. Delayed phase carotid 3D CE MRA. On this coronal MIP, significant enhancement of the jugular veins ("J") is seen because imaging was performed too late (i.e. after the period of preferential arterial enhancement). (Reprinted and adapted with permission from [7])

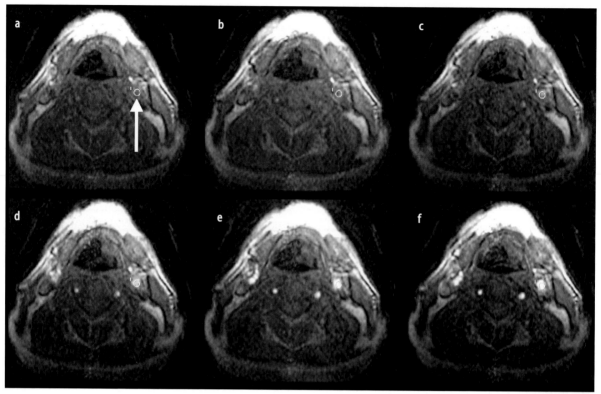

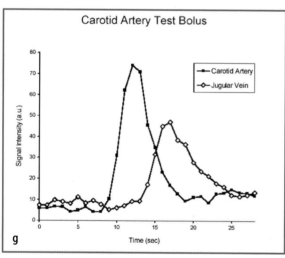

Fig. 6a-g. Carotid timing bolus scan. On axial fast spoiled gradient echo images (**a-f**) using a superior and inferior saturation bands, progressive enhancement of the carotid and vertebral arteries can be seen (compare top row with bottom row). Using an operator-defined region of interest, relative signal measurements in the carotid artery (arrow) and jugular vein (not shown) can be measured. Enhancement curves (**g**) can be plotted and the bolus arrival time can be estimated for CE MRA. In this case, the peak arterial enhancement of the test bolus occurs at 12 seconds. The preferential arterial phase window (i.e. period of selective arterial enhancement prior to venous contamination) is roughly 5 seconds. For optimum arterial depiction, the critical central k-space data should be timed to be acquired after 12 seconds but before significant venous enhancement (Reprinted and adapted with permission from [7])

on the other hand, will both minimize venous contamination and optimize arterial SNR and CNR resulting in improved diagnostic reliability and greater technical success rates. Moreover, by accurately timing the CE MRA examination, optimized arterial SNR and CNR can frequently be achieved with lower doses of contrast agent, thereby reducing overall examination costs. An additional benefit of using lower doses of contrast agent for CE MRA is that additional amounts can be used for other applications during the same examination period.

There are three methods for accurate timing. The most widely used method involves perform-

ing a test bolus scan to estimate the arrival of contrast in the target vascular bed [44-46]. This is usually achieved by administering a 1-2 mL dose of Gd-chelate contrast agent and measuring its arrival time in the vessel of interest. For optimal results it us advisable to administer the test bolus in a manner identical to that planned for the full dose during the CE MRA examination. Thus, it should be injected at the same rate and with sufficient saline flush (30 mL or more) to ensure that it arrives centrally and does not pool within the tubing set or a peripheral vein. Standardization of injections is easily afforded by use of an MR compatible injector.

Test bolus imaging should be performed using a fast two-dimensional (2D), T1-weighted spoiled gradient echo pulse sequence. Imaging parameters (e.g. repetition time, echo time, matrix, etc.) should be adjusted to yield a temporal resolution of approximately one image every 1-2 seconds. The field of view and matrix should also be adjusted to ensure proper visualization of the enhancing artery (e.g. aorta). If the intended image acquisition is perpendicular to the enhancing structure (e.g. axial for the abdominal aorta or carotid artery), then the use of inferior and superior saturation bands is recommended to minimize the normal signal variations that occur because of pulsatile inflow of spins (TOF effect) and to ensure that signal increases are due solely to the arrival of the contrast bolus. Image acquisition should be synchronized with the start of contrast agent injection. Thereafter the ideal contrast arrival time can be estimated based on the frame with the optimal arterial enhancement (Fig. 6).

More recently, real-time triggering for CE MRA has become commercially available. There are two main methods for real time synchronization of CE MRA. One early technique is referred to as automated bolus detection (e.g. MR SmartPrep, General Electric Medical Systems, Waukesha, WI, USA), in which monitoring for contrast bolus arrival and initiation of the MRA data acquisition are automated and integrated into a single pulse sequence [48-50]. This monitoring phase of the pulse sequence uses a high temporal resolution (400 msec) fast spin echo pulse sequence to monitor the arrival of contrast into an operator-defined volume of interest, typically a large vessel within the field of view. For example, the monitoring volume for a renal or abdominal CE MRA would be placed within the mid abdominal aorta. After a preliminary period (e.g. 10-20 sec) during which the baseline signal of the monitoring volume is determined, the pulse sequence informs the operator as to when to initiate the contrast administration

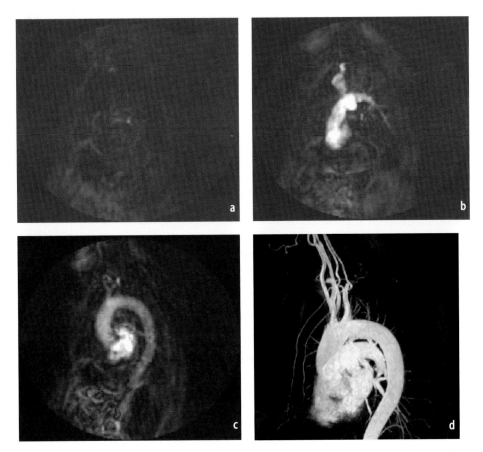

Fig. 7a-d. Arterial phase 3D CE MRA of the thoracic aorta timed using MR fluoroscopic triggering. During the monitoring mode, two-dimensional MR fluoroscopic viewing of the contrast bolus progression (**a**, pre-contrast; **b**, pulmonary artery enhancement; **c**, thoracic aortic enhancement) is shown. Upon seeing the arrival of the bolus in the thoracic aorta, the operator prompts the patient to hold his or her breath and then triggers the 3D MRA data acquisition to begin. The 3D CE MRA (**d**, sagittal MIP) in this 71-year-old man with aortic regurgitation demonstrates a mildly dilated ascending aorta, which measured 4.2 cm in maximum diameter, and normal arch vessels but no aneurysm. High spatial resolution imaging was facilitated on this CE MRA by using a torso phased-array coil and SENSE image processing (Reprinted and adapted with permission from [7])

while continuing its monitoring phase. Once the signal within the monitoring volume exceeds two pre-set thresholds (typically, two standard deviations and 20 percent rise over baseline signal), the pulse sequence automatically switches to its imaging phase. At the beginning of the imaging phase, the operator can also set a delay period (e.g. 3-5 sec) prior to the actual three-dimensional (3D) MRA data acquisition. The delay period provides an opportunity for the patient to initiate a breath hold prior to the actual 3D MRA data acquisition. A change in scanner sound (pitch) between the monitoring and imaging phases can serve as an audible cue for patients to alert them to the onset of the 3D MRA imaging acquisition.

The second method for real time CE MRA timing utilizes a fluoroscopic trigger (BolusTrak, Philips Medical Systems, Best, the Netherlands; Care Bolus, Siemens Medical Solutions, Erlangen, Germany; Fluoro Trigger, General Electric Medical Systems, Waukesha, WI, USA) [12, 13, 51]. Like the aforementioned automated triggering scheme, the real-time MR fluoroscopic technique also integrates a monitoring phase and an imaging phase into a single pulse sequence. However, with the MR fluoroscopic method, monitoring is performed by the operator visually using a continuous fast two-dimensional (2D) spoiled gradient echo pulse sequence with imaging centered over the vascular bed (Fig. 7). With this method, the operator is able to see the arrival of the contrast bolus and to manually initiate the imaging phase. Once again, a delay period can be selected to enable patient breath holding, which is generally preferable for most body applications.

All three methods for timing (test bolus scan, automated bolus detection and MR fluoroscopic trigger) permit reliable and time-efficient CE MRA acquisitions. For arteries such as the carotids in which very early enhancement of the veins occurs, bolus timing using a test bolus may provide good results without venous overlay even on scanners with less sophisticated gradient systems.

In general the actual method used varies from site to site, and typically depends on individual operator preference and equipment type. In all cases, however, it is important to ensure technical proficiency with the chosen method.

Imaging Parameters and Selections

Imaging parameters (e.g. TR, TE, flip angle, matrix, etc.) are critical for the determination of imaging speed (i.e. time required for image acquisition), vascular signal (i.e. vascular SNR and CNR) and spatial resolution. Typical parameters for the various operator selection choices for three common MR scanners are listed in Table 1.

TR, TE and Flip Angle

Since the key to CE MRA is T1 shortening, CE MRA is typically performed using a T1-weighted 3D fast gradient echo pulse sequence with radiofrequency spoiling (e.g. spoiled gradient echo (SPGR), General Electric Medical Systems, Waukesha, WI, USA; fast low angle shot (FLASH), Siemens Medical Solutions, Erlangen, Germany; T1-fast field echo (T1-FFE), Philips Medical Systems, Best, The Netherlands). The relative signal intensity (SI) for a 3D gradient echo pulse sequence is given by the equation [52]:

$$SI = [N(H) (1 - e^{-TR/T1})/(1-cos(\alpha)e^{-TR/T1})] sin(\alpha) \, e^{-TE/T2*}$$

in which $N(H)$ and α are proton density and flip angle, respectively. The SI is maximized when TR/T1 is large, thereby minimizing the value of $e^{-TR/T1}$. This can be achieved either by increasing TR or decreasing T1. For CE MRA, the arrival of contrast agent will significantly diminish the blood T1, thereby reducing the need for a long TR. Increasing TR, moreover, has the undesirable consequence of increasing scan time. In general, if time is available, it is more advantageous to increase the phase encoding steps (y resolution) for improved spatial resolution rather than to increase TR for improved signal for any given scan time. Typically, the shortest possible TR (e.g. <5-6 msec) and TE (e.g. 1-2 msec) should be selected.

As noted in the aforementioned equation, flip angle (α) also affects gradient echo signal intensity. The optimal flip angle (also called the Ernst angle or α_E) for any given combination of TR and T1 can be estimated by the equation [8]:

$$\alpha_E = cos^{-1}(e^{-TR/T1})$$

Using the above two equations, the relative signal intensity for any given combination of α and various T1 values can be predicted for a given TR. For CE MRA at 1.5 Tesla, a flip angle of 40 or 45 degrees is commonly used.

Receiver Bandwidth

Receiver bandwidth is another pulse sequence parameter. As with other applications, higher SNR can be achieved with narrower bandwidth, but generally at the expense of scan time. SNR is inversely related to the square root of the receiver bandwidth. Thus, a doubling of the receiver bandwidth results in a reduction of the SNR by the square root of 2. In patients with reduced breath holding capacity, a wider bandwidth (e.g. increase in "± kHz" on a General Electric MR scanner; less "water fat shift" on a Philips MR scanner; or more

Table 1. Typical Scanning Parameters for CE 3D MRA at 1.5 Tesla for Specific Vendors

Imaging Parameter	General Electric	Philips	Siemens
Pulse Sequence	3D FSPGR	3D FFE	3D FLASH
Imaging Options	Fast, GX	Contrast Enhancment - T1	
Repetition time (TR)	– (e.g. 4-6 msec)	Minimum (e.g. 4-6 msec)	Minimum (e.g. 3-5 msec)
Echo time (TE)	Minimum (e.g. 1-2 msec)	Minimum (e.g. 1-2 msec)	Minimum (e.g. 1-2 msec)
Flip Angle (FA)	45 degrees	40 degrees	25 degrees
Bandwidth	±32.25 kHz (option: ±62.5 kHz)	WFS = 0.9 (@ 448 matrix = ±57 kHz)	Variable (± 590 Hz/pixel)
Field of View (FOV)	30-40 cm (option: 0.8 FOV)	400 mm, RFOV = 0.75	400 mm
Matrix	256 or 512 x 192-256	448 x 258	256 - 512 x 192-384
Number of Partitions	40-60	40-60	60-80
Partition Thickness (true)	1.0-2.5 mm	1.0-2.5 mm	1.0-2.5 mm
K-space	• Elliptical Centric • Centric • Reverse Sequential (with partial Fourier or 0.5 NEX)	CENTRA Low_high Linear Half Scan (=partial Fourier)	• Elliptical Centric ± partial Fourier
Number of Excitations (NEX or NSA)	1 (option: 0.5)	1 (option: 0.5)	1 (option: 0.5)
Timing	SMARTPREP, Flouro Trigger or test bolus	BolusTrak or test bolus	Care bolus or test bolus
Misc. Options	ZIP x 2 ZIP 512 ASSET	Overcontiguous Slices Reconstruct 256, 512, 1024 SENSE	Reconstruct 256, 512, 1024 SENSE, GRAPPA

"Hz/pixel" on a Siemens MR scanner) will shorten scan time, but at the expense of diminished SNR. When using wider bandwidths, care must be taken to ensure sufficiently high vascular SNR (e.g. proper timing and adequate contrast agent dose) to provide a diagnostic study.

Spatial Resolution: Matrix, Partition Thickness and FOV

The remaining pulse sequence parameters which may be adapted in a given patient relate to spatial resolution. These parameters are matrix size, slice thickness and field of view (FOV). The actual parameters used depend greatly on the target vascular bed. In general, it is preferable that the structure of interest contains three pixels across its diameter [53]. Thus, for example, a 9 mm wide vessel will have at least three pixels across its width if a voxel dimension of 3 mm or smaller in any single dimension is used. The actual spatial resolution,

however, depends on the chosen FOV. The spatial resolution for the x, y and z dimensions of a 3D CE MRA can be calculated by:

$$\text{Spatial resolution}_x = \text{FOV}_x / N_x$$
$$\text{Spatial resolution}_y = \text{FOV}_y / N_y$$
$$\text{Spatial resolution}_z = \text{Partition thickness}$$

in which FOV_x and FOV_y are the frequency encoding dimensions of the field of view (x-axis) and phase encoding (y-axis) dimensions; and N_x and N_y are the number of frequency encoding and phase encoding steps, respectively.

In cases in which the anatomic region is much smaller in one dimension, a rectangular FOV can be used to reduce the overall scan time [54]. With a rectangular FOV the data in the phase direction is undersampled, causing a reduction of both the FOV and scan time. It is particularly important when using a rectangular FOV to pay particular attention to the anatomic region since too small a FOV or improper prescription of the volume can result in unwanted aliasing or "wrap around" arti-facts in which unwanted data from outside the FOV is included in the FOV. This can also happen if the venous line is placed in the direction of the FOV. The effects of a chosen FOV can easily be assessed on a pre-contrast MRA prior to the CE MRA.

A rectangular FOV is particularly useful for imaging the thoracic aorta. In this case, a sagittal 3D CE MRA is appropriate with the phase direction prescribed for the anterior-posterior plane. A 0.8 or 80% rectangular FOV will result in a reduction of the image anterior to the sternum and posterior to the spine. It is important that the sagittal acquisition is centered properly over the thorax. Importantly, it should be noted that anatomy in the periphery of the FOV in the phase encoding direction (i.e. outside of the rectangular FOV) will alias signal back into the 3D image set and degrade the resulting images. Care must therefore be taken to ensure that the FOV is sufficiently large as to avoid aliasing of signal over a vital vascular region of interest.

K-space Options

Another important concept concerning imaging parameters is the k-space acquisition order (Fig. 8) [7, 8, 12-14, 48-51]. As with all MR acquisitions, the resulting image contrast is dominated by data within the center of k-space (also called low spatial frequency data) (Fig. 9). Traditional k-space acquisition schemes are linear in that k-space data is acquired sequentially one line at a time from top to bottom (Fig. 10). The central k-space data are thus typically acquired during the middle of any given scanning period.

With the development of real-time timing methods for CE MRA, it is important for the central k-space data to be acquired early during the imaging period, as this ensures image acquisition when contrast is detected within the target vessel. Reliance on linear acquisition schemes in which central k-space data is centered within the imaging period (e.g. about 15 seconds into a 30 second acquisition) would necessitate placement of the signal monitoring volume or MR fluoroscopic image

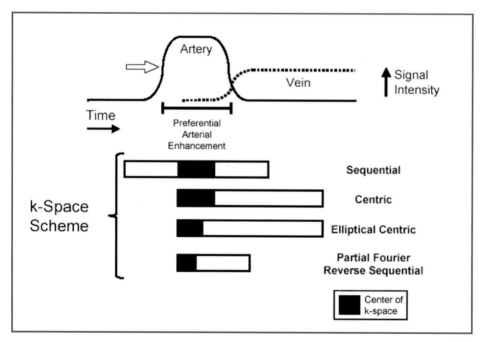

Fig. 8. Diagram illustrates the proper alignment of preferential arterial-phase enhancement for a variety of k-space schemes used for CE-MRA. The critical issue for all the schemes is that central k-space data (i.e. low spatial frequency data) be acquired during the plateau phase of arterial enhancement. In the conventional sequential k-space scheme, the central k-space data is acquired during the middle of the data acquisition period. In both the conventional centric and elliptical centric acquisition schemes, the central k-space data is obtained at the beginning of imaging. Note that with conventional centric acquisitions, k-space is only centric in k_y and that the high spatial frequency encodings in k_z are also acquired during each linear pass and thus the central k-space encodings in k_y and k_z are more efficiently gathered (i.e. acquired more quickly) in the elliptical centric acquisition scheme (see Fig. 2). Partial Fourier imaging with reverse sequential acquisition ordering can also provide a compact acquisition of low spatial frequency data during the beginning of image acquisition. Note that low spatial frequency data is best obtained during the plateau period of arterial enhancement. Acquisition of central k-space data prematurely during the rapid rise in arterial signal (*large hollow arrow*) can result in significant "ringing artifacts" (see Fig. 12) (Reprinted and adapted with permission from [7])

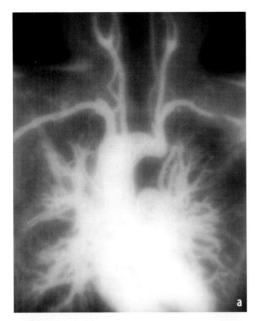

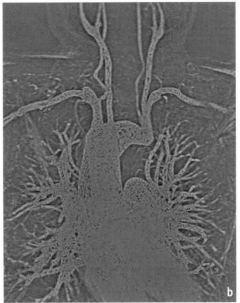

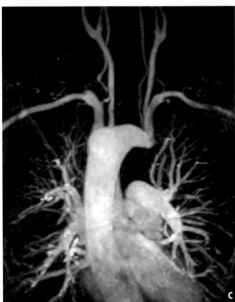

Fig. 9a-c. The influence of high and low frequency data on image appearance. Contrast is dominated by data within the center of k-space, also called low spatial frequency data (**a**). Reconstruction of an image using only these low frequency data results in an image that has high contrast, but in which details are missing. Conversely, if only high spatial frequency phase encoding steps at the edges of k-space are utilized (**b**) the image has low contrast and high detail visibility. Only if central and peripheral data are combined for reconstruction will the image (**c**) have both high contrast and high spatial resolution [Image courtesy of Dr. G. Schneider]

proximal (or "upstream") to the desired vascular bed. In addition to increasing the uncertainty for timing, this also introduces logistical problems related to proper localization as the center of the FOV for the monitoring volume and the 3D CE MRA may not be similar. Contrast agent arrival and imaging are best synchronized if the acquisition of central k-space data is more intimately timed to the actual bolus arrival within the target vessels. For this purpose, centric and more recently elliptical centric phase ordering schemes (Fig. 11) have been introduced for CE MRA. In centric phase ordering, the central lines of k-space are preferentially acquired early during the imaging period. With elliptical centric phase ordering the

most central points (i.e. radial distance from center) are acquired first, resulting in a shortened and more compact imaging period for the acquisition of central k-space data (Fig. 8).

One additional approach to the early acquisition of central k-space information is to use a partial Fourier acquisition scheme with reverse sequential ordering (Fig. 10) [7, 8, 54]. Partial Fourier imaging exploits the fact that one half of k-space closely mirrors the other half, and thus the entire k-space can be extrapolated from a little more than half the k-space data set. By acquiring the partial Fourier ordering in a reverse sequential manner, the central k-space data can be acquired early during the imaging period. Partial Fourier

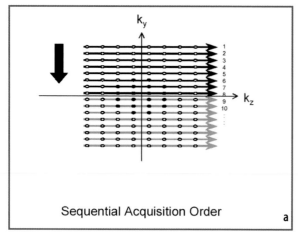

Sequential Acquisition Order **a**

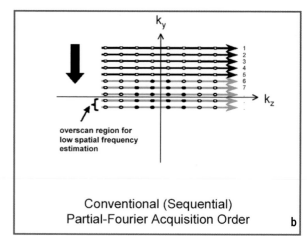

Conventional (Sequential)
Partial-Fourier Acquisition Order **b**

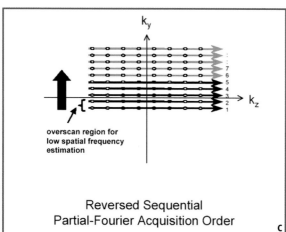

Reversed Sequential
Partial-Fourier Acquisition Order **c**

Fig. 10a-c. Conventional k-space acquisition schemes are sequential or linear (**a**). Consecutive lines of k-space data are acquired with the central lines during the middle of the acquisition period. Partial Fourier schemes enable faster image acquisition but at the expense of diminished signal to noise. Arterial signal, however, is uncommonly a concern on CE-MRA if imaging is properly timed for arterial phase imaging. Partial Fourier acquisitions also provide the added flexibility to place central k-space sampling either during the end (**b**, conventional sequential) or beginning (**c**, reverse sequential) of the imaging period. The darker dots represent the low spatial frequency views (center of k-space) in both the slice (k_z) and view (k_y) encoding directions. The black arrows represent the views acquired at the beginning; and the gray arrows, those at the end of the imaging period. Please note that not all k-space lines are drawn and only representative k-space data is shown (Reprinted and adapted with permission from [7])

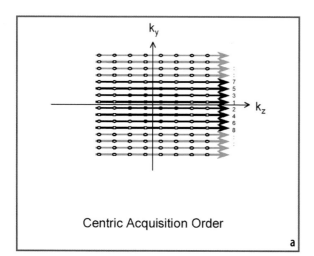

Centric Acquisition Order **a**

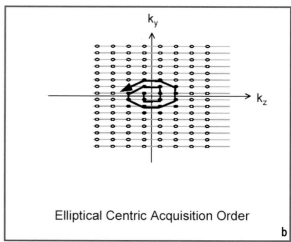

Elliptical Centric Acquisition Order **b**

Fig. 11a, b. Centric k-space acquisition schemes acquire central or low spatial frequency k-space data (represented by the central black dots in the k-space diagram) early in the imaging period. Conventional centric acquisitions (**a**) obtain data in a sequential or linear alternating fashion above and below $k_y=0$. Elliptical centric acquisitions (**b**) acquire data from the center out to the next most radial point–data acquisition is thus centrically acquired in both k_y and k_z. This results in the more efficient (i.e. compact) acquisition of low spatial frequency data by elliptical centric acquisitions (Reprinted and adapted with permission from [7])

imaging has the benefit of significantly decreasing acquisition time, but this comes at the expense of SNR.

Note that the number of phase encoding steps (y-resolution) can be partially sampled in several other ways, all of which reduce overall scan time, but affect SNR and spatial resolution to varying degrees [54]. Partial Fourier imaging (e.g. 0.5 acquisition or NEX; also known as "half scan") enables an asymmetric reduction of phase encoding steps. Although this approach reduces imaging time at the expense of SNR, it has the benefit of preserving spatial resolution. On the other hand, the homodyne reconstruction algorithm used for such acquisitions assumes a constant phase across the image volume, which may not be true in the presence of flow, and may lead to artifacts.

Time can also be saved by reducing the high spatial frequency phase encoding steps at the edges of k-space (i.e. number of phase encoding steps). This reduction, also known as symmetric reduction or scan %, results in lower spatial resolution in the phase encoding direction, but has the benefit of increasing the SNR. A general rule of thumb is to decrease the number of phase encodings until the spatial resolution in the y (phase) dimension is approximately equal to the z (slice or partition) thickness, thereby "balancing" the reso-lution in slice and phase. The individual options for k-space reduction vary depending on vendor, but most are capable of asymmetric (partial Fouri-er, 0.5 NEX or half scan) k-space sampling, which is particularly well suited for CE MRA. Properly timed, CE MRA will generally yield sufficient arte-rial SNR for successful arterial visualization using partial Fourier acquisition schemes.

An additional factor worthy of consideration with respect to k-space is the coordination with the contrast agent bolus itself. Ideally, the central k-space views should be timed with the more sta-ble (i.e. early plateau) phase of the contrast bolus – hence the short delay after contrast detection to al-low the contrast agent concentration to reach its peak. The acquisition of central k-space data dur-ing the rapid rise phase of Gd concentration (Fig. 8) will result in a "ringing artifact" (Fig. 12), which is recognized by the presence of alternating bright and dark lines that parallel the early enhancing vessel [55].

Zero Filled Interpolation

Zero filled interpolation (also known as sinc inter-polation, zero padding or filling, overcontiguous and ZIP), is an image reconstruction algorithm in

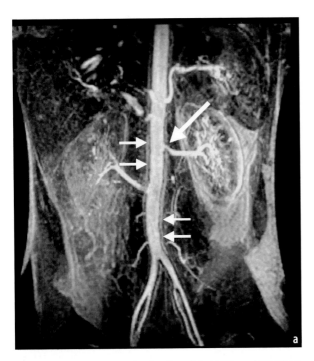
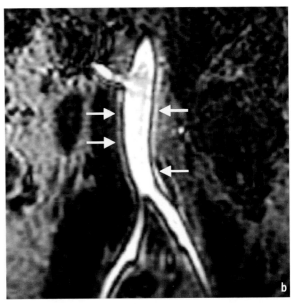

Fig. 12a, b. "Ringing artifact" on breath hold 3D renal CE-MRA in a 36-year-old man with left renal artery stenosis. This artifact is recog-nized by the presence of bright and dark lines (**a**, coronal MIP; **b**, coronal source image) that parallel the edge of the enhancing abdominal aorta (*small arrows*) and results from the premature acquisition of low spatial frequency data (central k-space) during the leading edge of the contrast bolus when arterial signal is rapidly rising. This artifact is more common with centric acquisition ordering which acquire cen-tral k-space data early. "Ringing artifact" can be avoided by timing such that low spatial frequencies are obtained during the plateau phase of the arterial enhancement (see Fig. 8). Note that despite the artifacts, the patient's left renal artery stenosis (**a**, *large arrow*) was well seen. (Reprinted and adapted with permission from [7])

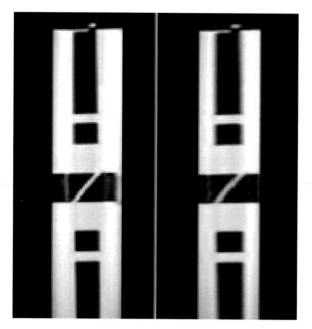

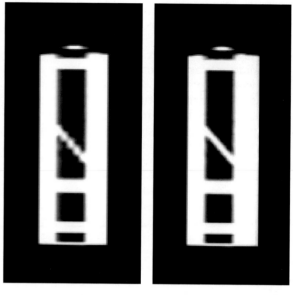

Fig. 13. Zero filled interpolation and spatial resolution. In these phantom images, images with true 2.0 mm section thickness and no zero filling (left, 32 sections of 2.0 mm without zero filling) appear sharper than those acquired using 4.0 mm section thickness zero filled to an apparent 2.0 mm section thickness (right, 16 sections of 4.0 mm with zero filled interpolated to yield 32 sections of an interpolated 2.0 mm interpolated thickness). Both acquisitions yielded 32 sections with seemingly equal "2.0 mm" thickness, but only the left image was acquired with 2.0 mm spatial resolution and only A offers true 2.0 mm spatial resolution [*Images courtesy of Thomas K.F. Foo, Ph.D*]

Fig. 14. Zero filled interpolation. Using phantoms, the relative benefits of zero filling are apparent when comparing an image from an acquisition without zero filling (left, 16 sections of 2.0 mm thickness) to a similar acquisition with zero filling (right, 16 sections of 2.0 mm thickness "zero filled" to yield 32 sections of 1.0 mm interpolated thickness). Note the smoother margins noted in the right side phantom images [*Images courtesy of Thomas K.F. Foo, Ph.D*]

which k-space data is zero "padded" or "filled" in the periphery prior to its fast Fourier transform [55, 56]. This results in the reconstruction of image data in smaller spatial steps than that of the acquired resolution, and the generation of smaller voxel sizes for the reconstructed data. It is important to note that zero filling does not actually improve the true spatial resolution (Fig. 13) of the data set, since this is determined by the acquired resolution. However, it does result in "higher resolution" interpolated image sets (Fig. 14) that will improve post-processing of the 3D data, especially for multi-planar reformation, MIP and VR oblique projections.

Parallel Imaging

One recent option that can be used quite successfully with CE MRA is parallel imaging (e.g. sensitivity encoding or SENSE [58]; and simultaneous acquisition of spatial harmonics or SMASH [59-61]). This approach requires the use of phased array coils, a sensitivity "reference" scan, and special-

ized software (SENSE, Philips Medical Systems, Best, The Netherlands; ASSET, General Electric Medical Systems, Waukesha, WI, USA; GRAPPA and SENSE, Siemens Medical Solutions, Erlangen, Germany). Each element of a phased array coil has its own sensitivity profile. Parallel imaging exploits the known sensitivities of each phased array coil element to reduce the density of the acquired k-space data, thereby reducing the imaging scan time. Effectively, this creates undersampled, heavily aliased datasets that can then be unfolded using spatial sensitivity maps. Individual sensitivity mapping of each coil element is determined by performing a preliminary reference scan. The subsequent CE MRA time can be reduced by a factor of 2 or more (acceleration factor or AF). The main compromise concerns the SNR, which is diminished by the square root of the acceleration factor plus a small additional amount related to the geometry of the coils and FOV. Parallel imaging strategies can be implemented to provide improved spatial resolution (Figs. 7, 15) or to reduce scan durations for patients with limited breath holding capacity (Fig. 16).

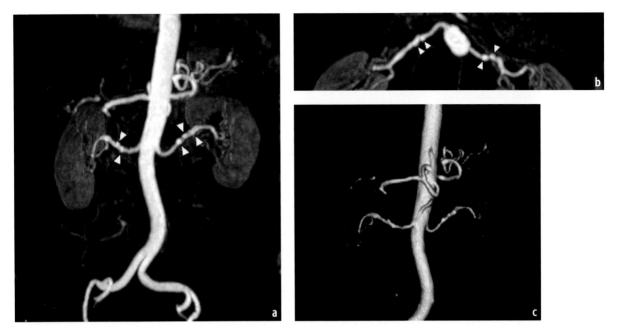

Fig. 15a-c. Fibromuscular dysplasia. Characteristic "string of beads" appearance (arrowheads) of fibromuscular dyslasia can be seen in both renal arteries on this optimized breath hold 3D CE MRA (**a**, coronal MIP; **b**, axial sub-volume MIP; **c**, coronal VR projection) using parallel imaging

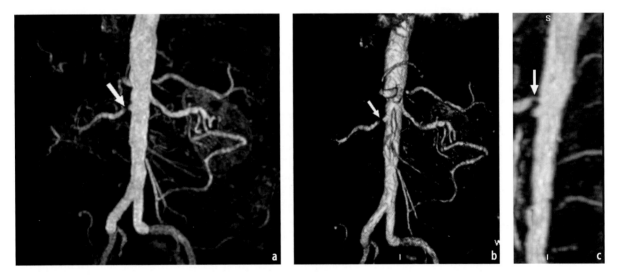

Fig. 16a-c. A fast 7-second renal 3D CE MRA performed during free breathing in a patient unable to hold his breath. Although the images are slightly blurred, the high-grade severe stenosis (arrow) of the right renal artery is clearly seen (**a**, coronal MIP; **b**, coronal VR; **c**, oblique sub-volume MIP). Review of the thinner sub-volume MIP is essential to identify continuity of the renal artery lumen across the lesion and to determine that there is a high-grade stenosis, rather than occlusion of the right renal artery

Scan Time: the Temporal vs. Spatial Resolution Dilemma

As with all MR applications, there is the classic dilemma of temporal resolution (i.e. scan time) versus spatial resolution, since higher spatial resolution imaging requires longer acquisition times. Optimization of these competing demands requires both an understanding of the minimal temporal and spatial requirements for the specific vascular territory, and familiarity with the options available for scan parameter modification that can meet those requirements. Imaging time and the various modifiable parameters for scan time reduction can be calculated by the equation:

$$\text{Scan time} = \text{TR} * N_z * N_y * (\text{k-space fraction}) * 1/\text{AF}$$

in which, N_Y is the number of actual phase encoding steps (y resolution); N_z is the number of partitions (z resolution); *(k-space fraction)* is the percentage of k-space views that are acquired (n.b. alternative k-space acquisition schemes such as partial Fourier and rectangular FOV will result in reductions in phase encoding steps and, as a result, in a comparable reduction in scan time); and *AF* is the acceleration factor if parallel imaging is implemented.

For CE MRA, scanning is typically performed during a breath hold, and thus the patient's breath hold will limit the acquisition time. Because most patients can hold their breath for 20-30 seconds, this is considered the typical upper limit acquisition time for most CE MRA examinations. In cases where breath holding is not required, such as carotid or peripheral CE MRA, longer acquisition times can be employed. The challenge is therefore to balance slice thickness and the number of phase encoding steps to ensure adequate spatial resolution for appropriate diagnosis with adequate anatomic coverage for the clinical indication.

Contrast Administration

CE MRA has traditionally been performed using one of the commercially available extracellular Gd-chelate contrast agents. The rate of injection affects the peak Gd concentration and thus the achievable arterial SNR. Generally, a faster injection rate will result in higher arterial SNR, but shorter bolus duration and earlier venous enhancement. Injection rates of 2 mL/sec are ideal for most CE MRA applications, with little benefit shown for higher rates [63]. Slower injection rates result in lower overall Gd concentrations, but extend the plateau phase of arterial enhancement and delay venous enhancement. Slower injection rates (e.g. 0.8-1.0 mL/sec [31, 32]) have generally been used for multi-station CE MRA in order to prolong the arterial phase and delay venous enhancement, both of which are desirable to ensure adequate arterial signal for multi-station coverage. Recently, biphasic (e.g. 0.8 mL/sec followed by 0.4 mL/sec (Fig. 17); 1.5 mL/sec followed by 0.5 mL/sec [38] or 2.0 mL/sec followed by 1.2 mL/sec [39]) injection protocols have become popular for multi-station peripheral bolus chase CE MRA examinations. The higher initial injection rate provides a greater early Gd concentration for improved visualization of the abdominal aorta, which may be enlarged by aneurysm and require more Gd for proper visualization. Biphasic injections may also be useful for imaging patients requiring assessment of regional venous structures, such as patients undergoing pre-operative planning for renal cell carcinoma removal. In these patients, the arterial supply as well as possible venous invasion by the renal carcinoma are important findings, especially given the current trend towards laproscopic or other less invasive interventions. The use of a biphasic injection for CE MRA helps provide proper arterial depiction and adequate venous signal for proper determination of potential venous invasion by the renal cell carcinoma. Similar techniques may be useful for assessment of the portal vein or central venous system.

For most CE MRA examinations, a dose of 0.15-0.2 mmol/kg (typically 20 - 30 mL) is sufficient. If timing is good, lower doses (0.1 mmol/kg) have also been found to be adequate [22]. In general, the use of a larger contrast agent dose has the benefit of prolonging the arterial phase and providing the operator with an additional buffer to compensate for errors in timing. For novice practitioners, it is suggested that they begin with an 0.2 mmol/kg dose, and then reduce the dose based on their mastery of timing for CE MRA. Unfortunately, aside from increased cost, larger contrast agent doses have the unwanted effect of increasing the likelihood of venous contamination and diminishing operator options should additional CE MRA or repeat acquisitions be desired during the same exam period. Hany et al [62] have estimated that a dose of at least 0.12 mmol/kg of Gd-chelate contrast agent is required for diagnostic CE MRA. This dose is very close to the "single dose" (single 20 mL vial) suggested by Rofsky et al [29] for CE MRA.

More recently, a new gadolinium contrast agent (gadobenate dimeglumine, Gd-BOPTA, Multi-Hance; Bracco Imaging SpA, Milan, Italy [64-67]) has become available in Europe and numerous other countries around the world. Compared with the gadolinium chelates traditionally used for CE MRA, this agent has improved T1 relaxivity due to weak interactions of the Gd-BOPTA chelate with serum proteins such as albumin. Knopp et al [64] have shown that the signal intensity increase with Gd-BOPTA is as much as 50% higher than with conventional gadolinium contrast agents at the same dose and injection rate making this agent particularly suitable for CE MRA. The relative benefits of Gd-BOPTA are more apparent in smaller vessels, which are better visualized using Gd-BOPTA than with traditional extracellular contrast agents [66, 67].

One final consideration for contrast administration is that of saline flush [68]. In practice, a large saline flush (at least 30 mL) should be used for all CE MRA examinations. A large flush will ensure that the entire contrast dose is administered beyond the tubing and that the bolus will travel through the peripheral veins into the right heart, ensuring sufficient Gd concentrations are delivered to the more distal arteries. The use of a large flush increases the slope of the enhancement

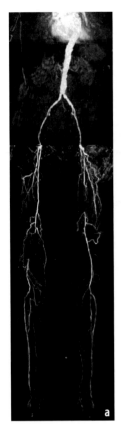
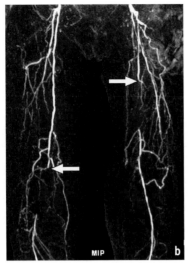
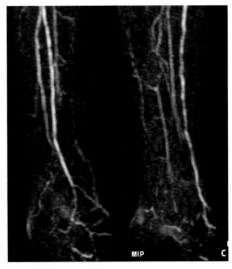

Fig. 17a-c. Multi-station 3D CE MRA (**a**, coronal large field of view MIP of overlapping three station exam) in a patient with severe peripheral vascular occlusive disease. Occlusions of both superficial femoral arteries (arrows) are clearly seen on the 3D MRA of the second station (**b**, coronal MIP). On this multi-station exam, distal run-off vessels were also well visualized (**c**, oblique MIP). Contrast was administered using a biphasic injection scheme whereby the initial half of the contrast dose was injected at 0.8 mL/sec and the remaining dose at 0.4 mL/sec

curve, increases the duration of the arterial phase of the bolus (up to 50% [68]), and delays significant venous enhancement, all of which are preferable for arterial CE MRA.

The CE MRA Protocol

A typical CE MRA examination includes several traditional pulse sequences (e.g. T1-weighted and T2-weighted fast spin echo pulse sequences). These images are particularly important for imaging not only concomitant visceral pathology, but also vessel wall abnormalities such as wall thickening (e.g. aortitis) or intramural hematoma [16]. These preliminary non-contrast pulse sequences are then usually followed by a localization scan for the CE MRA examination. These are typically performed using a bright blood pulse sequence such as TOF MRA or, more recently, steady state free precession (SSFP) pulse sequences (true FISP, Siemens Medical Solutions; Balanced FFE, Philips; FIESTA, GE Medical Systems).

For the CE MRA examination itself, the 3D MRA acquisition is usually performed three times. A pre-contrast 3D MRA acquisition is recommended to ensure proper anatomic coverage and precise positioning of the 3D volume. Unwanted

aliasing artifacts, for example, can easily be identified on the pre-contrast scan. It is also recommended that the pre-contrast 3D MRA acquisition be performed in an identical fashion to the actual CE MRA acquisition as this will familiarize the patient to both the breath holding procedure and the expected length for the breath hold. In addition, the pre-contrast acquisition can serve as a mask for subsequent image subtraction, if desired. For the CE MRA, acquisitions are typically performed in both the arterial and delayed phases. The addition of the second delayed phase acquisition will ensure proper visualization of vessels with slow flow or depiction of a late filling false channel in the case of an aortic dissection. Additionally, the second acquisition can often distinguish artifacts from true vascular findings (Fig. 4). Finally, the inclusion of the second post-contrast 3D MRA acquisition may provide additional venous depiction which may be of clinical importance in certain specific clinical situations.

Within this chapter, it is hoped that the reader has established a baseline understanding of the basic theory for CE MRA and improved his or her familiarity with the various terms and options available. In the chapters that follow, the different clinical indications for CE MRA will be discussed with specific technical suggestions for CE MRA.

References

1. Yucel EK, Anderson CM, Edelman RR et al (1999) AHA scientific statement. Magnetic resonance angiography: update on applications for extracranial arteries. Circulation 100(22):2284-22301
2. Koelemay MJ, Lijmer JG, Stoker J et al (2001) Magnetic resonance angiography for the evaluation of lower extremity arterial disease. A meta-analysis. JAMA 285(10):1338-1345
3. Nelemans PJ, Leiner T, de Vet HC et al (2000) Peripheral arterial disease: meta-analysis of the diagnostic performance of MR angiography. Radiology 217(1):105-114
4. Prince MR, Yucel EK, Kaufman JA et al (1993) Dynamic gadolinium-enhanced three-dimensional abdominal MR arteriography. J Magn Reson Imaging 3:877-881
5. Prince MR (1994) Gadolinium-enhanced MR angiography Radiology 191:155-164
6. Prince MR (1998) Contrast-enhanced MR angiography: theory and optimization. Magn Reson Imaging Clin N Am 6:257-267
7. Ho VB, Foo TKF, Czum JM et al (2001) Contrast-Enhanced Magnetic Resonance Angiography: Technical Considerations for Optimized Clinical Implementation. Top Magn Reson Imaging 12:283-299
8. Maki JH, Knopp MV, Prince M (2003) Contrast-enhanced MR angiography. Applied Radiology 32(supplement):3-31
9. Kaufman JA, MCCarter D, Geller SC et al (1998) Two-dimensional time-of-flight MR angiography of the lower extremities: artifacts and pitfalls. AJR Am J Roentgenol 171(1):129-135
10. Levy RA, Prince MR (1996) Arterial-phase three-dimensional contrast-enhanced MR angiography of the carotid arteries. AJR Am J Roetgenol 167:211-215
11. Isoda H, Takehara Y, Isogai S et al (1998) Technique for arterial-phase contrast-enhanced three-dimensional MR angiography of the carotid and vertebral arteries. AJNR Am J Neuroradiol 19:1241-1244
12. Huston J 3rd, Fain SB, Wald JT et al (2001) Carotid artery: elliptic centic contrast-enhanced MR angiography compared with conventional angiography. Radiology 218:138-143
13. Wilman AH, Riederer SJ, Huston J et al (1998) Arterial phase carotid and vertebral artery imaging in 3D contrast-enhanced MR angiography by combining fluoroscopic triggering with an elliptical centric acquisition order. Magn Reson Med 40:24-35
14. Foo TKF, Ho VB, Choyke PL (1999) Contrast-Enhanced Carotid Magnetic Resonance Angiography: Imaging Principles and Physics. Neuroimaging Clin N Am 9:263-284
15. Prince MR, Narasimham DL, Jacoby WT et al (1996) Three-dimensional gadolinium-enhanced MR angiography of the thoracic aorta. AJR Am J Roentgenol 166:1387-1397
16. Krinsky GA, Rofsky NM, DeCorato DR et al (1997) Thoracic aorta: comparison of gadolinium-enhanced three-dimensional MR angiography with conventional MR imaging. Radiology 202:183-193
17. Ho VB, Prince M (1998) Thoracic MR Aortography: Imaging Techniques and Strategies. RadioGraphics 18:287-309
18. Ho VB, Corse WR, Hood MN et al (2003) MRA of the Thoracic Vessels. Semin Ultrasound CT MR 24:192-216
19. Snidow J, Johnson MS, Harris VJ et al (1996) Three-dimensional gadolinium-enhanced MR angiography for aortoiliac inflow assessment plus renal artery screening in a single breath hold. Radiology 198:725-732
20. Prince MR, Schoenberg SO, Ward JS et al (1997) Hemodynamically significant atherosclerotic renal artery stenosis: MR angiographic features. Radiology 205:128-136
21. Wilman AH, Riederer SJ, King BF et al (1997) Fluoroscopically triggered contrast-enhanced three-dimensional MR angiography with elliptical centric view order: application to the renal arteries. Radiology 205:137-146
22. Lee VS, Rofsky NM, Krinsky GA et al (1999) Single-dose breath-hold gadolinium-enhanced three-dimensional MR angiography of the renal arteries. Radiology 211:69-78
23. Schoenberg SO, Bock M, Knopp MV, et al (1999) Renal arteries: Optimization of three-dimensional gadolinium-enhanced MR angiography with bolus-timing-independent fast multi-phase acquisition in a single breath hold. Radiology 211:667-679
24. Hood MN, Ho VB, Corse WR (2002) Three-dimensional phase-contrast magnetic resonance angiography: a useful clinical adjunct to gadolinium-enhanced three-dimensional renal magnetic resonance angiography? Mil Med 167:343-349
25. Ho VB, Corse WR (2003) MR Angiography of the Abdominal Aorta and Peripheral Vessels. Radiol Clin North Am 41:115-144
26. Snidow JJ, Johnson MS, Harris VJ et al (1996) Three-dimensional gadolinium-enhanced MR angiography for aortoiliac inflow assessment plus renal artery screening in a single breath hold. Radiology 198:725-732
27. Hany TF, Debatin JF, Leung DA et al (1997) Evaluation of the aortoiliac and renal arteries: comparison of breath-hold, contrast-enhanced, three-dimensional MR angiography with conventional catheter angiography. Radiology 204:357-62
28. Poon E, Yucel EK, Pagan-Marin H et al (1997) Iliac artery stenosis measurements: comparison of two-dimensional time-of-flight and three-dimensional dynamic gadolinium-enhanced MR angiography. AJR Am J Roentgenol 169:1139-1144
29. Rofsky NM, Johnson G, Adelman MA et al (1997) Peripheral vascular disease evaluated with reduced dose gadolinium-enhanced MR angiography. Radiology 205:163-169
30. Quinn SF, Sheley RC, Szumowski J et al (1997) Evaluation of the iliac arteries; comparison of two-dimensional time of flight magnetic resonance angiography with cardiac compensated fast gradient recalled echo and contrast-enhanced three-dimensional time of flight magnetic resonance angiography. J Magn Reson Imaging 7:197-203
31. Ho KY, Leiner T, de Haan MW et al (1998) Peripheral vascular tree stenoses: evaluation with moving-bed infusion-tracking MR angiography. Radiology 206:683-692
32. Meaney JM, Ridgeway JP, Chakraverty S et al (1999) Stepping-table gadolinium-enhanced digital subtraction MR angiography of the aorta and lower ex-

tremity arteries: preliminary experience. Radiology 211:59-67

33. Ho VB, Choyke PL, Foo TKF et al (1999) Automated bolus chase peripheral MR angiography: initial practical experiences and future directions of this work-in-progress. J Magn Reson Imaging 10:376-388

34. Ruehm SG, Hany TF, Pfammatter T et al (2000) Pelvic and lower extremity arterial imaging: diagnostic performance of three-dimensional contrast-enhanced MR angiography. AJR Am J Roentgenol 174:1127-1135

35. Leiner T, Ho KY, Nelemans PJ et al (2000) Three-dimensional contrast-enhanced moving-bed infusion-tracking (MoBI-Track) peripheral MR angiography with flexible choice of imaging parameters for each field of view. J Magn Reson Imaging 11:368–377

36. Schoenberg SO, Londy FJ, Licato P et al (2001) Multiphase-multistep gadolinium-enhanced MR angiography of the abdominal aorta and runoff vessels. Invest Radiol 36(5):283-291

37. Ruehm SG, Goyen M, Barkhausen J et al (2001) Rapid magnetic resonance angiography for detection of atherosclerosis. Lancet 357(9262):1086-1091

38. Shetty AN, Bis KG, Duerinckx AJ et al (2002) Lower extremity MR angiography: universal retrofitting of high-field-strength systems with stepping kinematic imaging platforms initial experience. Radiology 222(1):284-291

39. Maki JH, Ephron JH, Glickerman DJ et al (2000) Moving table Gd-enhanced MR angiography of the lower extremities: a combination 3D and 2D technique – preliminary results (abstr.). International Society for Magnetic Resonance in Medicine Eighth Scientific Meeting and Exhibition Program. Berkeley, Calif: ISMRM p. 1810

40. Hohenschuh E, Watson A (1997) Theory and mechanisms of contrast-enhancing agents. In: Higgins C, Hricak H, Helms C, eds. Magnetic Resonance Imaging of the Body. Philadelphia, Pa: Lippencott-Raven: 1439-1464

41. Marks B, Mitchell DG, Simelaro JP (1997) Breath-holding in healthy and pulmonary-compromised populations: Effects of hyperventilation and oxygen inspiration. J Magn Reson Imaging 7:595-597

42. Leiner T, de Weert TT, Nijenhuis RJ et al (2001) Need for background suppression in contrast-enhanced peripheral magnetic resonance angiography. J Magn Reson Imaging 14(6):724-733

43. Lee VS, Martin DJ, Krinsky GA et al (2000) Gadolinium-enhanced MR angiography: Artifacts and pitfalls. AJR Am J Roentgenol 175:197-205

44. Earls JP, Rofsky NM, DeCorato DR et al (1996) Breath-hold single dose Gd-enhanced three-dimensional MR aortography: usefulness of a timing examination and MR power injector. Radiology 201(3):705-710

45. Kim JK, Farb RI, Wright GA (1998) Test bolus examination in the carotid artery at dynamic gadolinium-enhanced MR angiography. Radiology 206:283-289

46. Hany TF, McKinnon GC, Leung DA et al (1997) Optimization of contrast timing for breath-hold three-dimensional MR angiography. J Magn Reson Imaging 7(3):551-556

47. Slosman F, Stolpen AH, Lexa FJ et al (1998) Extracranial atherosclerotic carotid artery disease: evaluation of non-breath-hold three-dimensional gadolinium-enhanced MR angiography. AJR Am J Roentgenol 170(2):489-95

48. Foo TK, Saranathan M, Prince MR et al (1997) Automated detection of bolus arrival and initiation of data acquisition in fast, three-dimensional, gadolinium-enhanced MR angiography. Radiology 203(1):275-280

49. Prince MR, Chenevert TL, Foo TK et al (1997) Contrast-enhanced abdominal MR angiography: optimization of imaging delay time by automating the detection of contrast material arrival in the aorta. Radiology 203(1):109-14

50. Ho VB, Foo TK (1998) Optimization of gadolinium-enhanced magnetic resonance angiography using an automated bolus detection algorithm (MR Smart-Prep). Original investigation. Invest Radiol 33(9):515-523

51. Riederer SJ, Bernstein MA, Breen JF et al (2000) Three-dimensional contrast-enhanced MR angiography with real-time fluoroscopic triggering: design specifications and technical reliability in 330 patient studies. Radiology 215:584-593

52. Hendrick R, Roff U (1991) Image contrast and noise. Chicago, IL: Mosby Yearbook

53. Hoogeeven RM, Bakker CJG, Viergever MA (1998) Limits to the accuracy of vessel diameter measurement in MR angiography. J Magn Reson Imaging 8:1228-1235

54. Lamb HJ, Doornbos J (2003) Clinical approach to cardiovascular MRI techniques. In: Higgins CB, de Roos A, eds. Cardiovascular MRI and MRA. Philadelphia, PA: Lippincott Williams & Wilkins 3-18

55. Maki JH, Prince MR, Londy FJ et al (1996) The effects of time varying intravascular signal intensity and k-space acquisition order on three-dimensional MR angiography image quality. J Magn Reson Imaging 6(4):642-651

56. Du YP, Parker DL, Davis WL et al (1994) Reduction of partial-volume artifacts with zero-filled interpolation in three-dimensional MR angiography. J Magn Reson Imaging 4(5):733-41

57. Saloner D (2003) MRA techniques. In: Higgins CB, de Roos A, eds. Cardiovascular MRI and MRA. Philadelphia, PA: Lippincott Williams & Wilkins 19-36

58. Weiger M, Pruessmann KP, Kassner A et al (2000) Contrast-enhanced 3D MRA using SENSE. J Magn Reson Imaging 12:671-677

59. van den Brink JS, Watanabe Y, Kuhl CK et al (2003) Implications of SENSE MR in routine clinical practice. Eur J Radiol, Apr 46(1):3-27

60. Maki JH, Wilson GJ, Eubank WB et al (2002) Utilizing SENSE to achieve lower station sub-millimeter isotropic resolution and minimal venous enhancement in peripheral MR angiography. J Magn Reson Imaging 15(4):484-491

61. Sodickson DK, McKenzie CA, Li W et al (2000) Contrast-enhanced 3D MR angiography with simultaneous acquisition of spatial harmonics: A pilot study. Radiology 217:284-289

62. Hany TF, Wegener R, Schmidt M et al (1998) Fixed contrast-dose scheme vs. fixed contrast-volume scheme for contrast-enhanced 3D MR angiography (abstr.). International Society for Magnetic Resonance in Medicine Sixth Scientific Meeting and Exhibition Program. Berkeley, Calif: ISMRM p. 768

63. Kopka L, Vosshenrich R, Rodenwaldt J et al (1998) Differences in injection rates on contrast-enhanced

breath-hold three-dimensional MR angiography. AJR Am J Roentgenol 170(2):345-348

64. Knopp MV, Schoenberg SO, Rehm C et al (2002) Assessment of Gadobenate Dimeglumine (Gd-BOPTA) for MR Angiography: Phase I Studies. Invest Radiol 37:706-715

65. Völk M, Strotzer M, Lenhart M et al (2001) Renal time-resolved MR angiography; quantitative comparison of gadobenate dimeglumine and gadopentetate dimeglumine with different doses. Radiology 220(2):484-488

66. Knopp MV, Giesel FL, von Tengg-Kobligk H et al (2003) Contrast-enhanced MR angiography of the run-off vasculature: intraindividual comparison of gadobenate dimeglumine with gadopentetate dimeglumine. J Magn Reson Imaging 17(6): 694-702

67. Wyttenbach R, Gianella S, Alerci M et al (2003) Prospective Blinded Evaluation of Gd-DOTA– versus Gd-BOPTA–enhanced Peripheral MR Angiography, as Compared with Digital Subtraction Angiography. Radiology 227:261-269

68. Boos M, Scheffler K, Haselhorst R et al (2001) Arterial first pass gadolinium-CM dynamics as a function of several intravenous saline flush and Gd volumes. J Magn Reson Imaging 13(4):568-576

I.3

Time-resolved MR Angiography

F. Scott Pereles and Vincent B. Ho

Introduction

Improvements in gradient performance and novel image acquisition schemes such as parallel imaging have greatly accelerated MR image acquisition. Until recently, these advancements have been used almost entirely for improving the spatial resolution of MR angiography (MRA). For most clinical applications, the goal of optimization of parameters for highest possible spatial resolution is advantageous for MRA, especially for contrast-enhanced (CE) MRA. High spatial resolution is often necessary for the confident visualization of smaller vessels, grading of arterial stenoses and proper identification of more subtle vascular pathologies such as penetrating ulcers.

However, faster imaging speed can also be used to improve the temporal resolution of CE MRA. The dynamic assessment of contrast media bolus progression through a vascular territory, or vascular lesion has long been an essential diagnostic tool for conventional x-ray angiography, especially x-ray digital subtraction angiography (DSA). The development of faster MR scanners and innovative software has enabled the performance of analogous dynamic viewing of Gd-chelate contrast media using fast two-dimensional (2D) and/or three-dimensional (3D) MRA acquisitions. Time resolved MRA is rapidly emerging as a valuable MRA tool in select diagnostic situations.

Until recently, time resolved imaging has primarily been available using two-dimensional (2D) pulse sequences for limited planar or "projectional" viewing. However, with the advent of ultrafast gradients (slew rates of faster than 100 T/m/s for "sub-second" 3D CE MRA [1]) and alternative k-space schemes (e.g. Time Resolved Imaging with Contrast Kinetics or TRICKS [2]), time-resolved imaging can now be achieved using three-dimensional (3D) MRA, for "4D" or time-resolved volumetric dynamic evaluations.

This chapter will explore some of the available techniques for time-resolved MRA and will highlight clinical scenarios in which high temporal resolution imaging can improve the diagnostic value for an MRA exam. Time-resolved imaging is a particularly helpful tool for multi-station MRA exams, identification of flow patterns associated with certain vascular pathologies and arterial-venous segmentation of complex vascular malformations or arrangements.

The Temporal vs. Spatial Resolution Dilemma Revisited

As mentioned in the preceding chapter, there is an inextricable link between temporal and spatial resolution. The relationship between achievable spatial and temporal resolution is to a great extent a simple inverse relationship, whereby improvements in spatial resolution result in lengthening of exam time (i.e. diminished temporal resolution) and vice versa [3]. For example, if all other parameters are being kept equal, higher spatial resolution imaging generally will increase the k-space data that will be required, which results in prolongation of overall scan time. Conversely if higher temporal resolution is desired, one must generally sacrifice spatial resolution – i.e. phase-encoding steps (k_y) or slice-encoding steps (k_z) – in order to reduce scan times for each temporal "phase" or time point of the dynamic evaluation.

Conventional high spatial resolution 3D CE MRA typically requires 20-30 seconds per scan. While these longer high spatial resolution 3D CE MRAs will often be sufficient to evaluate overall vascular morphology in a region, they may mask subtle vascular features that may only be appreciated by higher temporal resolution imaging. Long acquisition times may result in the temporal averaging of early and late filling effects, which may be critical for assessment of certain vascular pathologies. Details such as the direction of blood flow between channels or the source of a vascular leak may not be apparent on longer MRA acquisitions. Significant filling of structures can occur during the 20-30 second period during which the high spatial resolution MRA is being performed. Faster dynamic viewing (e.g. < 5 sec/frame) as provided by time resolved imaging may be necessary for proper identification of donor and recipient vascular channels. Time resolved MRA provides important supplemental information of contrast bolus progression (i.e. bolus kinetics) through the vascular region. High temporal resolution is particularly helpful for proper segmentation of arteries from veins in instances where blood flow is typically brisk and the vessels are overlapping, such as exist in the pulmonary circulation or in arterial-venous malformations.

Techniques for Time-resolved Imaging

2D Timing Scan

One of the first and arguably still the most widely used application for time-resolved imaging is for the estimation of the contrast arrival times–the bolus-timing scan–for arterial-phase 3D CE MRA [4]. As discussed previously, the success of CE MRA relies significantly on the proper synchronization of

low spatial frequency k-space data (also known as the center of k-space) with peak enhancement of the target vessel(s). The typical test bolus scan employs a T1-weighted, fast 2D gradient echo pulse sequence with a reasonably high frame rate of a single 2D image every 1-2 seconds. Information from these 2D images is typically limited to Gd-chelate contrast agent arrival time to a targeted vascular structure on a single slice. The practical issues related to this application of time resolved 2D imaging are that (1) the injection should be similar to that of the 3D CE MRA, (2) that it should be fast, and (3) that it uses a small amount of contrast material. The bolus timing scan merely serves as a planning tool for higher spatial resolution 3D CE MRA, which ultimately provides the morphologic detail necessary for vascular diagnosis. As such, a small dose (1-2 mL) of Gd-chelate contrast agent is usually used and an MR-compatible power injector is desirable to minimize differences between injections. Low doses of contrast minimize background tissue enhancement and enable the more judicious use of contrast agent for the achievement of high spatial resolution 3D CE MRA.

2D MR DSA

With further refinements, namely a good mask subtraction, fast 2D pulse sequences can also be used to provide 2D projectional angiograms similar to those of conventional x-ray digital subtraction angiography (DSA). Wang et al [5, 6] have successfully implemented 2D MR DSA using a specialized off-line complex subtraction algorithm. This technique is particularly helpful for illustration of distal run-off vessels [6, 7]. A series of relatively thick (8-10 cm) 2D projectional images are acquired during the intravenous injection of 6-10 mL of Gd-chelate contrast agent. During each injection, a series of 2D MR DSA is performed with

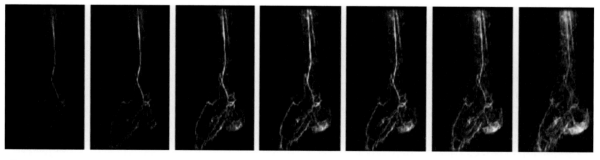

Fig. 1. 2D MR DSA of the ankle using complex subtraction. Projectional 2D subtraction images were obtained as a single slab, typically 80-100 mm thick, with spoiled gradient echo imaging using the standard head coil. 2D images were acquired repeatedly at 2-second intervals beginning simultaneously with the hand injection of a 7 mL bolus of Gd-chelate contrast media via a peripheral intravenous catheter at approximately 3 mL/sec. The contrast injection is followed by 20 ml of saline flush at the same rate. From these images the bolus timing for the thigh and knee stations can be determined and the timing for the abdomen-pelvis can be estimated. Typically the time to fill the abdomen pelvis is 2/3 the time required to reach the ankles. It is also possible to identify when veins begin to enhance so that the window of arterial enhancement without venous enhancement can be identified (Reprinted and modified with permission from [17])

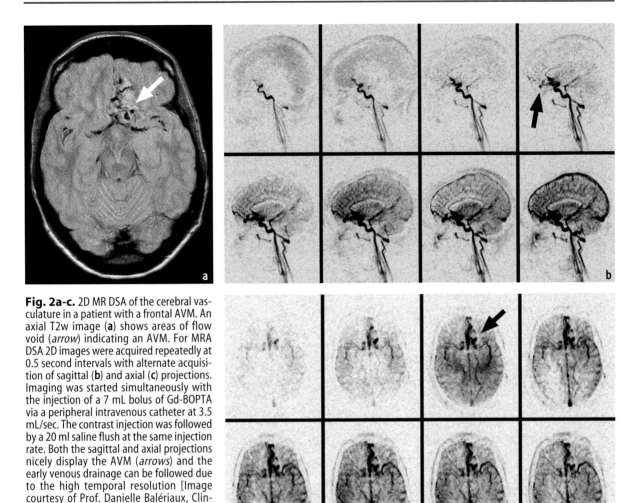

Fig. 2a-c. 2D MR DSA of the cerebral vasculature in a patient with a frontal AVM. An axial T2w image (**a**) shows areas of flow void (*arrow*) indicating an AVM. For MRA DSA 2D images were acquired repeatedly at 0.5 second intervals with alternate acquisition of sagittal (**b**) and axial (**c**) projections. Imaging was started simultaneously with the injection of a 7 mL bolus of Gd-BOPTA via a peripheral intravenous catheter at 3.5 mL/sec. The contrast injection was followed by a 20 ml saline flush at the same injection rate. Both the sagittal and axial projections nicely display the AVM (*arrows*) and the early venous drainage can be followed due to the high temporal resolution [Image courtesy of Prof. Danielle Balériaux, Clinique de Neuroradiologie, Hôpital Erasmus, Brussels, Belgium]

frame rates of every 2-3 seconds (Fig. 1). The technique, however, continues to be investigational with limited availability, nevertheless in imaging of cerebral AV-malformation it can already compete with catheter angiography (Fig. 2).

Ultrafast 3D MRA (including "sub-second" 3D MRA)

An additional method for time resolved imaging is to optimize the basic T1-weighted fast 3D gradient echo pulse sequence used for conventional high spatial resolution 3D CE MRA for faster acquisition times instead of highest spatial resolution. With newer high performance gradients, 3D MRA can be performed every 5-7 sec [8] on many commercial scanners enabling multi-phase 3D CE MRA during a single breath hold (Fig. 3). The main compromise is that of spatial resolution, as a reduction in phase-encoding (ky) and slice-encoding (kz) steps are generally required.

More recently, Finn et al [1] introduced a "sub-

second" time-resolved 3D MRA technique ("sub-second angiography" or "freeze-frame angiography") that uses an ultrafast 3D spoiled gradient echo pulse sequence with markedly reduced TR (e.g. 1.6 msec) and TE (e.g. 0.8 msec) times whereby individual 3D acquisition times are between 400 and 900 msec (i.e. "sub-second" 3D MRA). Tempo-

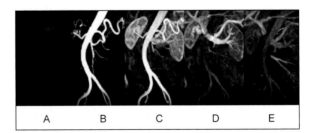

Fig. 3. Single breath-hold, multi-phase 3D CE MRA of the abdomen. Ultrafast 3D Multiphase CE-MRA (A-E, 5 phases, each 6.3 s; TR=3.2 ms, TE=1.1 ms, 40 degree flip angle) performed within a single breath hold after injection of 0.1 mmol/kg Gd-BOPTA (Bracco Diagnostics, Milan, Italy). Note the distinct vascular phases (B-E) with the arterial, late arterial, portovenous and delayed venous phases shown (Reprinted and modified with permission from [3])

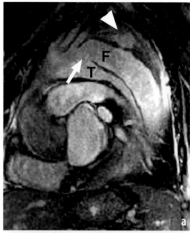

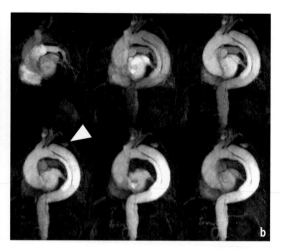

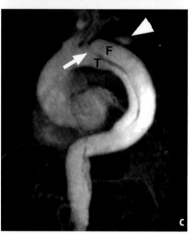

Fig. 4a-c. Sub-second 3D MRA in a patient with a Type B aortic dissection and extralumi-nal leak. Sagittal trueFISP image (**a**) demonstrates the true (T) and false (F) channels and in-timal tear (*arrow*) distal to the origin of the left subclavian artery. There is also a small region of bright signal (arrowhead) posterior to the aorta suspicious for extra-luminal blood, but its source is not clearly determined. On sagittal dynamic sub-second 3D MRA (**b**, 6 selected im-ages; **c**, single phase from dynamic study), the true and false channels as well as the intimal tear (*arrow*) are once again noted. On time resolved imaging, the aforementioned rounded area (*arrowhead*) is noted to enhanced at roughly the same time as the descending aorta consistent with a persistent communication with the aortic lumen

ral resolution was further facilitated with the im-plementation of partial Fourier and fractional FOV k-space schemes. The technique is typically obtained in coronal or sagittal orientation and is coupled with automated on-line image subtraction that can provide rapid generation of time resolved maximum intensity projections (MIPs) of the sub-tracted 3D CE MRA data sets for 3D MR DSA.

Most often it is advantageous to perform dy-namic sub-second 3D MRA prior to conventional 3D CE MRA of higher spatial resolution. Time re-solved imaging using sub-second 3D MRA can provide not only bolus timing information but al-so a wealth of information concerning the under-lying anatomy and its flow pattern (Fig. 4). Howev-er a few key concepts must be remembered, espe-cially if the sub-second angiogram is utilized as a replacement for timing runs prior to the 3D MRA.

First, sub-second angiography due to its inher-ently poor through plane resolution is usually best suited for interrogation of larger vessels, namely the aorta and pulmonary artery and their first or-der branches. If desired two consecutive sub-sec-ond MRAs may be performed in separate orienta-tions or projections (e.g. coronal and sagittal). Both acquisitions can occur virtually back-to-back without risk of image compromise.

Second, the sub-second angiogram as original-ly implemented uses a 6 mL Gd-chelate contrast bolus injection followed by an 18-20 mL saline flush, both injected at 6 mL/sec. One can tailor these parameters slightly in certain situations, like reducing contrast amount to 4 mL or decreasing injection rate to 4 mL/sec, however image quality will likely suffer, especially in vessels with slow flow or in areas with a large intravascular blood volume (e.g. aneurysms). Increasing rates beyond 6 mL/sec or using higher total volumes of contrast plus flush (>25 mL) are not advisable as most power injector and intravenous tubing setups are not capable of accurately delivering faster flow rates [9]. Furthermore, delivering higher total vol-umes at a rapid rate will likely increase risk for ve-nous extravasation. Anecdotally, in thousands of cases at Northwestern University there have been very few, if any, complications related to these low-volume, high-rate power injections. The injec-tions are typically administered safely via an 18-gauge venous catheter placed in the antecubital fossa or a large vein in the forearm proximal to the wrist, preferably of the right arm. Injection in-to the back of the hand is discouraged due to the size of veins and more importantly the risk of closed space extravasations and complications.

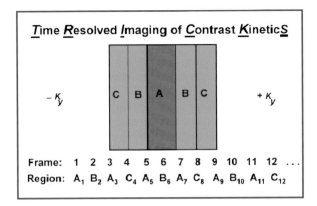

Fig. 5. K-space acquisition scheme for TRICKS [Image courtesy of Dr. F. Korosec, University of Wisconsin, Madison, WI; and Dr. T. Carroll, Department of Radiology, Northwestern University, Chicago, IL, USA]

Strengths of sub-second angiography include, as its name implies, the extremely high temporal resolution achievable (400-500 milliseconds), the very small 4-6 mL contrast dose necessary, and relative insensitivity to minor motion such as when patients are unable to perform a breath-hold. Disadvantages include the need for relatively high performance gradients with slew rates ≥100mT/m/msec. Images obtained are of low through-plane resolution and are therefore essentially projectional images. Hence, sub-second MRA often benefits from performance in two separate orientations or projections.

TRICKS

Korosec et al [2] described yet another method for time-resolved 3D MRA called TRICKS (Time-Re-solved Imaging with Contrast Kinetics). TRICKS is, however, vastly different than "sub-second" 3D MRA. The TRICKS algorithm consists of an alternative temporal k-space sampling scheme that repetitively samples low and high spatial frequency k-space views in a interleaved and slightly asymmetric fashion (Fig. 5). The low spatial frequency data (i.e. central k-space data) is updated at a much faster rate (i.e. higher temporal sampling) than the higher frequency data (i.e. peripheral k-space data). The resultant data is reconstructed to yield time resolved 3D data sets that have both high temporal and high spatial resolution. This is achieved by the sharing of k-space data, notably low spatial frequency data, across temporal 3D data sets. TRICKS and its iterative refinements of serial undersampling in multiple dimensions, such as PR TRICKS (Projection Reconstruction TRICKS [10]), used to suffer from inordinately long reconstruction times. However, improvements in reconstruction algorithms and computer processing speed have minimized these concerns, making this technique commercially available. The strength of TRICKS is that it continually samples k-space and upon reconstruction gives multiple 3D MRA phases of the contrast bolus as it passes through the desired area of evaluation. As mentioned previously this gives both a wealth of spatial and temporal resolution while eliminating the need for a timing run. Sub-second time resolved imaging can also be achieved using TRICKS, but as with traditional sub-second 3D MRA, imaging parameter adjustment typically results in a reduction in spatial resolution (Fig. 6) [11].

The performance of higher spatial resolution 3D TRICKS MRA with its relatively longer scan time requirements make its use for high spatial

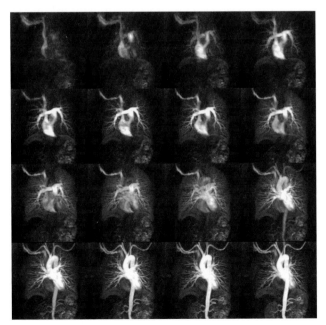

Fig. 6. Sub-second 4D MRA using TRICKS implemented with parallel imaging in a healthy volunteer. The technique, called 4D MR DSA, provides a high temporal resolution of 600 msec per 3D image set. Scan parameters include: TR, 3.1 msec; TE, 0.9 msec; Flip angle, 20 degrees; FOV, 42 x 42 cm; martrix, 256 x 128 matrix; partitions, 22; partition thickness, 5 mm; interpolation to 44 partitions. On these TRICKS images, the normal flow pattern from a right sided venous injection can be seen with enhancement of the right heart and pulmonary arteries (first two rows) followed by enhancement of the left heart and aorta (bottom two rows) [Images courtesy of Drs. M. Ookawa, N. Ichinose, S. Sugiura, Y Machida and M. Miyazaki, Toshiba Medical Systems, Otawara, Tochigi, Japan]

resolution thoracic of abdominal imaging somewhat more challenging as breath hold acquisition is generally preferred for best image quality. Proper timing, albeit less precise, is nonetheless required to ensure tolerable breath hold durations for the patient and adequate temporal coverage of the bolus to ensure arterial phase images.

Clinical Applications

Multi-station MRA

With the development of moving or stepped table techniques, multi-station MRA has become a clinical staple for the evaluation of the peripheral run-off vessels [12-17]. The stepping table technique, akin to that used for peripheral x-ray angiography, consists of the progressive movement of the imaging field of view in conjunction with the arterial transit of a Gd-chelate contrast bolus down the lower extremities. This technique also called bolus chasing has become a clinical standard for peripheral MRA and is now achievable on any new MR scanner, using scanner-specific software [12-14] and hardware or a third-party movable tabletop that mounts on the scanner bed [15, 16]. Bolus chase peripheral MRA is typically performed using three (or possibly more) overlapping contiguous 3D MRA acquisitions. The initial 3D MRA is either centered about the lower abdominal aorta (the aortoiliac segment) or the most distal part of the imaging volume (feet) with each subsequent 3D MRA prescribed in overlapping fashion for distal or proximal coverage. Improved distal anatomic coverage can be provided by the performance of a pre-contrast 2D TOF MRA of the most distal arterial segments (e.g. calves and feet) prior to the bolus chase.

Early iterations of this technique required the initiation of imaging to begin with arrival of contrast into the abdominal aorta (i.e. initial or first station) to continue with the rapid acquisition of subsequent distal 3D MRAs. Arterial phase timing was performed using any of the previously mentioned timing techniques (e.g. test bolus scan, MR fluoroscopic trigger, MR SMARTPREP). Since arterial phase timing was only performed for 3D MRA of the initial station, the arteries of the more distal stations, particularly the infrapopliteal arteries, are often unreliably visualized. Wang et al [6] reported obtaining diagnostic quality images of the infrapopliteal arteries in as few as 43% of cases as opposed to diagnostic quality images of the proximal two stations in 100% and 96% of cases, respectively. This is due in large part to the wide variation in bolus arrival times to the lower limbs, which hampers proper synchronization of imaging with arterial enhancement in the distal run-off

vessels. Differences in contrast arrival times are more significant distally, especially in patients with underlying vascular disease. Prince et al [18] reported arrival times to the distal tibial artery (at the ankle) that ranged from 18 to 64 sec and disparate flow (greater than 5 sec difference in contrast arrival times) between right and left lower legs in about a quarter of their 87 patients with peripheral vascular disease. These variations in contrast arrival understandably result in inconsistent arterial illustration of the infrapopliteal arteries using a single injection bolus chase method alone.

Time resolved imaging has been found to be particularly helpful for ensuring proper visualization of the infrapopliteal arteries as an adjunct to bolus chase MRA. One technique called the "hybrid technique" [19] integrates time-resolved imaging into a peripheral MRA exam (Fig. 7). This technique, developed at Northwestern University, is predicated on a basic 3D gradient echo pulse sequence (TR 3.5 msec / TE 1.2 msec / flip angle 25 degrees) and dedicated peripheral vascular coil utilization. In this hybrid technique, two separate bolus-timing scans are performed (one in the pelvis and the other in the calves). The pelvis and calf bolus timing scans utilize a relatively high (in-plane) spatial resolution 2D gradient echo scheme to acquire images in the axial plane every second for 40 seconds in the pelvis at the aortic bifurcation and for 80 seconds in the calves at the level of the posterior tibial and peroneal artery bifurcation. The timing sequence uses an image subtraction algorithm describe by Finn et al [19] where the first 3 images serve as a subtraction mask for all subsequent frames and the images are displayed on-line in near real time as the images are acquired. Each timing run is performed with a 2 mL bolus of Gd-chelate contrast media injected at 2 mL/sec followed by a 20 mL saline flush injected also at 2 mL/sec. Following the two bolus-timing scans, a pre-contrast mask 3D MRA acquisition is obtained in the distal station, which includes the calves and feet. Onset of distal station 3D MRA acquisition is based on the estimated arrival time of contrast media demonstrated on the initial 2D calf bolus timing scan. The actual calves/feet 3D MRA is performed with a 20 mL Gd-chelate contrast bolus injected at 2 mL/sec with two consecutive acquisitions obtained with no delay between acquisitions. Usually, each 3D MRA of the calves/feet are 22 seconds ±2 seconds in duration. If contrast arrival in each calf was demonstrated to be discrepant (i.e. asymmetric) by more than 10 seconds on the 2D calf bolus timing scan, then a third 3D MRA acquisition is performed at this station. The calves/feet 3D MRA slab is typically 80 mm thick with partition thickness of 1 to 1.2 mm each.

After the completion of the single station, multiphase 3D MRA of the calves/feet, the table is moved

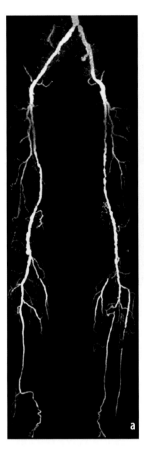
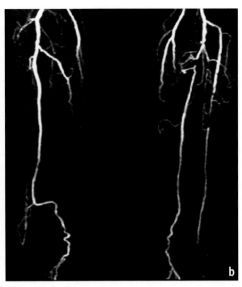

Fig. 7a, b. Hybrid 3D peripheral MRA. Patient with peripheral occlusive disease as shown by hybrid peripheral MRA. Coronal MIPs of the two injection MRA can be stitched together to provide an extended FOV (**a**) view of the run-off vessels. The initial dedicated high spatial resolution, arterial-phase 3D CE MRA of the infrapopliteal arteries (**b**) provides excellent visualization of this patient with bilateral distal run off disease. Visualization of the proximal vessels is provided by the subsequent bolus chase 3D MRA performed from the abdominal aorta through the knee during the second contrast injection

and mask 3D MRA acquisitions of the lower abdomen/pelvis and thigh stations are obtained. A second contrast infusion is performed with two-station moving table 3D MRA of the lower abdomen/pelvis (i.e. aortoiliac region) and thighs (i.e. superficial femoral/popliteal arteries). The start of the lower abdomen/pelvic acquisition is derived from the pelvic bolus timing scan. The thigh acquisition immediately follows that for the lower abdomen/pelvis with interval table translation in a manner similar to any other bolus chase technique. The general bolus profile utilized varies slightly based on patient weight but is as follows. The bolus chase through the lower abdomen/pelvis and thigh is performed using a biphasic contrast injection scheme (the first 20 mL at 2 mL/sec followed by the remaining 16 mL at 0.8 mL/sec, which yields a total pelvis and thigh contrast infusion time of 30 sec) for a total of 36 mL Gd-chelate contrast dose. The Gd-chelate contrast media injection is followed by a 20 mL saline flush injected at 2 mL/sec. The parameters (field of view, matrix size, number of partitions etc.) at each station are optimized to each patient body habitus to permit the most rapid scanning possible without clinically compromising through-plane resolution. Average scanning times for the lower abdomen/pelvis are 14-18 seconds for an 80 to 90 mm volume with partition thickness of 2.0-2.5mm each. If imaging times for the lower ab-

domen/pelvis are too long, one risks venous contamination in the thigh station that follows. Average scan time for the thigh station is approximately 14-18 seconds as well but with a thinner volume and partition thickness (44-60mm and 1.5-1.7mm respectively). For any patients in whom 60 mL of Gd-chelate contrast media dose exceeds 0.3 mmol/kg, the contrast dose should be reduced appropriately so that the initial calves/feet station is performed with 15 mL of contrast media and the lower abdomen/pelvis-thigh contrast infusion is reduced to the remaining amount of a 0.3 mmol/kg cumulative dose. For the lower abdomen/pelvis-thigh contrast infusion, the rate should continue to be biphasic (e.g. initial 15 mL injected at 1.5 mL/sec followed by the remaining contrast dose at 0.5-0.6 mL/sec). In the situation of reduced dose, if contrast is to be infused at 1.5 mL/sec rather than 2 mL/sec, then the initial bolus timing scans (i.e. pelvis and calf 2D bolus timing scans) should be accordingly adjusted to rates of 1.5 mL/second as well.

Wang et al [6] and Khilnani et al [7] have suggested a similar type of integration of time resolved imaging, but using a 2D projectional MR DSA method for the initial bolus timing scan. In their case, 6-10 mL of Gd-chelate contrast media are injected for each projectional 2D MR DSA for the infrapopliteal vessels first. This is followed by moving table 3D MRA of the proximal stations.

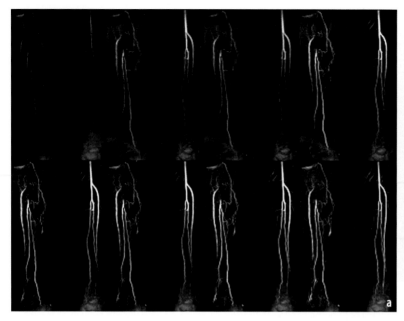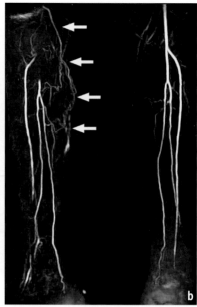

Fig. 8a, b. 3D TRICKS of the calf. Selected images (**a**) from a 3D TRICKS of the calf demonstrates fairly symmetric filling to the tibial and peroneal arterial segments despite an occlusion of the right popliteal artery. Note that the spatial resolution is sufficient to also see the many small collaterals about the right popliteal artery [Images courtesy of Dr. V. Laurent, CHU Nancy, Nancy, France]

The initial distal 2D MR DSA is thus used to approximate circulatory times for proper "bolus sharing" and planning of the multi-station bolus chase 3D MRA.

Hany et al [21] and Swan et al [22] have successfully implemented 3D TRICKS for peripheral MRA. In their original description, separate injections are used for each of the typical three stations, with cumulative contrast doses of 0.3 mmol/kg for each patient. TRICKS imaging of the infrapopliteal arteries (Fig. 8), appears to be particularly good and can be selectively used as described above as an initial lower station 3D MRA exam to be followed by a multi-station bolus chase 3D CE MRA exam for the proximal stations, thereby limiting the injections to two for a three station study.

Identification of Flow Patterns

Time resolved MRA can be critical for the proper identification of flow patterns (Fig. 4) within vascular lesions. Flow within various aortic pathologies is often faster than can be seen using slower high spatial resolution 3D CE MRA. Aneurysms and dissection, for example, often have important information revealed by watching their temporal filling patterns. The origin of the renal arteries, for example, may be misidentified as originating from the false lumen on conventional high spatial resolution 3D CE MRA. In these cases, time resolved imaging could often provide more conclusive information by revealing the actual filling pattern of

the renal arteries either early from the true lumen or late via the false channel.

Although endovascular stent grafts are typically characterized by CTA, to meet investigational requirements for many multi-center clinical trials, some may be well visualized by MRA. However, make no mistake–not all stent grafts can be seen well on MR because of their associated T2* susceptibility artifacts. Certain stent grafts composed of novel materials such as nitinol produce less susceptibility artifacts that both extraluminal and intraluminal areas of the stent graft can typically be evaluated by MRA and MRI. However, most stainless steel stent grafts produce significant signal loss and non-diagnostic images in the immediate vicinity of the stent graft. Other stents composed of elements and compounds such as nickel, and titanium are to a variable extent visualized on MR. Sub-second angiography may be a valuable tool in delineating collateral pathways (such as to lumbar arteries) of type 2 leaks [23]. To this end, sub-second 3D MRA may even reveal direction of flow ("entry versus leak site") within these endoleaks helping to decide the best means of correction if necessary.

Arterial-Venous Segmentation

Processes that derive some of the greatest benefit of time resolved imaging are circulatory beds with fast flow and short arterial venous windows, such as MRA of the pulmonary circulation, arteriovenous malformations or imaging in children.

Pulmonary MRA

Time resolved imaging can be useful for optimization of a pulmonary 3D CE MRA. Pulmonary 3D CE MRA has become particularly popular for pre-procedural pulmonary venous mapping in patients with paroxysmal atrial tachycardias in whom electrophysiological pulmonary venous ablation procedures are contemplated.

In this case, time resolved imaging can be used as a bolus timing scan to ensure proper timing of imaging for peak pulmonary venous imaging. This can be performed using a fast 2D or 3D technique. The 3D technique has the advantage of spatial coverage but for 3-5 sec temporal resolution provides insufficient spatial resolution for definitive pulmonary venous imaging. Time resolved 3D imaging can be performed using a sufficiently large 3D volume to cover the left atrium and proximal pulmonary veins with spatial resolution of the order of 2 x 2 mm in-plane, and 2.5 mm through plane. A contrast bolus of 12-15 mL is infused at 3 mL/sec is typically required. This relatively low spatial resolution sequence provides a series of images that can illustrate contrast bolus progression through the superior vena cava, right heart, pulmonary arteries, pulmonary veins, left heart, and aorta. From this preliminary time resolved scan, the optimum time for pulmonary venous imaging can be chosen for acquisition of a high-spatial resolution 3D CE MRA. The high spatial resolution pulmonary venous 3D CE MRA typically is acquired with a 1.2-1.5 mm through plane spatial resolution and an acquisition time of 10-15 seconds per 3D MRA. This high-resolution 3D CE MRA acquisition is obtained during the administration of approximately 30 mL of Gd-chelate contrast media injected at 3 mL/sec.

Arteriovenous Malformation

Arteriovenous malformations of large enough caliber can be well evaluated with sub-second resolution to sort out feeding arteries from draining veins (Fig. 9 a-e) [24]. This can be extremely helpful in pre-procedural or pre-operative planning for

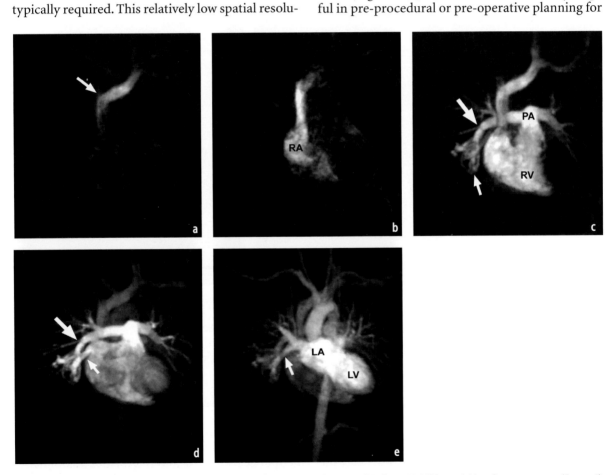

Fig. 9a-e. Sub-second 3D MRA of a Pulmonary AVM. Selected frames from a multi-phase 3D MRA acquisition demonstrates: **a** (Frame 4), Early filling of the superior vena cava from the left bracheocephalic vein (arrow); **b** (Frame 8), Progression of the bolus into the right atrium (RA); **c** (Frame 12), Contrast filling the right ventricle (RV), main pulmonary artery (PA) and its branches. More specifically, filling of the pulmonary AVM (*small arrow*) is noted via the right lower lobe pulmonary artery (large arrow); **d** (Frame 17), Persistent contrast filling of the right lower lobe pulmonary artery (*large arrow*) and AVM is noted with drainage via the right lower lobe pulmonary vein (*small arrow*) into the left atrium; **e** (Frame 22), The contrast bolus is seen still within the right lower lobe pulmonary vein (small arrow) with progression of the bolus into the left atrium (LA) and left ventricle (LV)

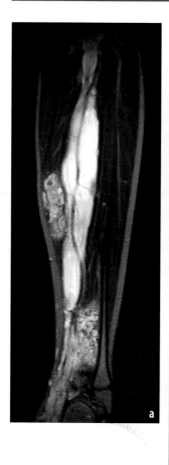

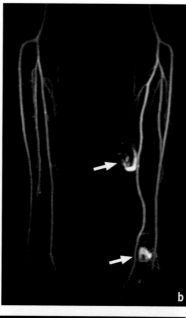

Fig. 10a-d. AV-malformation of the lower leg in an 8-year old boy. The T2w coronal image (**a**) shows high signal intensity lesions of the lower leg indicative of dilated vascular structures. Time resolved MRA (Gd-BOPTA, 0.1 mmol/kg, 1.5 ml/sec) was performed before surgery or embolization to further evaluate the vascular malformation. The different phases acquired (b-d) reveal early filling of the malformation (*arrows* in **b**) and early depiction of the draining veins (*arrow* in **d**), which were indicative of AV-malformations. These were treated successfully by catheter embolization [Image courtesy of Dr. G. Schneider]

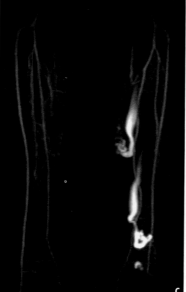

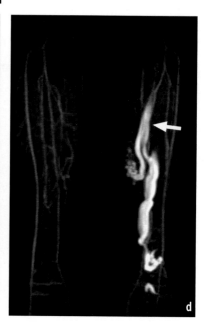

treatment of pulmonary AVM cases such as those encountered in Osler-Weber-Rendu disease, however since treatment of even 5mm large AVMs is recommended high spatial resolution imaging is necessary in addition. This technique is also applicable to other body AVM's and in practice should be applicable to intracranial AVM's as well (Fig. 2). Some centers are applying this technique to initial evaluation of dialysis fistulas prior to definitive interventional procedures. The MRA with its time resolved components has the capability to demonstrate whether the problem is arterial stenosis, venous stenosis, thrombosis, or a combination.

Especially in children, in which vascular malformations are quite frequent, time-resolved contrast enhanced MRI offers the possibility to no in-

vasively evaluate the vascular anatomy of a lesion and to plan further therapy without the risk of an interventional procedure (Fig. 10).

Congenital Heart Disease: Shunt Lesions

Lastly, time-resolved 3D MRA can often be helpful in the comprehensive evaluation of complex congenital heart disease and the various anatomic results and developmental complications of untreated or surgically corrected conditions [25].

The time resolved information gained with sub-second angiography often lays out such complex anatomy and physiology in exquisite detail (Fig. 11).

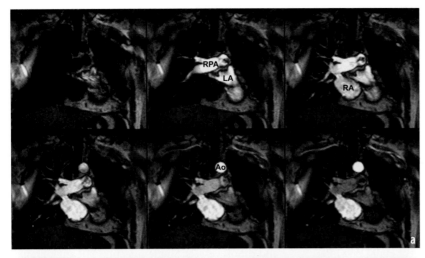

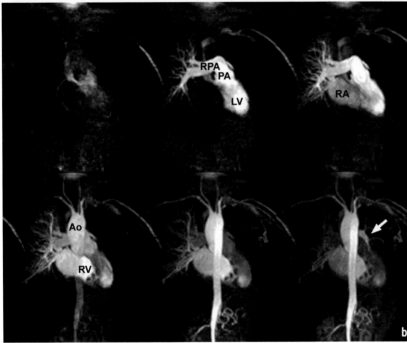

Fig. 11a, b. Time resolved imaging in a child with transposition of the great vessels s/p Mustard procedure. The post-operative chamber connections in this child with transposition of the great vessels following a Mustard procedure is abnormal. The Mustard procedure places an inter-atrial baffle that corrects for the ventricular inversion of a transposition by re-directing systemic venous return to the left ventricle which is connected to the pulmonary artery, and re-directing pulmonary venous return to the right ventricle which is connected to the aorta. On a dynamic coronal 2D time resolved acquisition (**a**, 6 select frames), contrast is noted initially filling the "left atrium" component of the baffle (LA) and right pulmonary artery (RPA). This is followed by pulmonary venous drainage of contrast into the "right atrium" (RA) and aorta (Ao). Note the diminished signal within each chamber with progression of the contrast bolus over each temporal frame. Similar but improved vascular detail can be achieved using dynamic sub-second 3D MRA (**b**). On an early sub-second 3D MRA (**b**, *top row*), enhancement of the left ventricle (LV), pulmonary artery (PA) and right pulmonary artery (RPA) are seen. On the same image, persistent enhancement of the superior vena cava and left bracheocephalic vein can also be seen–this represents the trailing edge of the contrast bolus. On a slightly later image, filling of the pulmonary veins, right atrium (RA) and right ventricle (RV) are noted. On late images (**b**, *bottom row*), progression of the bolus into the thoracic aorta (Ao) and abdominal aorta is seen. Note that due to decreased flow the left pulmonary artery (*arrow*) is displayed after the maximum enhancement of the aorta

References

1. Finn JP, Baskaran V, Carr JC et al (2002) Thorax: Low-dose contrast enhanced three-dimensional MR angiography with subsecond temporal resolution–initial results. Radiology 224:896-904
2. Korosec FR, Frayne R, Grist TM et al (1996) Time-resolved contrast-enhanced 3D MR angiography. Magn Reson Me 36:345-351
3. Ho VB, Foo TKF, Czum JM, Marcos H et al (2001) Contrast-Enhanced Magnetic Resonance Angiography: Technical Considerations for Optimized Clinical Implementation. Top Magn Reson Imaging 12:283-299
4. Earls JP, Rofsky NM, DeCorato DR et al (1996) Breath-hold single-dose gadolinium-enhanced three-dimensional MR aortography: usefulness of a timing examination and MR power injector. Radiology 201:705-710
5. Wang Y, Johnston DL, Breen JF et al (1996) Dynamic MR digital subtraction angiography using contrast enhancement, fast data acquisition, and complex subtraction. Magn Reson Med 36:551-556
6. Wang Y, Winchester PA, Khilnani NM et al (2001) Contrast-enhanced peripheral MR angiography from the abdominal aorta to the pedal arteries: combined dynamic two-dimensional and bolus-chase three-dimensional acquisitions. Invest Radiol 36:170-177
7. Khilnani NM, Winchester PA, Prince MR et al (2002) Peripheral vascular disease: combined 3D bolus chase and dynamic 2D MR angiography compared with x-ray angiography for treatment planning. Radiology 224:63-74
8. Schoenberg SO, Bock M, Knopp MV et al (1999) Renal arteries: Optimization of three-dimensional gadolinium-enhanced MR angiography with bolus-timing-independent fast multi-phase acquisition in a single breath hold. Radiology 211:667-679

9. Pereles FS, Hammelman B, Grouper S et al (2003) The efficacy of an MR compatible automated power injection system for intravenous gadolinium contrast injections (abstr). International Society for Magnetic Resonance in Medicine Eleventh Scientific Meeting and Exhibition Program. Berkeley, Calif: ISMRM 1352

10. Du J, Carroll TJ, Wagner HJ et al (2002) Time-resolved, undersampled projection reconstruction imaging for high-resolution CE-MRA of the distal runoff vessels. Magn Reson Med 48:516-522

11. Ookawa M, Ichinose N, Miyazaki M et al (2003) One-second temporal resolution 4D MR DSA with 3D TRICKS, elliptical centric ordering, and parallel imaging (abstr). International Society for Magnetic Resonance in Medicine Eleventh Scientific Meeting and Exhibition Program. Berkeley, Calif: ISMRM 324

12. Ho KYJAM, Leiner T, de Haan MW et al (1998) Peripheral vascular tree stenoses: Evaluation with moving-bed infusion-tracking MR angiography. Radiology 206:683-692

13. Meaney JM, Ridgeway JP, Chakraverty S et al (1999) Stepping-table gadolinium-enhanced digital subtraction MR angiography of the aorta and lower extremity arteries: preliminary experience. Radiology 211:59-67

14. Ho VB, Choyke PL, Foo TKF et al (1999) Automated bolus chase peripheral MR angiography: Initial practical experiences and future directions of this work-in-progress. J Magn Reson Imaging 10:376-388

15. Goyen M, Quick HH, Debatin JF et al (2002) Whole-body three-dimensional MR angiography with a rolling table platform: initial clinical experience. Radiology 224:270-277

16. Shetty AN, Bis KG, Duerinckx AJ et al (2002) Lower extremity MR angiography: universal retrofitting of high-field-strength systems with stepping kinematic imaging platforms initial experience. Radiology 222:284-291

17. Ho VB, Meaney JFM, Kent KC et al (2002) Bolus-Chase Peripheral MR Angiography: Technical Considerations. Applied Radiology 31:11-19

18. Prince MR, Chabra SG, Watts R et al (2002) Contrast material travel times in patients undergoing peripheral MR angiography. Radiology 224:55-61

19. Morasch MD, Collins J, Pereles FS et al (2003) Lower extremity stepping-table magnetic resonance angiography with multi-level contrast timing and segmented contrast infusion. J Vasc Surg 37:62-71

20. Finn JP, Francois CJ, Moore JR et al (2002) Lower extremity MRA with full prior specification of bolus transit times (abstr). International Society for Magnetic Resonance in Medicine Tenth Scientific Meeting and Exhibition Program. Berkeley, Calif: ISMRM 266

21. Hany TF, Carroll TJ, Omary RA et al (2001) Aorta and runoff vessels: Single-injection MR angiography with automated table movement compared with multiinjection time-resolved MR angiography–Initial results. Radiology 221:266-272

22. Swan JS, Carroll TJ, Kennell TW et al (2002) Time-resolved three-dimensional contrast-enhanced MR angiography of the peripheral vessels. Radiology 225:43-52

23. Lookstein RA, Goldman J, Pukin L et al (2004) Time-resolved magnetic resonance angiography as a noninvasive method to characterize endoleaks: Initial results compared with conventional angiography. J Vasc Surg 39:27-33

24. Goyen M, Ruehm SG, Jagenburg A et al (2001) Pulmonary arteriovenous malformation: characterization with time-resolved ultrafast 3D MR angiography. J Magn Reson Imaging 13:458-460

25. Mutupillai R, Vick GW 3rd, Flamm SD et al (2003) Time-resolved contrast-enhanced magnetic resonance angiography in pediatric patients using sensitivity encoding. J Magn Reson Imaging 17:559-564

I.4

Image Processing in Contrast-Enhanced MR Angiography

Philippe C. Douek, Marcela Hernández-Hoyos and Maciej Orkisz

Introduction

Magnetic resonance angiography (MRA) is a medical imaging modality used to reveal the shape of vessels for diagnosis and therapeutic purposes. This technique receives much attention because it is non-invasive and provides three-dimensional (3D) data sets as opposed to the planar or two-dimensional (2D) projections of conventional x-ray digital subtraction angiography (DSA) [1-7]. Like DSA, contrast-enhanced MRA (CE MRA) uses contrast agents to enhance the vascular lumen.

The term post-processing refers to a vast number of image manipulation techniques that facilitate the assessment of arterial and venous structures at an independent console. It refers to all operations from data transfer and image visualization to automatic quantification of vessel lesions. For accurate image interpretation, knowledge of the available image processing tools is mandatory. A variety of reformatting techniques are now available, and it is advantageous to be well versed in as many of these as possible. Each technique has its own strengths and weaknesses, which can lead to pitfalls and artifacts in inexperienced hands. The main challenges for MRA image processing include proper visualization of vessel lumen, optimized thresholding of vessel-to-background image contrast, and arterial-venous separation. The most widely available methods for post-processing MRA data sets are multiplanar reformatting (MPR), maximum-intensity projection (MIP), subvolume MIP, surface-rendering (SR), volume-rendering (VR) and virtual intraluminal endoscopy (VIE).

This article will focus on the three main areas of the MRA post-processing systems: data handling, image visualization and vascular analysis (Fig. 1).

Data Handling

Any post-processing system for medical images should be compatible with the DICOM (Digital Imaging and Communications in Medicine) standard [8-12]. DICOM defines a complex communication protocol and requires that two connected workstations agree on the exchanged services. The unit requesting a service is called a "Service Class User" (SCU) and the unit supplying the requested service is called the "Service Class Provider" (SCP). Typically, a SCU (a post-processing workstation) performing a "Query/Retrieve" on a SCP (an imag-

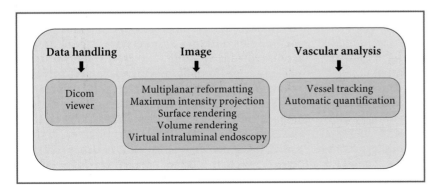

Fig. 1. Tools for the MRA post-processing

ing unit) first asks for a list of patients; then, once the patient is locally selected, the SCU asks for a set of images (series). Thereafter, the SCP initiates transfer through the network and the SCU locally stores the received files on a local hard disk. DICOM also defines the file format in which the images are encoded, allowing local visualization and post–processing of the data with no loss of quality. A DICOM file consists of two parts: 1) a header containing a set of Data Elements (Patient Name, Acquisition Protocol, Image Matrix, Pixel Size, etc.), and 2) the original pixel/voxel data.

Initially, DICOM functions were limited to the exchange of data between proprietary workstations. Recently, however, some DICOM-compliant applications have become available on personal computers and their easier diffusion allows medical institutions or laboratories to perform specific post-processing tasks (measurements, MPR, MIP, archiving) with lower investment. Some of these applications can provide SCP/SCU functions [13].

Many general purpose post-processing systems are commercially available. There is a great variety of programs called "Dicom Viewers" which include the data handling and the image visualization functions (e.g. eFilm Workstation [13], DicomEye [36], Osiris [37], MediMatic Dicom Viewer [38], DicomWorks etc.). More sophisticated post-processing algorithms are available on independent workstations (e.g. Vitrea [21], Advantage Windows [39], Leonardo Workstation [40], EasyVision [41], etc.). However, none of those was designed specifically for use on standard office personal computers. Few of the available software packages, moreover, include dedicated quantitative vascular analysis tools.

In response to the specific medical need for MRA-targeted image analysis software, we have developed our own post-processing program called MARACAS (MAgnetic Resonance Angiography Computer ASsisted analysis). It is an interactive software package for visualization and analysis of blood vessels using 3D MRA data which provides automated quantification of the arterial stenosis.

Image Visualization

Although assessment of source images acquired by the scanner gives access to a precise local information on vessel diameter, area, etc., mental reconstruction of the global morphology and appreciation of spatial relationships is often difficult. Moreover, this local information may not be available when the slices are not perpendicular to the vessel of interest [14]. Several post-processing techniques are available to improve rendering of the overall morphology and/or the spatial relationships of the

anatomical structures. Their purpose is to allow the user to simultaneously view the MRA data sets in different display formats such as maximum intensity projections, multiplanar reformats, surface and volume rendered images and virtual intraluminal endoscopic views. This section briefly explains the principles of these techniques and discusses their principal advantages and disadvantages.

Re-sampling and Editing Approaches

Re-sampling mainly involves reformatting the image data produced from the original reconstruction process in an orientation other than that which was originally produced. The process of re-sampling and editing is called multiplanar reconstruction or reformation (MPR). The reformatting process does not alter the MRA voxels in any way; instead it presents them in off-axis views and displays the images produced from the original reconstruction process in a new orientation.

For example MPR displays planar sections in any orientation through a 3D data volume (Fig. 2). Whereas some systems extract slices only in the planes perpendicular to the native slices i.e. sagittal, or coronal, other more sophisticated programs allow for interactive real time extraction of oblique planes. MPR should not be confused with a thick projection like subvolume MIP. Rather, it represents a single voxel section through the volume. Thus, oblique MPR can be performed but requires interpolation of image data, as in effect, it rearranges the data into a different coordinate system. For example, axially acquired MRA data can be reformatted or rearranged into sagittal MPR images.

On most systems MPR views of a 3D MRA data set are primarily obtained in the standard orthogonal planes (i.e. axial, sagittal, and coronal views). Using a center point of interest, the operator is able to "slide" through the volume along these standard orientations. Using MPR, the operator can simultaneously visualize the arterial lumen and the adjacent structures in a localized region and interactively view features that may not be readily apparent on the native "source images" [15]. However, the MPR requires a trained operator, who must mentally reconstruct a three-dimensional picture from two-dimensional views. Some software packages additionally permit curved reformation of image data according to an irregular orientation in space. This is particularly useful for reformations of the coronary arteries. Curved reformatting is based on two operations: interpolation and re-sampling, which enable signal intensities to be assigned to voxels located "somewhere between" the actual data points. It is then possible to sample a

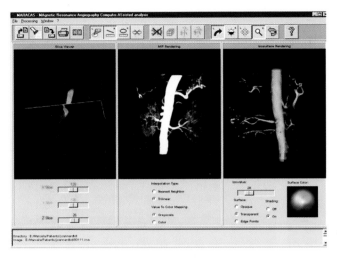

Fig. 2. 3D visualization techniques: MPR according to three orthogonal axes (*left*), oblique MIP (*middle*), surface rendered (*right*)

3D MRA data set along a curved plane. The technique is especially useful for visualizing stenoses in tortuous blood vessels.

Subtraction of a precontrast data set from the arterial-phase data is a classical means of re-sampling data. This is performed routinely in x-Ray angiography (Digital Subtraction Angiography, DSA) and is now widely used in 3D CE MRA, especially for peripheral MRA of the lower extremities when subtraction of mask images is necessary to eliminate background structures and provide better visualization of smaller vessels. However, this technique is more problematic in the abdomen, where discrepancies in breath holding between acquisitions may result in misregistration artifacts. In practice, arterial-phase CE MRA images of the abdomen are almost always diagnostic without subtraction as long as good bolus timing has been achieved.

The Maximum Intensity Projection

Maximum intensity projection (MIP) post-processing is the most common means of displaying MRA data as the views are comparable to those yielded by conventional x-ray angiography. To obtain a MIP reconstruction, parallel rays are cast through the 3D data set (i.e. volume) with each pixel of the projection image plane representing the maximum signal intensity encountered along the corresponding ray. With this technique, a ray is projected through the 3D data set in the desired direction, and the highest voxel value along the ray becomes the pixel value of the two-dimensional MIP image. Thus, the MIP algorithm does not simply add up the signal intensities from slice to slice along the projected axis. Instead, it finds the highest signal intensity value (i.e. maximum intensity) along a projection line. In this way 3D data can be collapsed into a 2D projection image. MIP process-

ing of 3D CE MRA data permits clear visualization of vessel enhancement, producing views that closely resemble those of conventional x-ray angiography. For this reason MIP reconstructions tend to be clinically popular for viewing and interpretation of 3D CE MRA. This method is particularly well suited for image interpretation of arterial-phase CE MRA, in which the arterial-to-background signal difference (i.e. contrast-to-noise ratio or CNR) is high. Most MR scanner manufacturers now include options for automated MIP processing of data in pre-determined orientations (e.g. axial, sagittal and coronal) at the end of the image acquisition process. This allows a rapid assessment of the vessels while the patient is still in the scanner.

Unfortunately, some disadvantages are associated with automated MIP algorithms that typically include all data within the entire volume (Fig. 3). First, full volume MIP reconstructions tend to misrepresent anatomic spatial relationships since depth information is not displayed [16]. Eccentrically located stenoses may remain undetected and superimposition of structures may erroneously simulate the presence of a stenosis [17]. Second, full volume MIP reconstructions tend to increase the mean signal intensity of the background [18] [19]. Consequently, vessels with low signal intensity, which may be seen on individual source images, may be partially or completely imperceptible on full volume MIP images [20]. Since the MIP algorithm does not differentiate the etiology of signal intensity, it may not project a vessel sufficiently if its signal intensity is equivalent to that of its background. Regions of high signal intensity are invariably seen on CE MRA. Since the pulse sequence is T1-weighted, tissue with short T1 times such as fat or bone marrow might degrade MIP viewing of CE MRA acquisitions. The likelihood of increasing background signal (i.e. maximum intensity signal along the ray in non-vascular tissue), increases

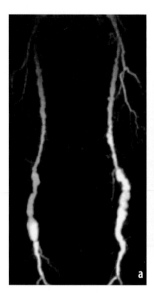
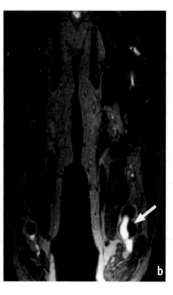

Fig. 3a–c. MIP of lower limb arteries (**a**), corresponding coronal "source image" (**b**) and axial MPR (**c**). The dark thrombus (*arrows*) in the left popliteal artery aneurysm is well visualized on the coronal source image and the axial MPR image, but is not appreciated on the coronal MIP image

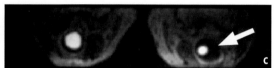

with the inclusion of additional non-vascular regions. Thus, a vessel which may be seen on an individual source image may not be apparent on a full volume MIP reconstruction if there is a lot of spurious high signal tissue overlying the region (e.g. subcutaneous fat above and behind the vessel). Furthermore, full volume MIP images obtained from the entire 3D data set are frequently contaminated by wraparound or edge artifacts, which can limit the visibility of vessels. On full volume MIP reconstructions, overlapping vessels, whether arterial or venous, may mask an arterial stenosis or occlusion thereby making evaluation impossible. Finally, depth information is not represented on MIP reconstructions. Therefore, it is often difficult to tell the relationship between stray intensities and blood vessel or to separate the signals from two overlapping vessels. In order to compensate for the loss of the depth information on standard full volume MIP images, post-processing systems provide such solutions as: 1) enabling MIP reconstructions of a sub-volume of interest, instead of projecting the whole volume, and 2) varying the projection angle (interactive rotation).

Although the generation of rotational sub-volume MIP images is often routinely performed by the technologist at many sites, this alone is rarely sufficient for final diagnosis. Therefore more intricate additional post-processing of the 3D data set by the investigating radiologist is often required for confident diagnosis. Although image quality can almost always be improved by obtaining sub-volume MIP images or by manually editing the entire data set, source images or thin-section reformatted images should also be examined routinely since small vessels, arterial dissections (Fig. 4) and non-occlusive thrombi may easily be missed on MIP images alone.

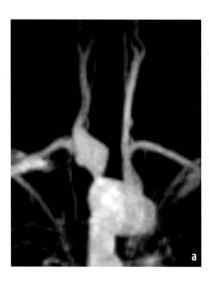
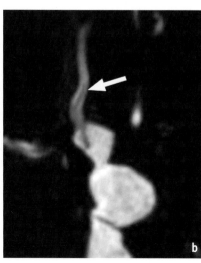

Fig. 4a, b. a Coronal MIP projection **b** Coronal source image from the 3D CE MRA acquisition reveals a right carotid artery dissection (*arrow*) not seen on the MIP projection

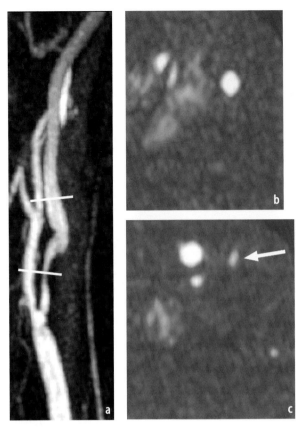

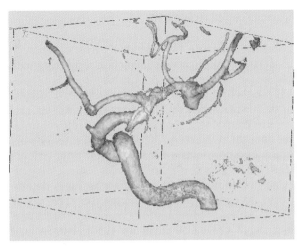

Fig. 6. Surface rendered view of MRA of internal carotid artery. The voxel size is 500 microns

Fig. 5a-c. The MIP reconstruction (**a**) clearly demonstrates a carotid artery stenosis. However, quantification of stenosis is best performed on MPR images (**b**, **c**) perpendicular to the vessel axis (*arrow* in **c**, stenosis of internal carotid artery in the axial plane)

The loss of image contrast on MIP reconstructions is most apparent at the edge of vessels. The signal intensity near the wall of a vessel is less than that at the center since pixels at the edge are partially volume averaged with the low intensity background. If the vessel is small (i.e. less than 4 times the voxel size) it will appear artificially narrowed. Vessel diameter is thus best measured on the individual partitions rather than on the projections (Fig. 5).

Surface Rendering

Surface rendering (Fig. 6) uses the boundary voxels between the object to be displayed and the background to create a 3D surface. Hence, it requires preliminary segmentation. Accurate segmentation methods capable of precisely delineating the vascular structures and of separating them from other tissues are still being developed. However, for an approximate visualization, segmentation may be achieved by simple thresholding. In surface rendering, the voxels located at the edge of a structure are thus identified and possibly en-

hanced with morphologic filtering or connectivity, and then displayed. The remaining voxels in the image are usually invisible. This approach can be useful for examining tubular structures such as blood vessels. The thresholding assignment of the voxels that will be visible is both critical and sometimes difficult to define reproducibly. If the thresholding process is too aggressive, actual protruding structures can be lost from view because of partial volume effects. On the other hand, if the thresholding process is too lax, tissue materials can also be rendered which may lead to vessel structures becoming obscured. Surface rendering is also called shaded surface display (SSD) because the intensity of each pixel in an SSD image is calculated using the local orientation of the surface with respect to a virtual lighting source. In contrast to the MPR and to the MIP, the SSD better renders the three-dimensional aspect of MRA data. The surface representation accurately captures and represents the position and shape of the relevant vascular structures, and can be visualized and manipulated interactively. However, it requires user intervention in order to select the appropriate thresholding value to optimally extract the surface of the vessel of interest. This can sometimes be difficult, especially if boundaries are not well defined either because of noise or low contrast data. The threshold-based SSD should not be used for quantification since vessel diameters are threshold-dependent and thus can lead to under- or over-estimation of stenoses. As a result, surface rendering should always be displayed simultaneously with at least one complementary visualization mode to assess the appropriateness of the threshold choice [16].

Volume Rendering

Volume rendering (VR) (Figs. 7, 8) has replaced most earlier applications of surface rendering with the notable exception of interior vessel analysis. VR is a technique that displays all of the 3D data at once. It works directly on the voxel intensities, and creates translucent renderings of the full volumetric data set. Objects with high signal intensity are opaque and objects with low signal intensity are transparent. As commonly implemented, VR generates an image in the following way. First, it computes color and partial opacity for each voxel. Then, it blends contributions made by voxels projecting to the same pixel on the picture plane (along a line from the viewer's eye through the data set). In most cases, the user manually sets color, opacity and brightness corresponding to different voxel intensities. In volume rendering, the signal intensity values that make up the image are assigned to be either visible or invisible, to be displayed with varying colors, and often to be displayed with varying opacity levels (transparency). The assignment of these characteristics to the voxels can be defined for specific imaging protocols and organ systems such as standard arterial-phase CE MRA alone or display of arterial-phase and venous-phase data together in different colors. Some systems use standard preset settings [21]. However, these settings are much more difficult to establish for MRA than for CTA images. The main advantage of this technique is the ability to generate images without explicitly defining surface geometry. It reveals internal structures that would nor-

mally be hidden or omitted when using surface rendering techniques. VR thus appears very interesting for the study of arterial plaques.

Vendors have developed independent workstations and software that can display these three-dimensional images quickly, and which generally have some flexibility in terms of thresholding parameters (i.e. which voxels become visible). However, color maps and transparency levels may be more difficult to control for individual cases. Frequently, 3D VR image displays of vascular anatomy provides excellent anatomic information for surgical planning.

Virtual Intraluminal Endoscopy

Virtual intraluminal endoscopy (VIE) is a recently developed technique for assessing the inside of the vascular wall (Fig. 9). It combines the features of endoscopic viewing and cross-sectional volumetric imaging and involves the generation of a sequence of perspective views calculated from points (flight path) located within the vascular lumen. These views can be computed using both surface rendering and volume rendering algorithms. In the most current systems, the flight path is automatically calculated, based on a preliminary extraction of the vessel centerline. Despite being a high-level method of image post-processing, VIE is not yet a popular application. Most errors and artifacts are related to the somewhat arbitrary nature of data thresholding. The goal of VIE is to define a set of thresholds that will perfectly define the

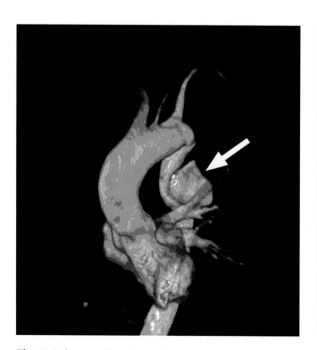

Fig. 7. Volume rendered view of a pseudo aneurysm of the descending aorta

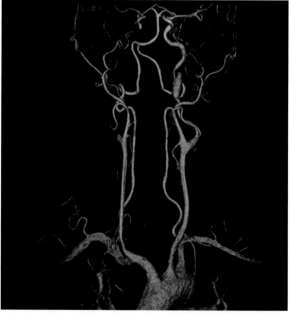

Fig. 8. Volume rendered view of the aortic arch and branches

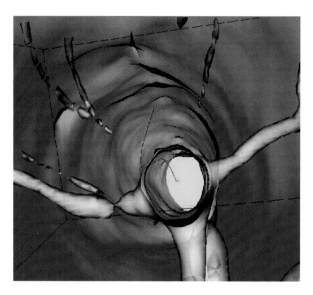 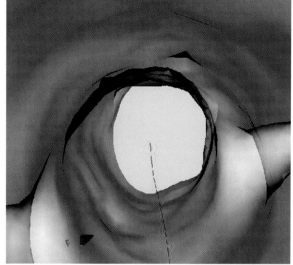

Fig. 9. Virtual endoscopy of the abdominal aorta guided by the vessel centerline (red line)

edge of the vessel while excluding everything else. This is most likely to occur when the 3D data set is optimal (i.e. signal intensity within the vessel is uniformly high and signal intensity outside the vessel uniformly low). The most common error is trying to generate VIE images from suboptimal data sets with threshold problems. This leads to two typical problems: holes in vessel walls, which can be mistaken for the origins of small vessels such as accessory renal arteries, and floating shape artifacts within the vessel lumen. As yet there is no corresponding clinical technique and no clear evidence that this form of data presentation provides any advantages over traditional methods. Nevertheless, MR-generated VIE can produce striking endovascular images, and its potential importance as a clinical tool should not be underestimated. The technique is still relatively new, and important clinical applications may yet be demonstrated.

Vascular Analysis

The purpose of vascular analysis is to allow the clinician to perform quantitative assessment of vessel morphology in order: 1) to decide on the appropriate approach to treatment (surgical or pharmacological) according to the degree of stenosis, and 2) to monitor the progress of the disease. Intraluminal diameters and cross-sectional areas are needed to accurately quantify the degree of stenosis. Traditionally, only diameters were used for the estimation of stenosis, with the degree of stenosis calculated according to the following equation:

$$Stenosis = \frac{D_{distal} - D_{min}}{D_{distal}} \times 100\ \%$$

where D_{min} = the smallest diameter within the stenosis and D_{distal} = the diameter of the normal vessel beyond the diseased segment. Unfortunately, for non-elliptic or amorphous stenoses, estimation of the smallest (as well as of the largest) diameter is not clear. Moreover, some authors argue that, in this case, cross-sectional area reduction better correlates with the hemodynamic impact of the stenosis than diameter reduction. For these reasons, vessel cross-sectional area has been proposed as a more accurate parameter for stenosis calculation [22].

Most post-processing systems provide interactive operator tools to manually perform these measurements. These tools considerably increase the accuracy of stenosis quantification compared to a purely visual appreciation. However, manual tracing of the lumen centerline as well as delineation of vessel boundaries are time-consuming tasks and are subject to variability between operators. These major drawbacks have thus been the motivation for the development of new techniques for automatic quantification of the vascular morphology.

In terms of image processing, the first step necessary to quantitatively evaluate a vessel is to separate it from surrounding structures. This procedure is called "segmentation". Two main approaches to vessel segmentation have been suggested. The first approach relies on purely photometric criteria and focuses mainly on thresholding and region-growing techniques [23-26]. The major advantage of this technique is that it is reasonably easy to implement. However, an additional modeling step is necessary to extract meaningful measurements from the segmented images.

The second approach exploits the geometrical specificity of the vessels, in particular their orien-

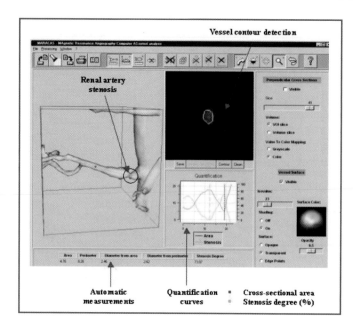

Fig. 10. Automatic quantification along the vessel centerline

tation and tubular shape. Techniques that use this approach tend to use vessel-tracking [27-31] and (often implicitly) a generalized-cylinder model, *i.e.* an association of an axis (centerline) and a surface (vessel wall) [32-33]. Consequently, the segmentation process involves two tasks: centerline extraction and vessel contour detection in the planes perpendicular to the axis. This procedure results in a stack of 2D contours along the vessel (Fig. 10) which allow quantitative cross-sectional measurements and visualization by means of triangulation-based surface rendering. Other recent approaches have looked at using 3D models of the vessel surface [34, 35].

Summary

Image post-processing is a fundamental aspect of all MRA procedures to the extent that accurate diagnosis of vascular disease would be impossible without it. Accordingly, a great deal of time and effort has gone into the development of post-processing algorithms in order to facilitate and improve the diagnostic process both in terms of the variety of available techniques, and in terms of their speed, access and ease of application. Today, the clinician has a wide variety of robust post-processing techniques available with which to visualize, diagnose and quantify all manner of vascular lesions. With the ongoing development of more intricate, less time-consuming procedures, even sophisticated image post-processing promises to become a readily available, user-friendly feature of clinical routine.

References

1. Lee VS, Doug JM, Krinsky GA, Rofsky NM (2000) Gadolinium-enhanced MR angiography: artifacts and pitfalls. AJR Am J Roentgenol 175:197-205
2. Barbier C, Lefevre F, Bui P et al (2001) Contrast-enhanced MRA of the carotid arteries using 0.5 Tesla: comparison with selective digital angiography. J Radiol 82(3 Pt 1):245-249
3. Vanninen RL, Manninen HI, Partanen PK, et al (1996) How should we estimate carotid stenosis using magnetic resonance angiography? Neuroradiology 38(4):299-305
4. Young GR, Humphrey PR, Nixon TE, Smith ET (1996) Variability in measurement of extracranial internal carotid artery stenosis as displayed by both digital subtraction and magnetic resonance angiography: an assessment of three caliper techniques and visual impression of stenosis. Stroke 27(3):467-473
5. Ruehm SG, Goyen M, Barkhausen et al (2001) Rapid magnetic resonance angiography for detection of atherosclerosis. Lancet 357(9262):1086-1091
6. Wong KS, Lam WW, Liang E et al (1996) Variability of magnetic resonance angiography and computed tomography angiography in grading middle cerebral artery stenosis. Stroke 27(6):1084-1087
7. Elgersma OE, Wust AF, Buijs PC et al (2000) Multidirectional depiction of internal carotid arterial stenosis: three-dimensional time-of-flight MR angiography versus rotational and conventional digital subtraction angiography. Radiology 216(2):511-516
8. Clunie DA (2000) DICOM Structured Reporting. Bangor: PixelMed Publishing
9. Philips Medical Systems. DICOM Cook Book. Available at: ftp://ftp-wjq.philips.com/medical/interoperability/out/DICOM_Information/CookBook.pdf
10. Horii SC (1997) Primer on computers and information technology. Part four: A nontechnical introduction to DICOM. Radiographics 17:1297-1309

11. ACR and NEMA Digital Imaging and Communications Standards Committee. The DICOM V3.0 standard. Available at http://medical.nema.org/Dicom/Geninfo/brochure/BROCH95.DOC

12. NEMA's official DICOM web page. http://medical.nema.org/dicom.html

13. eFilm Workstation by eFilm Medical Inc. http://www.efilm.ca

14. Zhao M, Charbel FT, Alperin N et al (2000) Improved phase-contrast flow quantification by three-dimensional vessel localization. Magn Reson Imaging 18(6):697-706

15. Gutberlet M, Hosten N, Beier J et al (1999) Quantification of the degree of a stenosis using multiplanar reformation (MPR) of a magnetic resonance angiography (MRA) data set and 2-dimensional MR images compared with MR-flow measurement in patients with coarctation. In CARS'99 Computer Assisted Radiology and Surgery. H.U. Lemke, M.W. Vannier, K. Inamura and A.G. Farman (Eds) Amsterdam, The Netherlands. Elsevier 124-128

16. Calhoun PS, Kuszyk BS, Heath DG et al (1999) Three-dimensional volume rendering of spiral CT data: theory and method. Radiographics; 19:745-764

17. Hany TF, Schmidt M, Davis CP, et al (1998) Diagnostic impact of four postprocessing techniques in evaluating contrast-enhanced three-dimensional MR angiography. AJR Am J Roentgenol 170:907-912

18. Anderson CM, Saloner D, Tsuruda JS et al (1990) Artifacts in maximum intensity projection display of MR angiograms. AJR Am J Roentgenol 154(3):623-629

19. Orkisz M, Bresson C, Magnin IE et al (1997) Improved vessel visualization in MR angiography by nonlinear anisotropic filtering. Magn Reson Med 37:914-919

20. Anderson CM (1993) Postprocessing and display. In: CM Anderson, RR. Edelman and P. Turski, (Eds) Clinical magnetic resonance angiography. New York: Raven Press 83-98

21. Vitrea by VitalImages. http://www.vitalimages.com

22. Wise SW, Hopper KD, Ten Have T, Schwartz T (1998) Measuring carotid artery stenosis using CT angiography: the dilemme of artifactual lumen eccentricity. AJR Am J Roentgenol 170(4):919-923

23. Hu X, Alperin N, Levin DN et al (1991) Visualization of MR angiographic data with segmentation and volume-rendering techniques. J Magn Reson Imaging 1(5):539-546

24. Wilson DL, Noble JA (1997) Segmentation of cerebral vessels and aneurysms from MR angiography data. In Information Processing in Medical Imaging. (Lecture Notes in Computer Science). G. Goos, J. Hartmanis and J.van Leeuwen, Eds. Springer-Verlag, Heidelberg, Germany 1230:423-428

25. Masutani Y, Schiemann T, Höne KH (1998) Vascular shape segmentation and structure extraction using a shape-based region-growing model. In MICCAI'98 Medical Image Computing & Computer-Assisted Intervention (Lecture Notes in Computer Science). A. Colchester, W.M. Wells and S. Delp, Eds. New York: Springer-Verlag 1496:1242-1249

26. Chung ACS, Noble JA (1999) Statistical 3D vessel segmentation using a Rician distribution. In: Taylor C, Colchester A. (Eds) MICCAI'99 Medical Image Computing & Computer-Assisted Intervention (Lecture Notes in Computer Science). Springer Berlin Heidelberg, New York, pp 1679:82-89

27. Verdonck B, Bloch I, Maître H et al (1996) Accurate segmentation of blood vessels from 3D medical images. In ICIP'96 IEEE Int. Conf. On Image Processing. Lausanne vol. III:311-314

28. Nazarian B, Chédot C, Sequeira J et al (1996) Automatic reconstruction of irregular tubular structures using generalized cylinders. Revue de CFAO et d'informatique graphique 11:11-20

29. Lorenz C, Carlsen IC, Buzug TM et al (1997) Multiscale line segmentation with automatic estimation of width, contrast and tangential direction in 2D and 3D medical images. In: Trocazz J, Grimson E, Mösges R (Eds) CVRMed/MRCAS'97, (Lecture Notes in Computer Science). Springer Berlin Heidelberg, New York, pp 233-242

30. Wink O, Niessen WJ, Viergever MA (1998) Fast quantification of abdominal aorta aneurysms from CTA volumes. In: Colchester A, Wells WM, Delp S (Eds) MICCAI'98 Medical Image Computing & Computer-Assisted Intervention (Lecture Notes in Computer Science). Springer Berlin Heidelberg, New York, pp 1496:138-145

31. Wang KC, Dutton RW, Taylor CA (1999) Improving geometric model construction for blood flow modeling. IEEE Eng Med Biol Mag 18(6):33-39

32. Swift RD, Ramaswamy K, Higgins WE (1997) Adaptive axes generation algorithm for 3D tubular structures. In ICIP'97 IEEE Int. Conf. On Image Processing. Sta Barbara vol. II:136-139

33. Orkisz M, Hernández-Hoyos M, Douek P, Magnin I (2000) Advances of blood vessel morphology analysis in 3D magnetic resonance images. Machine Graphics & Vision 9:463-471

34. Frangi AF, Niessen WJ, Hoogeveen RM et al (1999) Model-Based quantitation of 3-D magnetic resonance angiographic images. IEEE Trans Med Imaging 18(10):946-956

35. Bulpitt AJ, Berry E (1998) An automatic 3D deformable model for segmentation of branching structures compared with interactive region growing. In: Berry E (Ed) Proceedings of Medical Image Understanding and Analysis'98. pp 189-192

36. DicomEye by ETIAM. http://www.etiam.com

37. Osiris by the University Hospital of Geneva. http://www.expasy.ch/www/UIN/html1/projects/osiris/osiris.html

38. MediMatic Dicom Viewer by MediMatic. Http://www.medimatic.com

39. MRI Flex Trial by General Electric. http://apps.gemedicalsystems.com/geCommunity/aw/FlexTrial/awmr_flextrial_home.jsp

40. Leonardo Workstation by Siemens. http://siemensmedical.com/

41. EasyVision by Philips. http://www.philips.com/ms

42. Marchand B, Hernández-Hoyos M, Orkisz M, Douek P (2001) Diagnostic des Sténoses de l'Artère Rénale en Angiographie par Résonance Magnétique et Appréciation du Degré de Sténose. J Mal Vasc 25:(5) 312-320 (in French)

43. Hernández-Hoyos M, Anwander A, Orkisz M et al (2000) A deformable vessel model with single point initialization for segmentation, quantification and visualization of blood vessels in 3D MRA. In MICCAI'00 Medical Image Computing & Computer-Assisted Intervention (Lecture Notes in Computer Sci-

ence). S.L. Delp, A.M. Digioia and B. Jaramaz Eds. Berlin, Germany: Springer-Verlag 1935:735-745

44. Hernández-Hoyos M, Orkisz M, Roux JP, Douek P (1999) Inertia-based vessel axis extraction and stenosis quantification in 3D MRA images. In CARS'99 Computer Assisted Radiology and Surgery. H.U. Lemke, M.W. Vannier, K. Inamura and A.G. Farman (Eds) Amsterdam, The Netherlands. Elsevier.; 189-193

45. McInerney T, Terzopoulos D (1996) Deformable models in medical image analysis: a survey. Med Image Anal 1(2):91-108

46. Kass M, Witkin A, Terzopoulos D (1988) Snakes: active contour models. IJCV 1:321-331

47. Cohen LD (1991) On Active Contour Models and Balloons. CVGIP 53(2):211-218

48. Renaudin CP, Barbier B, Roriz R et al (1994) Coronary Arteries: New Design for Three-dimensional Arterial Phantoms. Radiology 190:579-582

49. Sato Y, Nakajima S, Atsumi H et al (1997) 3D Multiscale line filter for segmentation and visualization of curvilinear structures in medical images. In CVRMed/MRCAS'97, (Lecture Notes in Computer Science) J. Trocazz, E. Grimson and R. Mösges (Eds) Berlin. Germany: Springer-Verlag 213-222

50. Prinet V, Monga O (1997) Vessel representation in 2D and 3D angiograms. In CARS'97 Computer Assisted Radiology and Surgery. HU Lemke, MW Vannier and K. Inamura Eds. Amsterdam, The Netherlands. Elsevier 240-255

SECTION II

Contrast Agents

II

Contrast Agents for MR Angiography: Current Status and Future Perspectives

Michael V. Knopp and Miles A. Kirchin

Introduction

Techniques and applications for contrast-enhanced magnetic resonance angiography (CE-MRA) have developed rapidly in recent years, due largely to advances in hard- and software design. The advent of innovative new contrast agents with properties distinct from those of the traditional, extracellular gadolinium agents promises to further expand the clinical applicability of CE-MRA, making this the modality of choice for diagnostic imaging of the vasculature. With few exceptions, most of the commercially available contrast agents are not approved directly for CE-MRA [1, 2]. The present review summarizes the properties and imaging applications of currently available contrast agents which are in routine use in CE-MRA. Described also are those agents in clinical development which may one day find utility in CE-MRA.

Classification of Contrast Agents for CE-MRA

Contrast agents for CE-MRA fall into two broad categories, those based on gadolinium which are predominantly paramagnetic in nature, and those based upon iron oxide particles which are superparamagnetic in nature. Agents in the former category can be sub-classified further into agents with no capacity for interaction with intravascular proteins and those with either weak or strong capacity for protein interaction. Similarly, agents in the latter category can be sub-divided on the basis of the size and coating of the iron oxide particles present. A summary of contrast agents that are either available or in advanced stages of development is given Fig. 1. A brief outline of these agents has been given elsewhere [3].

Paramagnetic Contrast Agents: First Pass Gadolinium Agents

Currently, seven gadolinium contrast agents are approved in one or more countries of the world and an eighth is in the final stages of the approval process (Fig. 2). Although all are suitable for use in first-pass CE-MRA, few agents are actually approved specifically for this indication. Six of these seven agents possess no capacity for interaction with serum proteins and can be considered "conventional" first generation gadolinium chelates (Fig. 1, column 1; Fig. 2a-f). The seventh agent, gadobenate dimeglumine (Fig. 2g), possesses elevated T1-relaxivity in blood due to a unique capacity among currently available agents for weak, transient interaction with serum albumin. This agent is the first representative of a new class of second generation gadolinium agents (Fig. 1, column 2).

Gadolinium Contrast Agents with no Capacity for Protein Interaction

The group of "conventional" gadolinium agents includes the first compounds to be developed for MRI some 12–15 years ago (i.e. gadopentetate dimeglumine, gadoterate meglumine, gadoteridol and gadodiamide) plus two newer agents (gadoversetamide and gadobutrol). Among these agents five are available as 0.5 Molar formulations and one, gadobutrol, as a 1.0 Molar formulation. Although differences exist between these agents in terms of molecular structure and chemical and physical properties (Table 1) [4], all are non-specific and extracellular in nature and all are excreted unchanged through the kidneys by glomerular filtration. Furthermore, the T1 relaxation rates of these agents are comparable, falling in the range between 4.3 and 5.6 L/mmol $\cdot$ s^{-1} [4-7]. The similar concentrations and relaxation properties of these

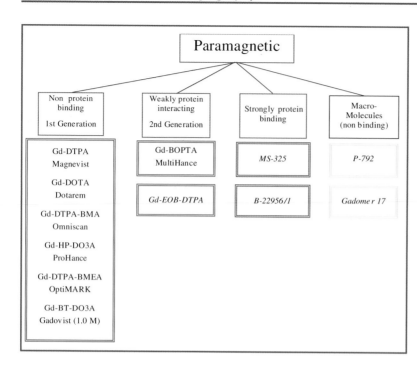

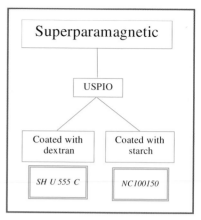

Fig. 1. Classification scheme for "vascular" MR contrast agents. The paramagnetic gadolinium chelates can be classified according to their degree of protein interaction. The ultra small iron oxide particles are "blood pool agents" which demonstrate long intravascular enhancement. (n.b. The products in italics are still in the developmental phase at the time of writing)

Table 1. Physicochemical characteristics of commercially-available first pass gadolinium-based MR contrast agents

Characteristic	Magnevist (0.5 mol/L)	Dotarem (0.5 mol/L)	ProHance (0.5 mol/L)	Omniscan (0.5 mol/L)	Gadovist (1.0 mol/L)	OptiMARK (0.5 mol/L)	MultiHance (0.5 mol/L)
Molecular structure	Linear, ionic	Cyclic, ionic	Cyclic, non-ionic	Linear, non-ionic	Cyclic, non-ionic	Linear, non-ionic	Linear, ionic
Thermodynamic stability constant ($\log K_{eq}$)	22.1	25.8	23.8	16.9	21.8	16.6	22.6
Osmolality (Osm/kg)	1.96	1.35	0.63	0.65	1.6	1.11	1.97
Viscosity (mPa · s at 37°C)	2.9	2.0	1.3	1.4	4.96	2.0	5.3
T1 relaxivity (L/mmol · s^{-1}), plasma	4.9	4.3	4.6	4.8	5.6	N/A	9.7

N/A = not available

agents generally translate into similar vascular imaging performance when injected at equivalent dose, and, until recently, the choice of which to use was dictated largely by non-radiological factors.

That certain of the "conventional" gadolinium agents might be considered preferable over others for CE-MRA has emerged from the observations of Prince et al. [8] and others [9, 10] who confirmed earlier work [11, 12] in noting that gadodiamide and gadoversetamide interfere with the colorimetric test for serum calcium, resulting in spurious hypocalcemia in routine clinical laboratory investigations. This was shown to be due to the relatively low stability of these agents compared to the other available gadolinium agents (Table 1)

and, pertinently, was shown to be a greater problem with higher doses and in patients with renal insufficiency [13]. Notably, high doses of conventional gadolinium agents of up to 0.3 mmol/kg have been routinely used in numerous CE-MRA protocols, particularly those involving large vascular territories such as the run-off vessels [9], and those involving MR angiography of the renal arteries – a frequent procedure among patients with renal insufficiency [14-16].

Another recent observation related to gadolinium chelate stability which may influence the choice of contrast agent for MRI procedures in general concerns the issue of gadolinium retention within the body following possible transmetalla-

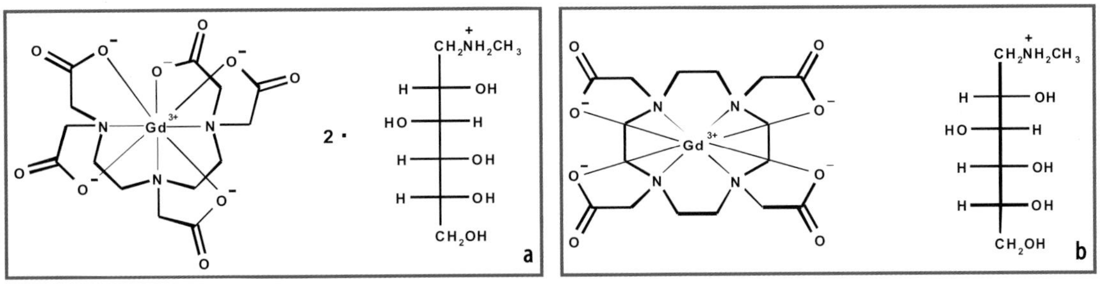

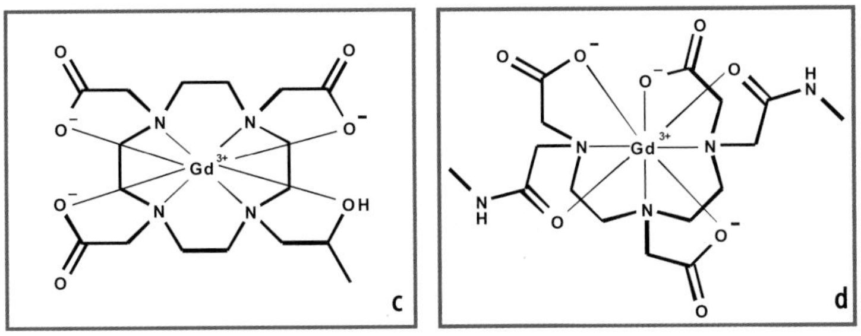

Fig. 2a-h. Molecular structures of first pass gadolinium contrast agents. **a** gadopentetate dimeglumine (Gd-DTPA, Magnevist); **b** gadoterate meglumine (Gd-DOTA, Dotarem); **c** gadoteridol (Gd-HP-DO3A, ProHance); **d** gadodiamide (Gd-DT-PA-BMA, Omniscan); **e** gadoversetamide (Gd-DTPA-BMEA, OptiMARK); **f** gadobutrol (Gd-BT-DO3A, Gadovist); **g** gadobenate dimeglumine (Gd-BOPTA, MultiHance); **h** gadotexetate disodium (Gd-EOB-DT-PA, not yet available)

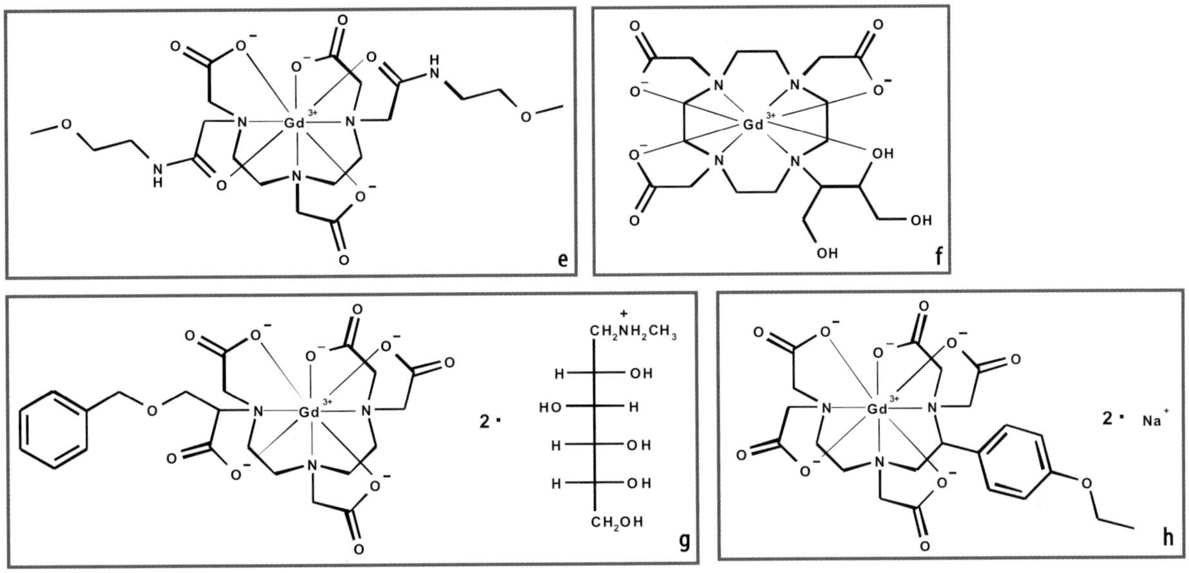

tion and the release of free gadolinium[3+] ion. In a study of 18 human subjects undergoing hip joint replacement at 3 to 8 days after the administration of a clinical 0.1 mmol/kg dose of either gadoteridol or gadodiamide, Gibby et al. [17] found as much as 4.2 times more gadolinium in the bone samples of patients given gadodiamide than in the samples of patients given gadoteridol (1.90 µg/g versus 0.45 µg/g, respectively, by ICP-Mass Spectroscopy). Given that free gadolinium is highly toxic and is not readily eliminated from the body, the potential for release from the less stable agents could be considered a cause for concern particularly for patients undergoing frequent contrast-enhanced procedures or contrast procedures at high doses.

Due to the long-standing and comparatively widespread availability of the majority of non-protein interacting agents formulated at 0.5 M, much of the published literature on CE-MRA is based on studies conducted with these agents and most CE-

MRA examinations in routine practice are performed with these agents. However, the frequent need for high doses of up to 0.3 mmol/kg has prompted the development of newer agents with preferential properties for CE-MRA.

A first departure from the traditional 0.5 M formulation is gadobutrol (Fig. 2f) which is the only agent at present to be prepared commercially as a 1.0 M formulation. Like an early non-commercial 1.0 M formulation of gadoteridol [18], on which the molecular structure of gadobutrol is based, the 1.0 M formulation of gadobutrol is feasible due to a satisfactorily low viscosity of the Gd-BT-DO3A chelate. The principal advantage of gadobutrol in CE-MRA is that twice the concentration of gadolinium can be delivered to the vessel of interest per unit volume resulting in a greater intravascular signal than is achievable with an equivalent dose of a conventional 0.5 M agent. Alternatively, a lower overall dose can be given enabling a smaller,

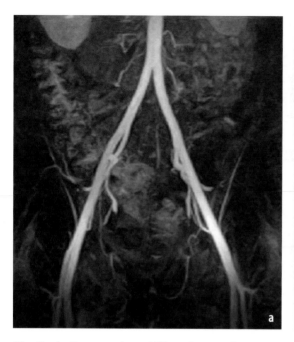 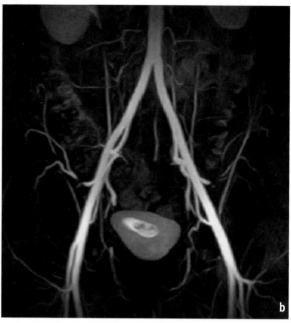

Fig. 3a, b. Contrast-enhanced MR-angiograms of a 31-year-old male volunteer of 78 kg after (**a**) Magnevist and (**b**) Gadovist 1.0. Both contrast agents were administered at a dose of 0.13 mmol/kg bodyweight although the injection rate of the Gadovist-enhanced exam (0.8 ml/s) was half that of the Magnevist-enhanced exam (1.6 ml/s) to ensure identical overall injection times. Both images reveal diagnostic image quality, but the Gadovist 1.0 exam illustrates better delineation of smaller vessels [Images courtesy of Dr. Mathias Goyen, Dept. of Diagnostic and Interventional Radiology, University Hospital Essen, Germany]

more compact bolus which is preferable for maintaining a greater, more prolonged SNR enhancement [19]. Initial studies have shown that gadobutrol is safe [20] and that it may have advantages over conventional agents for total body MRA [21] and for the improved visualization of smaller vessels in the pelvic vasculature [22, 23] (Fig. 3). However, a recent multicenter study to evaluate gadobutrol for the detection of peripheral vascular disease has suggested that whereas comparable image quality to that seen with DSA is achievable in the pelvis and thigh, imaging of the calf muscles with gadobutrol may still be compromised by spatial resolution and technical limitations [24]. On the other hand, many of these problems may be overcome with the use of midfemoral venous compression techniques [25]. Finally, the anticipated benefits of using smaller bolus volumes for improved time-resolved multiphasic pulmonary MRA [3], have not yet been borne out in clinical practice: a recent study comparing gadobutrol with gadopentetate dimeglumine reported no relevant advantages for the former agent and it was concluded that the absence of a significant benefit may have been due to T2/T2* effects caused by the high intravascular concentration at the high injection rate used (5.0 mL/second) [26]. T2/T2* effects may also explain the observed absence of any benefit of gadobutrol over gadopentetate dimeglumine in time-resolved multiphasic MRA of the abdomen [27].

Gadolinium Contrast Agents with weak Protein Interaction

A second and more innovative departure from the conventional first generation non-protein interacting gadolinium chelates is gadobenate dimeglumine (Fig. 2g). This agent differs from the other available gadolinium agents in that it possesses a higher T1 relaxivity in blood (9.7 L/mmol · s^{-1}) due to weak and transient interactions between the Gd-BOPTA chelate and serum proteins, particularly albumin [4, 28]. This higher T1 relaxivity manifests as a significantly greater intravascular signal intensity enhancement compared to that achieved with conventional gadolinium chelates at equivalent dose [29, 30], with the benefits noted in particular for the visualization of smaller vessels (Fig. 4). Preliminary dose-finding studies in the pelvic and abdominal/renal vasculature established that the optimum dose needed to obtain images of high diagnostic quality was 0.1 mmol/kg bodyweight [31, 32]. A recent intra-individual crossover study in the renal vasculature has demonstrated that the image quality achieved with gadobenate dimeglumine at this dose is equivalent to that achieved with gadopentetate dimeglumine at a double dose of 0.2 mmol/kg bodyweight [33] (Fig. 5). The need for only a single 0.1 mmol/kg dose of gadobenate dimeglumine is clearly beneficial in this group of patients with potential renal insufficiency.

The clinical advantages of the increased relax-

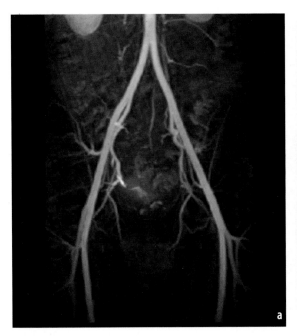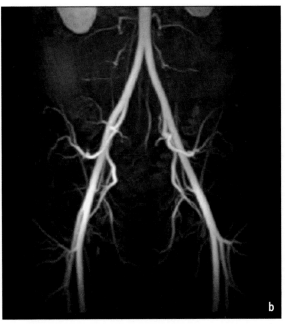

Fig. 4a, b. Contrast-enhanced MR-angiograms of a 24-year-old male volunteer of 81 kg after (**a**) Magnevist and (**b**) MultiHance. Both contrast agents were administered at a dose of 0.1 mmol/kg bodyweight and at an injection rate of 1.6 ml/s. Both images reveal diagnostic image quality, but the MultiHance exam shows improved delineation of distal vascular segments and smaller vessels in the lower abdomen and pelvis [Images courtesy of Dr. Mathias Goyen, Dept. of Diagnostic and Interventional Radiology, University Hospital Essen, Germany]

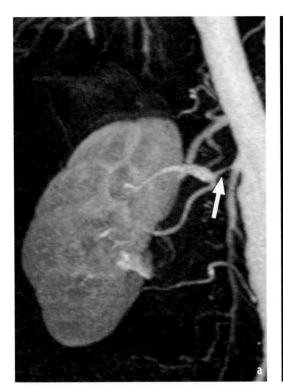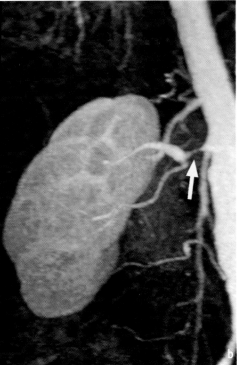

Fig. 5a, b. Maximum intensity projection (MIP) reconstructions of the right renal artery after the administration of (**a**) MultiHance at 0.1 mmol/kg bodyweight and (**b**) Magnevist at 0.2 mmol/kg bodyweight. Both images reveal a severe proximal stenosis (*arrows*). The two-fold higher T1-relaxivity of MultiHance compared to that of Magnevist permits images of equivalent diagnostic quality at a standard dose of 0.1 mmol/kg

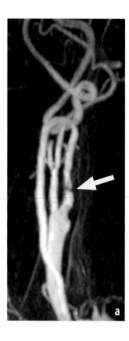
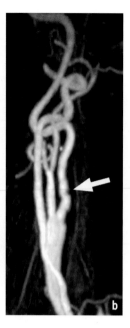
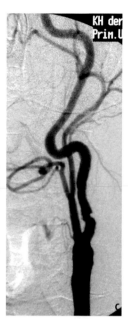

Fig. 6a-c. Stenosis of the left carotid artery. The MR-angiogram after 18 ml (0.13 mmol/kg) gadodiamide (Omniscan) (**a**) reveals a severe stenosis (*arrow*) of the left internal carotid artery. Conversely, the MR-angiogram after 14 ml (0.1 mmol/kg) gadobenate dimeglumine (MultiHance) (**b**) reveals only a moderate stenosis (*arrow*) of the left internal carotid artery. Conventional digital subtraction angiography (**c**) confirms the presence of only a moderate stenosis of the internal carotid artery [Images courtesy of Prof. Siegfried Thurnher, Dept. of Radiology and Nuclear Medicine, Hospital Brothers of St. John of God, Vienna, Austria]

ivity have been demonstrated for all vascular territories from the carotid vasculature [34, 35] to the distant run-off vessels [36, 37]. In the carotid arteries gadobenate dimeglumine – enhanced MRA has been shown to be superior to unenhanced MRA and at least as accurate as conventional DSA for the depiction of carotid artery stenosis [35] (Fig. 6). A major advantage of gadobenate dimeglumine compared to other gadolinium agents, however, is in imaging of the peripheral vasculature and other vascular territories for which a large field of view is required. In imaging of the peripheral run-off vessels, gadobenate dimeglumine has been shown to be superior to both gadopentetate dimeglumine and gadoterate meglumine, particularly for visualization of the vessels of the lower legs [36-38]. It is possible that the benefit with gadobenate dimeglumine in more distal vessels is due not only to the increased relaxivity of this agent but also to a reduced rate of extravasation compared to that occurring with other agents due to the weak interaction of the Gd-BOPTA molecule with serum proteins. The weak interaction has previously been postulated to explain a tendency towards increased signal-to-noise (SNR) and contrast-to-noise (CNR) with gadobenate dimeglumine compared to gadopentetate dimeglumine on descending the abdominal aorta [33].

In addition to improved MRA of the vessels of the lower extremities, gadobenate dimeglumine has also been shown to be effective for MRA of the upper extremities [39] and for whole body CE-MRA [40-43]. The higher relaxivity of gadobenate dimeglumine is again beneficial for this latter application in that a dose of only 0.2 mmol/kg body-weight is needed to achieve high quality images from the carotid arteries to the distal run-off vessels [41, 43]. Like the conventional non-protein interacting gadolinium chelates, gadobenate dimeglumine has an excellent safety profile with a very low incidence of adverse events noted for the clinical development program as a whole and for CE-MRA applications in particular [44].

A second agent with elevated T1 relaxivity (8.2 L/mmol $\cdot$ s^{-1}) in human plasma is gadotexetate disodium (Fig. 2h) [45]. Although not yet approved anywhere for contrast-enhanced MR imaging, it is conceivable this agent may also have advantages over conventional gadolinium agents for CE-MRA. However, all available developmental information concerns the potential of this agent for liver imaging: no data are as yet available concerning its potential for CE-MRA applications.

Paramagnetic Contrast Agents: "Blood Pool" Contrast Agents

The so-called paramagnetic "blood pool" contrast agents are agents for which the intra-vascular residence time is considerably extended compared to the conventional "first pass only" gadolinium agents. With these agents the intravascular signal remains high for an extended period of time thereby permitting MR imaging during a more prolonged "steady-state" timeframe in addition to conventional first pass CE-MRA. There are two principal types of paramagnetic "blood pool" contrast agent: those whose intravascular residence time is prolonged due to a capacity of the gadolinium chelate for strong interaction with serum proteins, and those that have a macro-molecular structure whose large size limits the extent of extravasation compared to the first pass gadolinium agents. As yet none of these agents are approved for clinical use.

Gadolinium Contrast Agents with strong Protein Interaction

Currently, two agents with strong affinity for serum proteins are undergoing clinical development. The agent furthest along the developmental process is gadofosveset trisodium (MS-325) which has completed Phase II and III clinical trials and has been submitted for FDA approval for use in CE-MRA at a dose of 0.03 mmol/kg bodyweight. This agent has been reported to be 88-96% noncovalently bound to albumin in human plasma and to exhibit a relaxivity at 0.5T that is 6 to 10 times that of gadopentate dimeglumine [46-49]. Studies have shown that this agent can be utilized both for first pass CE-MRA and for steady-state CE-MRA of a number of vascular territories, including the carotid arteries [50], the aortoiliac vasculature (Fig. 7) and the peripheral run-off vessels [48]. Other studies suggest MS-325 may also prove beneficial for CE-MRA of the coronary arteries [51, 52].

The second agent with strong affinity for serum proteins is gadocoletic acid (B22956). This agent has completed Phase I trials and is currently undergoing Phase II trials for enhanced coronary MRA. B22596 has been shown to have even stronger affinity for serum albumin than MS-325 (approximately 94% bound noncovalently) and to have a similarly long intravascular residence time [53, 54]. Preliminary studies have shown that a dose of 0.075 mmol/kg B22596 is able to markedly improve visualization of both the left and right coronary artery systems compared to that achievable with state-of-the-art unenhanced 3D coronary MRA techniques [55-57] (Fig. 8). Like MS-325, B22956 can be used to acquire conventional high quality first pass dynamic images in addition to delayed steady state vascular images.

Both these agents appear very promising and have excellent safety profiles.

Gadolinium Contrast Agents with Macro-molecular Structures

Examples of gadolinium-based blood pool agents with macromolecular structures are P792 [58, 59] and gadomer-17 [60, 61]. These agents differ from the currently available low molecular weight gadolinium agents in possessing large molecular structures that prevent extravasation of the molecules from the intravascular space following injection. The molecular weights of P792 and gadomer-17 are 6.5 kDa and 35 kDa, respectively [59, 61], which compare with weights of between approximately 0.56 and 1.0 kDa for the purely first pass gadolinium agents. Whereas the structure of P792 is based on that of gadoterate substituted with four large hydrophilic spacer arms [62], gadomer-17 is a much larger polymer of 24 gadolinium cascades [61]. In addition to differences in molecular weight and structure, these two agents appear to differ in terms of their rates of clearance, with P792 considered a rapid clearance blood pool agent [59, 62]. Despite these differences, both agents are currently under investigation for possible applications in CE-MRA of the coronary arteries [59, 61].

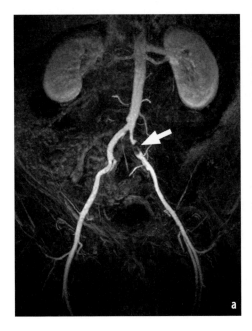
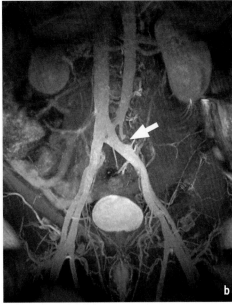

Fig. 7a, b. MR-angiograms of the pelvic arteries obtained (**a**) during the first pass of MS-325 and (**b**) on steady state MR angiography. The presence of pelvic artery stenoses (*arrows*) is evident on both images. [Images courtesy of EPIX Medical, Cambridge, Massachusetts, USA, Schering AG, Berlin, Germany; Mathias Goyen, University Hospital Essen, Essen/Germany, and Steven D. Wolff, Cardiovascular Research Foundation, New York, USA]

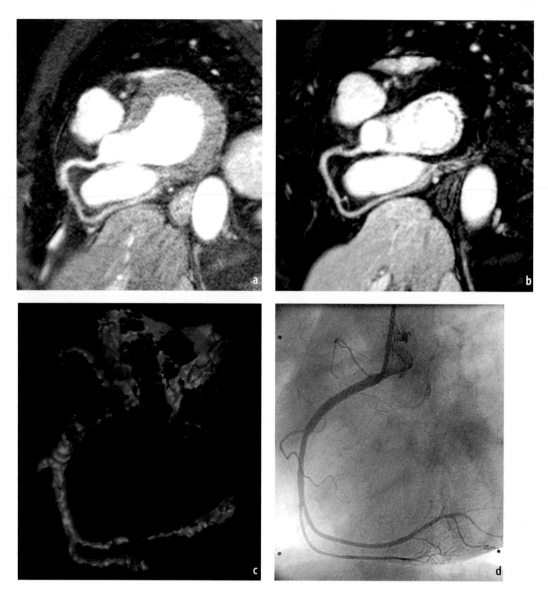

Fig. 8a-d. Coronary MRA of RCA. **a** T2 prep coronary artery imaging (standard sequence). **b** Intravascular contrast enhancement using B22956 in combination with an inversion-recovery sequence. **c** 3D volume rendered MRA of the RCA (**d**) conventional x-ray angiography. Multiplanar reformatted 3 D images ("soap-bubble reconstruction") showing the effect of intravascular contrast enhancement (**b**) in comparison with the standard, non-contrast enhanced imaging approach (**a**). Note the postcontrast increase in vessel sharpness, visible vessel length and the highly efficient suppression of signal from surrounding tissue, thereby facilitating clear visualization of the RCA. 3 dimensional volume rendered coronary MRA of a non-diseased RCA (**c**) in comparison with conventional x-ray angiography (**d**). The intense signal from the coronary artery lumen due to intravascular contrast enhancement allows visualization of the RCA far beyond the crux and improves visibility of coronary side branches. [Images (**a**), (**b**) and (**d**) courtesy of Dr. Eike Nagel, Clinic of Internal Medicine/Cardiology, German Heart Institute, Berlin, Germany. Image (**c**) courtesy of Dr. I. Paetsch, Clinic of Internal Medicine/Cardiology, German Heart Institute, Berlin, Germany]

Superparamagnetic Iron Oxide Agents

The second major group of potential contrast agents for MRA comprises the superparamagnetic agents based on ultrasmall particles of iron oxide (USPIO). To date, two USPIO agents have undergone preliminary clinical development, SH U 555 C [63] which is a subfraction of SH U 555 A, a USPIO molecule coated in dextran which is currently ap-

proved in Europe for liver-specific imaging, and NC100150 [64–66], a USPIO molecule coated with starch. Other USPIO molecules to have undergone preliminary investigative studies include SH U 555 A itself which has been evaluated for CE-MRA of the upper abdomen [67] and AMI 227 [68].

Of the USPIO molecules to be evaluated for CE-MRA, the agent to have undergone the greatest early development was NC100150. As with the gadolinium blood pool agents, the potential advantages of this agent include a long intravascular half-life with minimal leakage into the interstitial space, thereby permitting steady-state vascular imaging. Preliminary evaluation on this agent was performed for coronary MRA [65] and for other MR applications such as renal perfusion [66].

Unfortunately, a major drawback of NC100150 and other USPIO molecules for CE-MRA appears to be a high T2* effect compared to the T1 effect they deliver. This high T2* effect, particularly at higher contrast agent doses, results in a loss of vascular signal leading to decreased vessel sharpness and size. This limitation would appear to have curtailed the further development of the USPIO molecules at the present time and it remains to be seen whether technological advances will improve the prospects of these agents.

Future Perspectives

The future generation of contrast agents for MRA will include agents with targeted properties for imaging vessel walls or atheroschlerotic plaque. With increasing regulatory emphasis on the demonstration of improved efficacy and safety compared to currently available agents, the future generations of MRA contrast agents are likely to be highly effective with excellent safety profiles, facilitating the further acceptance of CE-MRA as the diagnostic imaging modality of choice for vascular disease.

References

1. Runge VM, Knopp MV (1999) Off-label use and reimbursement of contrast media in MR. JMRI 10:489-495
2. Knopp MV, Lodemann KP, Kage U et al (2001) Administration of MR contrast agents outside of approved indications (off-label use). Radiologe 41:296-302
3. Knopp MV, von Tengg-Kobligk H, Floemer F et al (1999) Contrast agents for MRA: future directions. JMRI 10:314-316
4. de Haën C, Cabrini M, Akhnana L et al (1999) Gadobenate dimeglumine 0.5M solution for injection (MultiHance"): pharmaceutical formulation and physicochemical properties of a new magnetic resonance imaging contrast medium. J Comput Assist Tomogr 23 (Suppl. 1):S161-S168
5. Grossman RI, Rubin DL, Hunter G et al (2000) Magnetic resonance imaging in patients with central nervous system pathology. A comparison of OptiMARK (Gd-DTPA-BMEA) and Magnevist (Gd-DTPA). Invest Radiol 35:412-419
6. Benner T, Reimer P, Erb G et al (2000) Cerebral MR perfusion imaging: first clinical application of a 1M gadolinium chelate (gadovist 1.0) in a double-blinded dose-finding study. J Magn Reson Imaging 12:371-380
7. Tombach B, Bremer C, Reimer P et al (2001) Renal tolerance of a neutral gadolinium chelate (gadobutrol) in patients with chronic renal failure: results of a randomized study. Radiology 218:651-657
8. Prince MR, Erel HE, Lent RW et al (2003) Gadodiamide administration causes spurious hypocalcemia. Radiology 227:630-646
9. Doorenbos CJ, Ozyilmaz A, van Wijnen M (2003) Severe pseudohypocalcemia after gadolinium-enhanced magnetic resonance angiography. N Engl J Med. 349:817-818
10. Kang HP, Scott MG, Joe BN et al (2004) Model for Predicting the Impact of Gadolinium on Plasma Calcium Measured by the o-Cresolphthalein Method. Clin Chem. 50:141-146
11. Normann PT, Froysa A, Svaland M (1995) Interference of gadodiamide injection (OMNISCAN) on the colorimetric determination of serum calcium, Scand J. Clin Lab Invest; 55:421-426
12. Lin J, Idee JM, Port M et al (1999) Interference of magnetic resonance imaging contrast agents with the serum calcium measurement technique using colorimetric reagents. J Pharm Biomed Anal. 21:931-43
13. Goyan M, Ruehm SG, Debatin JF (2000) MR Angiography: the role of contrast agents. Eur J Radiol 34:247-256
14. Hany TF, Schmidt M, Hilfiker PR, et al (1998) Optimization of contrast dosage for gadolinium-enhanced 3D MRA of the pulmonary and renal arteries. Magn Reson Imaging 16:901-906
15. Dong Q, Schoenberg SO, Carlos RC et al (1999) Diagnosis of renal vascular disease with MR angiography. Radiographics 19:1535-1554
16. Leung DA, Hagspiel KD, Angle JF et al (2002) MR angiography of the renal arteries. Radiol Clin North Am 40:847-865
17. Gibby WA, Gibby KA, Gibby WA (2004) Comparison of Gd DTPA-BMA (Omniscan) versus Gd HP-DO3A (ProHance) retention in human bone tissue by Inductively Coupled Plasma Atomic Emission Spectroscopy. Invest Radiol 39:138-142
18. Tweedle M (1992) Physicochemical properties of gadoteridol and other magnetic resonance contrast agents. Invest Radiol 27(Suppl 1):2-6
19. Leung DA, Hagspiel KD, Angle JF et al (2002) MR angiography of the renal arteries. Radiol Clin North Am 40:847-865
20. Balzer JO, Loewe C, Davis K et al (2003) Safety of contrast-enhanced MR angiography employing gadobutrol 1.0 M as contrast material. Eur Radiol 13:2067-2074
21. Goyen M, Herborn CU, Vogt FM, et al (2003) Using a 1 M Gd-chelate (gadobutrol) for total-body three-dimensional MR angiography: preliminary experience. J Magn Reson Imaging 17:565-571
22. Goyen M, Lauenstein T, Herborn C et al (2001) 0.5 M Gd chelate (Magnevist) versus 1.0 M Gd chelate (Gadovist): dose-independent effect on image quality of pelvic three-dimensional MR-angiography. J Magn Reson Imaging 14:602-607
23. Herborn C, Lauenstein T, Ruehm S et al (2003) Intraindividual comparison of gadopentetate dimeglumine, gadobenate dimeglumine and gadobutrol for pelvic 3D magnetic resonance angiography. Invest Radiol 38:27-33
24. Hentsch A, Aschauer MA, Balzer JO, et al (2003) Gadobutrol-enhanced moving-table magnetic reso-

nance angiography in patients with peripheral vascular disease: a prospective, multi-centre blinded comparison with digital subtraction angiography. Eur Radiol 13:2103-2114

25. Herborn CU, Ajaj W, Goyen M et al (2004) Peripheral vasculature: whole-body MR angiography with midfemoral venous compression–initial experience. Radiology 230:872-878

26. Fink C, Bock M, Kiessling F et al (2004) Time-resolved contrast-enhanced three-dimensional pulmonary MR-angiography: 1.0 M gadobutrol vs. 0.5 M gadopentetate dimeglumine. J Magn Reson Imaging 19:202-208

27. von Tengg-Kobligk H, Floemer F, Knopp MV (2003) [Multiphasic MR angiography as an intra-individual comparison between the contrast agents Gd-DT-PA, Gd-BOPTA, and Gd-BT-DO3A] Radiologe 43:171-178. In German

28. Cavagna F, Maggioni F, Castelli P et al (1997) Gadolinium chelates with weak binding to serum proteins. A new class of high-efficiency, general purpose contrast agents for magnetic resonance imaging. Invest Radiol 32:780-796

29. Knopp M, Schoenberg S, Rehm C et al (2002) Assessment of Gadobenate Dimeglumine (Gd-BOPTA) for MR Angiography: Phase I Studies. Invest Radiol 37:706-715

30. Völk M, Strotzer M, Lenhart M et al (2001) Renal time-resolved MR angiography: quantitative comparison of gadobenate dimeglumine and gadopentetate dimeglumine with different doses. Radiology 220:484-488

31. Wikström J, Wasser MN, Pattynama PM, et al (2003) Gadobenate dimeglumine-enhanced magnetic resonance angiography of the pelvic arteries. Invest Radiol 38:504-515

32. Kroencke TJ, Wasser MN, Pattynama PM et al (2002) Gadobenate dimeglumine-enhanced MR angiography of the abdominal aorta and renal arteries. AJR Am J Roentgenol 179:1573-158

33. Prokop M, Schneider G, Vanzulli A et al (2005) Contrast-enhanced MR angiography of the renal arteries: blinded multicenter crossover comparison gadobenate dimeglumine and gadopentetate dimeglumine. Radiology (in press)

34. Pediconi F, Fraioli F, Catalano C et al (2003) Gadobenate dimeglumine (Gd-DTPA) vs gadopentetate dimeglumine (Gd-BOPTA) for contrast-enhanced magnetic resonance angiography (MRA): improvement in intravascular signal intensity and contrast to noise ratio. Radiol Med 106:87-93

35. Anzalone N, Scomazzoni F, Castellano R et al (2005) Carotid artery stenosis: intra-individual correlations of unenhanced 3D-TOF-MR Angiography, contrast-enhanced MR Angiography, and digital subtraction angiography versus rotational angiography for detection and grading. Radiology (in press)

36. Knopp MV, Giesel FL, von Tengg-Kobligk H et al (2003) Contrast-enhanced MR Angiography of the Run-off Vasculature: Intraindividual comparison of gadobenate dimeglumine with gadopentetate dimeglumine. J Magn Reson Imaging 17:694-702

37. Wyttenbach R, Gianella S, Alerci M et al (2003) Prospective Blinded Evaluation of Gd-DOTA– versus Gd-BOPTA–enhanced Peripheral MR Angiography, as Compared with Digital Subtraction Angiography. Radiology 227:261-269

38. Herborn CU, Goyen M, Lauenstein TC, et al (2003) Comprehensive time-resolved MRI of peripheral vascular malformations Am J Roentgenol 181:729-735

39. Winterer JT, Scheffler K, Paul G et al (2000) Optimization of contrast-enhanced MR angiography of the hands with a timing bolus and elliptically reordered 3D pulse sequence J Comput Assisted Tomogr 24:903-908

40. Ruehm SG, Goyen M, Barkhausen J et al (2001) Rapid magnetic resonance angiography for detection of atherosclerosis. Lancet 357:1086-1091

41. Goyen M, Herborn CU, Lauenstein TC et al (2002) Optimization of contrast dosage for gadobenate dimeglumine-enhanced high-resolution whole-body 3D magnetic resonance angiography Invest Radiol 37:263-268

42. Goyen M, Quick HH, Debatin JF et al (2002) Whole-body three-dimensional MR angiography with a rolling table platform: initial clinical experience. Radiology 224:270-277

43. Goyen M, Herborn CU, Kröger K et al (2003) Detection of atherosclerosis: systemic imaging for systemic disease with whole-body three-dimensional MR angiography – initial experience. Radiology 227:277-282

44. Kirchin MA, Pirovano G, Venetianer C et al (2001) Safety assessment of gadobenate dimeglumine (Multihance,): extended clinical experience from phase I studies to post-marketing surveillance. J Magn Reson Imaging 14:281-294

45. Huppertz A, Balzer T, Blakeborough A et al (2004) European EOB Study Group. Improved detection of focal liver lesions at MR imaging: multicenter comparison of gadoxetic acid-enhanced MR images with intraoperative findings. Radiology 230:266-275

46. Lauffer R, Parmelee D, Dunham S et al (1998) MS-325: albumin-targeted contrast agent for MR angiography. Radiology 207:529-538

47. Grist T, Korosec F, Peters D et al (1998) Steady-state and dynamic MR angiography with MS-325: initial experience in humans. Radiology 207:539-544

48. Perreault P, Edelman MA, Baum RA et al (2003) MR angiography with gadofosveset trisodium for peripheral vascular disease: phase II trial. Radiology 229:811-820

49. Caravan P, Cloutier NJ, Greenfield MT et al (2002) The interaction of MS-325 with human serum albumin and its effect on proton relaxation rates. J Am Chem Soc. 124:3152-3162

50. Bluemke D, Stillman A, Bis K et al (2001) Carotid MR angiography: phase II study of safety and efficacy of MS-325. Radiology 219:114-122

51. Stuber M, Botnar RM, Danias PG et al (1999) Contrast agent-enhanced, free-breathing, three-dimensional coronary magnetic resonance angiography. J Magn Reson Imaging 10:790-799

52. Kraitchman DL, Chin BB, Heldman AW et al (2002) MRI detection of myocardial perfusion defects due to coronary artery stenosis with MS-325. J Magn Reson Imaging 15:149-158

53. Cavagna FM, Anelli PL, Lorusso V et al (2001) B-22956, a new intravascular contrast agent for MR coronary angiography. Proc of the Int. Soc. for Magnetic Resonance in Medicine, p 519 (Abstract)

54. La Noce A, Stoelben S, Scheffler K et al (2002) B22956/1, a new intravascular contrast agent for

MRI: first administration to humans–preliminary results. Acad Radiol 9 [Suppl]:S404-406

55. Cavagna FM, La Noce A, Maggioni F, et al (2002) MR Coronary Angiography with the New Intravascular Contrast Agent B-22956/1: First Human Experience. Proc of the Int. Soc. for Magnetic Resonance in Medicine, p 114 (Abstract)

56. Huber M, Paetsch I, Schnackenburg B, et al (2003) Performance of a new gadolinium-based intravascular contrast agent in free-breathing inversion-recovery 3D coronary MRA. Magn Reson Med 49:115-121

57. Paetsch I, Huber M, Bornstedt A et al(2004) Improved 3D free-breathing coronary MRA using gadocoletic acid (B-22956) for intravascular contrast enhancement. J Magn Reson Imaging 20:288-293

58. Gaillard S, Kubiak C, Stolz C et al (2002) Safety and pharmacokinetics of p792, a new blood-pool agent: results of clinical testing in nonpatient volunteers. Invest Radiol 37:161-166

59. Taupitz M, Schnorr J, Wagner S et al (2001) Coronary magnetic resonance angiography: experimental evaluation of the new rapid clearance blood pool contrast medium P792. Magn Reson Med 46:932-938

60. Dong Q, Hurst D, Weinmann H et al (1998) Magnetic resonance angiography with gadomer-17. An animal study original investigation. Invest Radiol 33:699-708

61. Herborn CU, Barkhausen J, Paetsch I et al (2003) Coronary arteries: contrast-enhanced MR imaging with SH L 643A–experience in 12 volunteers. Radiology 229:217-223

62. Port M, Corot C, Raynal I et al (2001) Physicochemical and biological evaluation of P792, a rapid-clearance blood-pool agent for magnetic resonance imaging. Invest Radiol 36:445-454

63. Reimer P, Bremer C, Allkemper T et al (2004) Myocardial perfusion and MR angiography of chest with SH U 555 C: results of placebo-controlled clinical phase I study. Radiology 231:474-481

64. Weishaupt D, Ruhm S, Binkert C et al (2000) Equilibrium-phase MR angiography of the aortoiliac and renal arteries using a blood pool contrast agent. Am J Roentgenol 175:189-195

65. Taylor A, Panting J, Keegan J et al (1999) Safety and preliminary findings with the intravascular contrast agent NC100150 injection for MR coronary angiography. J Magn Reson Imaging 9:220-227

66. Bachmann R, Conrad R, Kreft B et al (2002) Evaluation of a new ultrasmall superparamagnetic iron oxide contrast agent Clariscan, (NC100150) for MRI of renal perfusion: experimental study in an animal model. J Magn Reson Imaging 16:190-195

67. Reimer P, Allkemper T, Matuszewski L et al (1999) Contrast-enhanced 3D-MRA of the upper abdomen with a bolus-injectable SPIO (SH U 555 A). J Magn Reson Imaging 10:65-71

68. Mayo-Smith W, Saini S, Slater G et al (1996) MR contrast material for vascular enhancement: value of superparamagnetic iron oxide. Am J Roentgenol 166:73-77

SECTION III

Head and Neck Vessels

III.1

MR Angiography of Extracranial Carotid and Vertebral Arteries

Kenneth R. Maravilla and Baocheng Chu

Introduction

The advantages for using MRA as a noninvasive method for evaluating the extracranial carotid and vertebral vasculature are obvious. MRA is safer, faster and cheaper than traditional x-ray angiography, and avoids the complications inherent to invasive catheterization. Nowhere in the body is this more important than in evaluation of the supraaortic vessels. Catheterization of the carotid and vertebral arteries can lead to cerebral complications, resulting in major neurologic disability or even death. Over the past fifteen years, a number of different MRA approaches have been explored for imaging the extracranial carotid and vertebral arteries. These include 3D time-of-flight (TOF), 3D phase contrast and 2D TOF imaging. Each has its advantages and disadvantages as will be discussed in the subsequent passages. Recently, arterial-phase bolus contrast enhanced MRA has rapidly evolved to the point where it is now the preferred method for cervical vascular evaluation. However, even this method has its limitations, resulting in its frequent combination with one or more of the above-mentioned techniques.

Indications

The indications for MRA of the extracranial vessels can be divided into four major categories. These include atherosclerosis evaluation, suspected carotid or vertebral vessel dissection, evaluation of head and neck tumors and post treatment evaluation.

Atherosclerosis

Patients presenting for evaluation of known or suspected atherosclerotic disease comprise the single most common indication for neck MRA. These include patients who have signs and/or symptoms of cerebral vascular insufficiency as well as asymptomatic patients who are at high risk for atherosclerotic disease or who have known carotid vascular disease on one side and need evaluation for possible significant disease on the contralateral side. In these cases, the goal of diagnostic MRA is to evaluate the degree of vessel stenosis, most commonly occurring at the common carotid artery bifurcation. Criteria for definition of stenosis is usually based on the NASCET criteria that compares lumen diameter at the site of maximal stenosis in the proximal internal carotid artery with the lumen diameter of the cervical internal carotid artery at a level distal to the carotid bulb where the walls of the internal carotid artery are parallel and represent luminal diameter above the level of atherosclerotic plaque [1].

Arterial Dissection

Cervical vessel dissections fall into two broad categories. First is traumatic dissection that occurs in patients who have had recent blunt trauma to the head or neck or who have had minor trauma such as chiropractic manipulation. The second major category is spontaneous dissection, which arises in patients with genetically determined vessel wall disease or without known etiologic cause [2].

Head and Neck Tumor Evaluation

MRA is infrequently used to evaluate head and neck tumors for degree of vascularity but more commonly, it is used for surgical treatment planning to determine whether or not major vessels such as the carotid artery have been encased or if there has been vascular wall invasion by adjacent tumor. In either case this may render the tumor inoperable [3, 4].

Post-Treatment Surveillance

Finally, post treatment follow up is important in patients who have had prior endarterectomy and who are being evaluated for post treatment restenosis. Also patients who have had prior carotid or vertebral artery dissection and are currently on anticoagulant therapy need follow up evaluation to determine if the vessel wall is healing and the lumen patency is reestablished in order to define the end point for anticoagulant therapy [5].

Normal Anatomy and Anatomic Variations

The aortic arch and great vessel origins are best shown on the CE MRA. They are also seen to relatively good advantage on the 2D TOF images although "stairstep" artifact is usually quite noticeable in this region due to a combination of vessel pulsation and respiratory motion at the level of the aortic arch. This motion degradation is minimized with CE MRA due to the rapid acquisition and the averaging of pulsatile motion across the entire 3D data acquisition set.

The common carotid arteries bifurcate into internal and external carotid arteries and are also well shown on neck MRA (Figs. 1, 2). The common carotid artery bifurcations most commonly occur at approximately the level of C4 (Fig. 3). Occasionally, one or both carotid bifurcations occur either higher or lower in the neck. This variation can present a problem in visualization when using a targeted 3D TOF technique to provide better vessel detail over a limited length of coverage. However, this is not a problem for 2D TOF or for contrast enhanced MRA since the entire length of the vessels is typically defined with high detail.

Both vertebral arteries throughout their length are also well shown with CE MRA. However, depending on the thickness of coverage of the coronal 3D slab for contrast enhanced MRA and the degree of cervical lordosis present, there may be a slight cutoff of the most posterior portion of the distal loop of the vertebral arteries at C1-2 just prior to their entry into the foramen magnum at the skull base.

The aortic arch generally gives rise to three separate origins of the great vessels of the neck (Fig. 4). These include the right innominate artery, the left common carotid artery, and the left subclavian artery. The right innominate artery courses slightly superiorly and laterally prior to giving rise to the right common carotid artery. Just a few mil-

limeters distal to this origin is the origin of the right vertebral artery. The left common carotid artery most often arises as a separate branch from the aortic arch and courses superiorly and slightly leftward through the base of the neck. It gives off no branches until it reaches the common carotid bifurcation. The left subclavian artery courses superiorly and turns laterally. Generally in the region at or just proximal to the lateral turn of the left subclavian artery one can find the origin of the left vertebral artery.

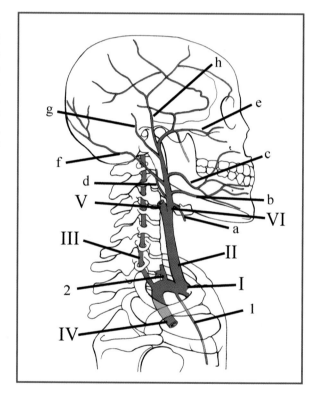

Fig. 1. Normal anatomy of the head and neck vessels
I   Brachiocephalic trunk (innominate artery)
II Right common carotid artery
III Right vertebral artery
IV Right subclavian artery
V   Right internal Carotid artery
VI Right external Carotid artery

1 Right mammarian artery
2 Right thyrocervical trunk
a Right superior Thyroid artery
b Right lingual artery
c Right facial artery
d Right ascending Pharyngeal artery
e Right maxillary artery
f Right occipital artery
g Right posterior Auricular artery
h Right superficial Temporal artery

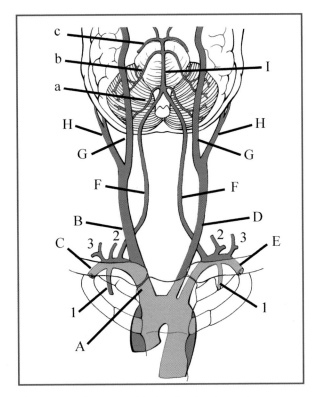

Fig. 2. Normal anatomy of the head and neck vessels

A Brachiocephalic trunk (innominate artery)
B Right common carotid artery
C Right subclavian artery
D Left common Carotid artery
E Left subclavian artery
F Vertebral arteries
G Internal carotid arteries
H External carotid artery
I   Basilary artery

1 Internal mammarian arteries (internal thoracic artery)
2 Thyrocervical trunk
3 Costocervical trunk

a Posterior inferior cerebellar artery
b Anterior inferior cerebellar artery
c Superior cerebellar artery

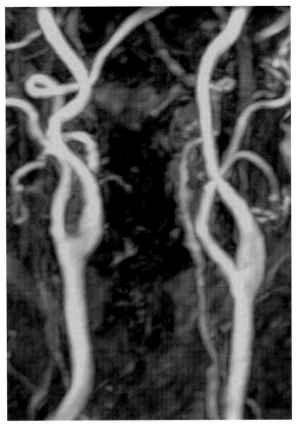

Fig. 3. Normal common carotid artery bifurcations are well demonstrated on CE MRA. Note the excellent contrast together with smooth vessel outlines without stairstep artifact

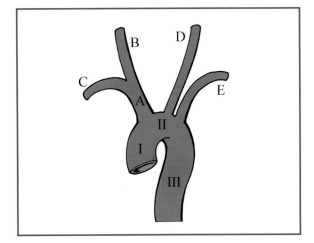

Fig. 4. Normal antomy of the aortic arch

I   Ascending aorta
II Aortic arch
III Descending aorta

A Brachiocephalic trunk (innominate artery)
B Right common carotid artery
C Right subclavian artery
D Left common carotid artery
E Left subclavian artery

Normal Variations

There are a number of common variations in the anatomy of the great vessels that generally occur at the level of the origins from the aortic arch (Figs. 5, 6). A common anomaly is that of the so-called bovine arch. In this anomaly the right common carotid artery and the left common carotid artery essentially arise together and branch just distal to their origin from the aortic arch. In this anomaly, there is a common ostium for the right inominate artery and the left common carotid artery. The right inominate artery and the left common carotid artery arise together and bifurcate immediately above the aorta (Fig. 7a-c). This is a rather common finding and is seen in approximately 30% of normal individuals.

In another commonly seen variation, the left vertebral artery arises as a separate branch from the aortic arch rather than as a branch of the left subclavian artery. This occurs in approximately 10% of normal individuals. In these cases, the separate origin of the left vertebral artery arises between the ostea of the left common carotid artery and the left subclavian artery (Fig. 8).

Additionally, the right common carotid artery may have an anomalous origin from the descending aorta. In these cases, rather than arising as a branch of the right innominate artery, the anomalous right common carotid artery is the last branch of the neck vessels arising separately from the descending aortic arch just distal and posterior to the left subclavian artery origin. The anomalous right common carotid artery then courses right-ward and crosses the midline behind the trachea and the esophagus prior to turning superiorly and ascending in the right neck. This anomalous configuration forms a partial vascular ring around the trachea and esophagus. Similarly in case of a lusorian artery the right subclavian artery arises separately from the descending aortic arch distal to the left subclavian artery origin with the right common carotid artery branching directly from the aorta as the first vessel of the aortic arch (Fig. 9).

The size of the vertebral arteries between right and left is often asymmetric. In approximately 70% of cases the left vertebral artery is dominant in size relative to the right vertebral artery. There is a wide variation in the caliber of the vertebral arteries from symmetrical left and right vertebral artery size (approximately 10 % of population) to that of an extremely hypoplastic right vertebral artery and a large dominate left vertebral artery. In approximately 20% of cases the right vertebral artery is the dominate vessel. A distinction must be made between naturally occurring asymmetry due to normal anatomic variation and pathologic narrowing of a vertebral artery due to atherosclerosis or vessel dissection. In the case of normal variations cited above, the hypoplastic vertebral artery has a uniform and diffuse narrow size from origin to skull base. In pathologic cases due to atherosclerotic stenosis or narrowing from vessel dissection, there is generally focal reduction(s) in caliber between the proximal vertebral artery and that of the vertebral artery distal to the site of stenosis or dissection.

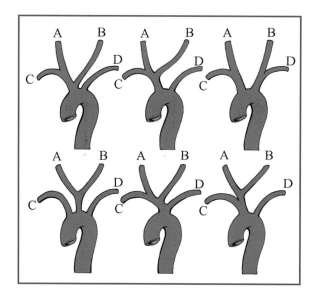

Fig. 5. Common variations of the supraaortic vessels and the arch

A Right common carotid artery
B Left common carotid artery
C Right subclavian artery
D Left subclavian artery

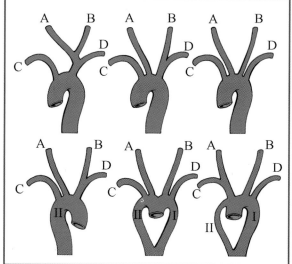

Fig. 6. Common variations of the supraaortic vessels and the arch

I   Left aortic arch
II Right aortic arch

A Right common carotid artery
B Left common carotid artery
C Right subclavian artery
D Left subclavian artery

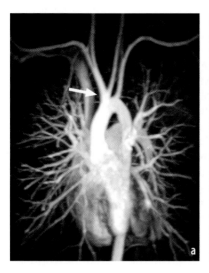
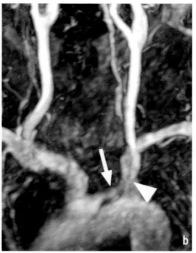
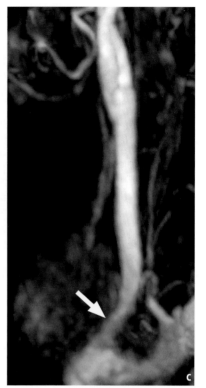

Fig. 7a-c. Bovine type aortic arch is seen in approximately 30% of normal individuals. **a** Incidental finding of a bovine type arch in a 14-year old boy. Note the common ostium (*arrow*) of the right innominate artery and the left common carotid artery [Image courtesy of Dr. G. Schneider]. **b** Bovine type aortic arch in an elder patient with arteriosclerotic disease. The right innominate artery and the left common carotid artery arise from a common ostium. Due to vessel elongation in arteriosclerosis the left common carotid artery courses almost horizontally leftward across the mediastinum (*arrow*) before ascending along the left side of the neck. Note there is also a mild narrowing of the proximal left common carotid artery (*arrowhead*). **c** Targeted MIP image of the left common carotid artery confirms narrowing of the proximal left common carotid artery (*arrows*)

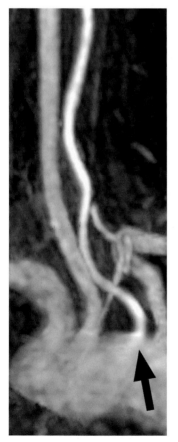

Fig. 8. Normal variation illustrating separate origin of the left vertebral artery, which arises directly from the aortic arch (*arrow*) rather than from the left subclavian artery. This is seen in approximately 10% of normal individuals

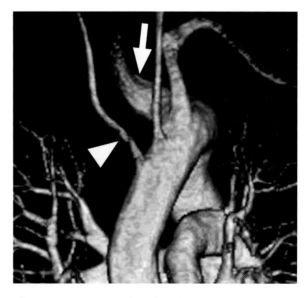

Fig. 9. Lusorian artery. The right subclavian artery arises separately from the descending aortic arch (*arrow*) distal to the left subclavian artery origin with the right common carotid artery branching directly from the aorta as the first vessel of the aortic arch (*arrowhead*)

Technique

The typical cervical MRA examination should encompass the top of the aortic arch, inferiorly, and the skull base, superiorly. The extracranial course of both carotid and both vertebral arteries should be included in this field-of-view (FOV). The radio frequency (RF) imaging coil should ensure adequate visualization of this large area of coverage while still maintaining a high signal-to-noise (SNR) ratio, which is required for proper visualization of vessel detail. Dedicated phased array neurovascular RF coils are available from a number of manufacturers and are the preferred imaging coil design for this purpose. These coils allow head/brain examinations that are comparable in quality to dedicated head coil MR imaging exams while, at the same time, also provide high SNR images of the neck and thoracic inlet, including the top of the aortic arch. These neurovascular RF coils allow extracranial MRA, intracranial MRA and brain MRI exams to be acquired during the same MR study without the need to move the patient or to change coils during the examination.

A number of different pulse sequences are available for cervical MRA imaging. Each has its own advantages and disadvantages. The 2D TOF technique using an inferior "walking" saturation pulse that moves with each serially acquired slice was originally devised and popularized by Keller, et al [6]. This technique has the advantage that it can encompass any length of coverage that is needed by merely prescribing an adequate number of slices. Axial 2D TOF acquisitions can provide fairly uniform vessel visualization throughout the neck since each 2D slice is acquired separately. The use of thin slices will minimize flow saturation effects if blood flow is brisk. The in-plane resolution on axial 2D TOF MRA is very good; but the longitudinal resolution is limited to about 1.5 – 2 mm due to the limitations imposed by the minimum slice thickness the MR scanner can generate together with the traditional practical consideration of imaging time. The disadvantages of this technique include a limited SNR due to the fact that each slice is acquired as a separate thin 2D acquisition rather than averaging the entire volume of slices in a 3D acquisition. This technique also has the disadvantage of overestimating the degree of stenosis when higher grade vessel narrowing and/or slow flow is present [7, 8]. In addition, 2D TOF technique is highly sensitive to even small amounts of patient motion that can lead to the so-called "stairstep" artifact due to misregistration of adjacent slices. This artifact can be seen even with small amounts of motion that may be produced through normal quiet breathing and certainly is heightened by swallowing (Fig. 10). An additional limitation of this

technique is the poor temporal resolution, which can take as long as 8-12 minutes to acquire the total number of slices needed, which usually number 80-100 slices of 1.5mm thickness. However, despite these limitations, this technique remains a viable alternative for cervical vessel MRA.

Another major technique is 3D TOF MRA. This can be acquired either as a single 3D volume of images or as a series of multiple overlapping 3D volumes, which can be combined to provide a single longitudinal segment of coverage. In either case, the major limitation of this technique is that it generally cannot be used to visualize the entire length of coverage needed for a complete evaluation of the cervical vasculature. Thus, this technique is most often used as a supplemental imaging technique to evaluate the common carotid artery bifurcations in more detail or to better estimate the degree of stenosis. Unlike 2D TOF, the 3D TOF technique is much more robust for accurately determining the degree of stenosis [7, 9, 10]. These targeted 3D TOF sequences also generally require less time to image compared with the 2D TOF MRA of the entire neck. They are also less affected by minor degrees of motion such as that caused by quiet breathing although they are significantly degraded by major degrees of motion such as swallowing or gross patient movement of the head and neck.

Contrast enhanced 3D MRA (CE 3D MRA) is the preferred method (Fig. 11) for total evaluation of the extracranial cervical vasculature [11-13]. This method utilizes a rapid T1-weighted fast 3D gradient echo pulse sequence. Imaging is typically performed in the coronal plane during the first pass of contrast following an intravenous bolus injection of a gadolinium-chelate contrast agent. Acquisition time for this sequence is generally between twenty and forty seconds and this rapid acquisition time results in far fewer motion artifacts when compared with either traditional 2D TOF or 3D TOF imaging sequences. These rapid imaging sequences are best acquired with elliptical centric k-space phase encoding that allows the low spatial frequency data (i.e. center of k-space) for each of the phase encoding axes to be acquired at the beginning of the pulse sequence so that maximal contrast weighting occurs early in the image acquisition. This results in both increased resistance to breathing artifacts and a good separation of arteries from veins even with acquisition times of forty seconds or longer [14].

Another emerging technique utilizes time-resolved imaging whereby only a portion of the k-space phase encoding steps are selectively repeated with each subsequent temporal phase. 3D TRICKS (Time-Resolved Imaging of Contrast Kinetics) is one such technique [15] and it utilizes the periodic refreshing of the high contrast (lower order)

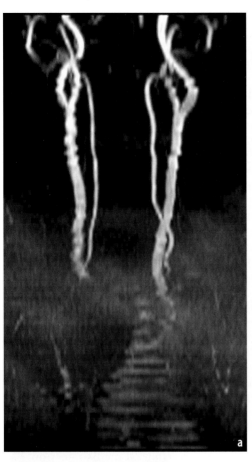

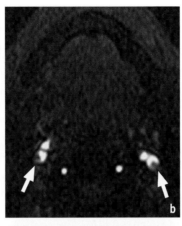

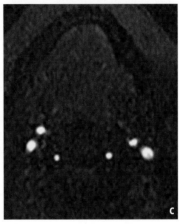

Fig. 10a-c. 2D TOF MRA of the neck in a normal individual. **a** The normal neck vessels are visualized from the level of the aortic arch to just below the skull base. Note the normal appearance of the common carotid artery bifurcations on both sides. The vertebral arteries are also well shown. Also note the marked "stairstep" artifacts present due to slight patient motion between individual axial source images. This artifact is most pronounced within the lower portion of the MRA at the level of the aortic arch and origin of the great vessels. Combination of normal pulsation motion and breathing motion causes severe stairsteping with resultant loss of signal and detail. **b** Axial source images at the level of the common carotid artery bifurcations show a flow artifact along the posterior wall of both internal carotid artery bulbs (*arrows*). This is due to signal loss from turbulence and high velocity flow. This type of artifact is accentuated with higher degrees of stenosis and can lead to overestimation of stenosis. **c** Axial source images a few millimeters above B now shows that the vessel outlines are well demonstrated in both internal and external carotid branches as well as in both vertebral arteries

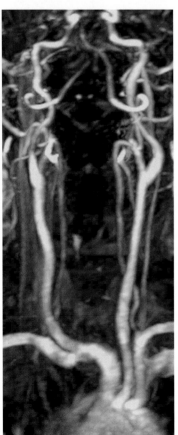

Fig. 11. CE MRA in a normal individual. Coronal CE MRA obtained during the first pass of a bolus of contrast material shows visualization of the neck vessels from the aortic arch to the skull base. There is good visualization of the great vessel origins as well as the carotid and vertebral arteries. This is the same patient as illustrated in Fig. 10. Note the greatly improved appearance of the aortic arch and great vessel origins. Note also the uniformly smooth vessel outlines without stairstep artifact. It is for this improved visualization that this is the preferred neck MRA technique

phase encoding steps interleaved with higher order phase steps that are combined for high spatial resolution images with high temporal resolution. Elements of this method include an increased sampling rate for centric k-space lines, temporal interpolation of k-space views, and zero filled interpolation in the slice-encoding dimension. By sharing vital k-space data, this technique results in the generation of multiple high resolution 3D data sets representing 4-9 second time points for dynamic visualization of arterial wash-in and venous wash-out of the contrast bolus.

In order to obtain high quality images with arterial-phase CE MRA the timing of the contrast bolus and the rate of injection is crucial [16]. The period of preferential carotid enhancement is typically brief (e.g. as short as 5 seconds). Imaging too late can result in significant jugular venous contamination of the images and poor carotid visualization. There are a number of options for contrast bolus timing with the start of the image acquisition that are available with different manufacturers and MR scanner models. The simplest technique and one that is very reliable is to deliver a small test injection of contrast (usually a 2 cc bolus) while serially imaging a fixed region of interest in the neck, generally the common carotid artery just below the bifurcation [17]. Using this method a time versus contrast enhancement curve is plotted that shows the time-of-arrival post injection of peak contrast enhancement. This time delay is then used to program the start of the CE MRA acquisition following the start of injection of the contrast bolus. Since the time delay following start of injection and the rate of contrast injection are both critical for obtaining good quality CE MRA that is reproducible across different subjects, an automated contrast injection using an MR compatible injector is essential.

An alternate method for triggering the start of the CE MRA sequence utilizes automated detection of contrast arrival [18]. This method generally involves placing a region-of-interest (ROI) over a vessel on the scout image in which signal intensity is sampled on rapid serially acquired measurements. Pre-determined thresholds are set for an amount of signal intensity change within this preselected monitoring ROI and when this threshold is detected the start of the CE MRA sequence is automatically triggered. While this method may seem useful and time efficient by allowing one to bypass the need to acquire and analyze a test bolus injection, in the cervical region at least, this method is has several pitfalls. The reasons for this are several fold and include improperly set thresholds, variations in the degree of contrast enhancement among different patients and, possibly most importantly, sporadic detection errors caused by partial volume effects due to the small size of the

neck vessels relative to the chosen ROI. If the ROI is too small, low SNR in the monitoring volume or slight patient motion may limit detection of small amounts of enhancement. On the other hand, if the sampling volume is too large, averaging of the vessel with surrounding non-enhancing tissues may also yield poor contrast material detection. In either case, the result may be unreliable detection of contrast bolus arrival. In our experience, automated triggering has proved too unreliable for cervical vessel MRA and we have discarded its use in favor of test injections.

More recently, MR fluoroscopic triggering has been used for carotid CE MRA [19]. This method uses serial rapidly acquired and instantaneously displayed low-resolution 2D images (i.e. MR fluoroscopy) of the area of interest to detect the time of arrival of the full contrast bolus. When the contrast bolus is visually detected on the serial images, the sequence is then triggered manually by the observer. This technique, although available only on newer MR scanners, is the most rapid and reliable technique.

As already indicated, an automated MR-compatible contrast injector is a very important piece of equipment if one is to obtain optimized and reproducible carotid CE MRA. Timing of the injection relative to triggering of the start of the CE MRA sequence is important, as is an accurate and reproducible rate of contrast media injection. The optimal rate of contrast media injection has been shown to be approximately 2 mL per second [16]. If the contrast bolus is injected too rapidly it can result in signal loss from T2* effects and an increased blurring of vessel outlines due to the short bolus duration of gadolinium which does not cover a large segment of k-space when injected too rapidly [16]. These artifacts are generally seen at contrast injection rates in excess of 4 mL per second. In addition high injection rates may result in a retrograde filling of the jugular vein, which than causes venous overlay on arterial phase images with poor carotid visualization.

The total dose of contrast used for neck MRA is a full 20 mL vial of Gd-chelate contrast agent (minus the 2 mL used for a test injection if needed). Injection of this 18-20 mL bolus of contrast material is followed immediately by a 20 mL bolus of normal saline injected at the same rate (2 mL/sec) in order to flush the contrast agent rapidly through the arm veins and superior vena cava. This helps to ensure that the full dose of contrast reaches the cervical vessels in a uniform bolus.

Mistiming of a contrast bolus can result in poor MRA images. If the imaging starts too early relative to bolus arrival then there is poor vessel contrast since the high contrast-weighted phase encodings are acquired early in the elliptical centric ordered image acquisition. On the other hand, if

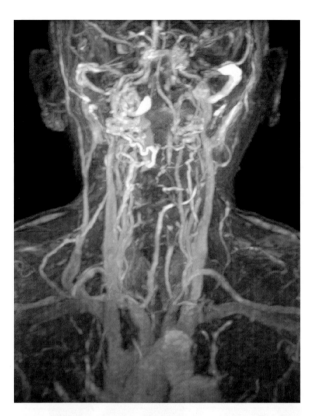

the image acquisition is delayed relative to arrival of a contrast bolus in the neck vessels, this will result in overlap between arteries and veins making diagnostic interpretation of the CE MRA difficult and less sensitive (Fig. 12).

Post processing of the images is done following acquisition of the MRA. This is done whether the sequences are acquired as 2D TOF, 3D TOF or CE MRA. Maximum intensity projection (MIP) images are obtained of the entire volume of images. These can generally be performed automatically by the MR scanner as part of its standard image post-processing , whereby a series of longitudinal radial projections of the neck vessels are projected from multiple different angles of rotation around the neck (Fig. 13a-c). In addition, we also generally acquire targeted MIP images where the ipsilateral carotid and vertebral arteries are isolated from

Fig. 12. CE MRA demonstrates overlap between arterial and venous phases. The acquisition was mistimed and started a few seconds after arrival of the contrast bolus. There is simultaneous visualization of both arteries and veins filled with contrast. This results in obscuring of arterial vessel details and greatly interferes with diagnostic interpretation

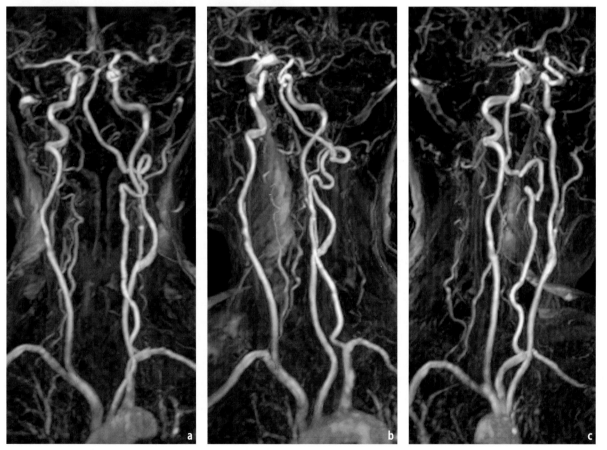

Fig. 13a-c. Normal contrast enhanced 3D MRA. **a-c** Direct coronal view of the first pass 3D MRA acquired with elliptical centric phase encoding technique. Note good visualization of all of the major vessels as well as many smaller vessels within the neck. Also note good separation of arteries and veins, the latter not being visible. **b** and **c** The 3D MRA can be rotated in different projections as illustrated

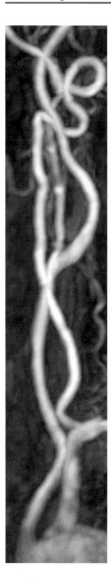

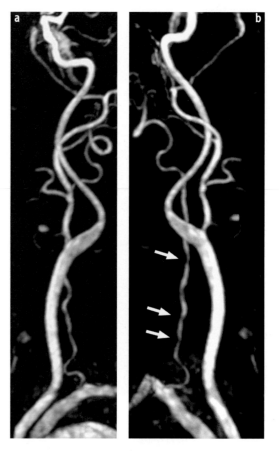

Fig. 14. CE 3D MRA can also be edited such that only selected portions of the vessel system are displayed using a targeted MIP algorithm. Note here that this view shows only the left carotid and left vertebral arteries while other vessels have been selectively removed in order to improve visualization without overlap and interference from other vessels

Fig. 15a, b. Edited MIP projection of the left carotid and left vertebral arteries obtained from a CE MRA. Two representative projections illustrate good demonstration of the left common carotid artery bifurcation, which is normal in appearance as well as a small left vertebral artery. Note irregular narrowing at several points in the left vertebral artery caused by extrinsic compression from vertebral osteophytes. Also note good demonstration of the origin of the left vertebral artery using the edited MIP technique. **a** Vessels demonstrated in LAO projection. **b** Vessels demonstrated in RAO projection

the contralateral vessels using a targeted region of interest (Fig. 14). By selecting or editing the region of interest the MIP algorithm is not only restricted to the vessels of one side of the neck but also much of the anatomical structures and high signal intensity subcutaneous fat is excluded as well. These edited MIP images (also called sub-volume MIPs) of isolated vessels render a much higher quality MRA image that is unencumbered by overlapping vessels from the opposite side or by artifacts caused by high intensity background structures such as bone marrow fat or subcutaneous fat (Fig. 15a, b). The latter may result in additional noise on the full FOV MIP images. The targeted MIP images can be done either on the MR scanner operator console or using an offline independent computer workstation where generally there are additional tools that allow one to color the vessels and to introduce 3D shading to provide an improved visual impression of vessel anatomy.

The MIP images provide angiographic-like views that readily display anatomical configuration and location, and are thus easy to interpret. However, it is also imperative to review the individual source images that make up the entire MRA volume. This is important since the maximum intensity projection algorithm sets arbitrary thresholds for including or rejecting pixels. Thus, some areas of shading that actually represent the vessel lumen may be excluded on the MIP projection while other high signal intensity non-vascular structures (i.e. fat, hemorrhage, etc.) may be projected onto the vessel outline and appear as part of the vessel. In either case, this can result in misdiagnosis. These potential pitfalls can be avoided and the true vessel lumen better appreciated when visualizing the actual cross sectional source images. This is especially critical when evaluating the 2D TOF and 3D TOF images. It appears to be less crucial, although still important and advisable, when evaluating the CE MRA images. The latter is less critical probably due to the fact that the source images for the CE MRA are acquired in coronal projection, parallel to the vessel of interest rather than presenting cross sectional pictures of the vessel of interest.

Clinical Examples

Atherosclerosis

The most common indication for cervical MRA is for evaluation of atherosclerotic disease of the extracranial cerebral vasculature. Cerebrovascular insufficiency, whether symptomatic or asymptomatic, is generally diagnosed and its severity expressed as the degree of (percent) stenosis within the proximal internal carotid artery at the carotid bifurcation. This is the most common site of stenotic atherosclerotic plaque formation although it should be noted that plaque formation and stenosis can occur anywhere along the extracranial cerebral circulation between the common carotid origin from the aortic arch and the distal internal carotid artery at the skull base. In addition, significant intracranial internal carotid stenosis secondary to atherosclerotic plaque formation occurs less commonly but these will be discussed in the intracranial MRA section.

MRA is a non-invasive alternative technique to invasive diagnostic catheter angiography. Catheter angiography has a long history of utilization for diagnosis of vascular pathology and has an established track record of high accuracy for the diagnosis of vessel stenosis. Thus, in evaluating MRA, catheter angiography provides the reference gold standard against which MRA is generally compared. It should be noted, however, that since catheter angiography is an invasive procedure there are measurable risks and complications associated with it. Clinical series have shown that reversible complications occur in 1 – 14% of catheter angiograms and that significant and often irreversible complications with severe morbidity or mortality occur in between 0.5 and 1% of cases [20, 21]. This should be kept in mind when comparing efficacy of catheter angiography with non-invasive techniques such as MRA and CT angiography (CTA). Although there may be slight differences or discrepancies in diagnosis between invasive versus noninvasive vascular imaging, minor decreases in sensitivity, specificity or accuracy may be tolerated in the case of noninvasive vessel imaging if the number and types of misdiagnoses potentially cause less harm than the number of patients who would have been significantly injured due to the known complication rate of invasive catheter angiography [22].

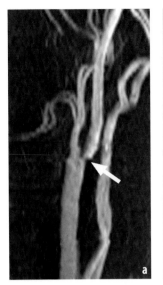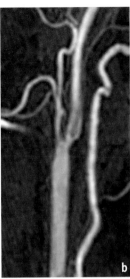

Fig. 16a, b. Overestimation of stenosis on 2D MRA. **a** 2D TOF MRA of the carotid bifurcation shows what appears to be severe narrowing at the origin of the internal carotid artery (*arrow*). **b** CE MRA of the same patient obtained in approximately the same projection now shows only moderate narrowing (measuring less than 50% in degree of stenosis) of the internal carotid artery origin. Both images are viewed from the projection that shows maximum degree of narrowing

There have been a large number of studies comparing sensitivity and specificity of MRA with that of catheter angiography. Variations in results can be attributed to differences in the type of MRA technique used for carotid imaging. In the case of 2D TOF the major discrepancy is that of overestimation of vessel stenosis (Fig. 16a, b). This overestimation in stenosis becomes more significant with increasing levels of stenosis [8]. With increased stenosis that approaches, but does not reach, the critical stenosis level of 70% determined by the NASCET study to be the threshold for treatment of patients with surgical endarterectomy, there is an increasing possibility of miscategorizing the lesion. Miscategorizing a lesion due to overestimation could result in a patient undergoing invasive endarterectomy when in actuality the degree of stenosis was somewhat less than 70% if evaluated by catheter angiography. Another potential pitfall would involve patients with severe high-grade stenosis that result in a flow void on the MRA that is misdiagnosed as total vessel occlusion when in reality the vessel is patent [23, 24]. Despite this limitation, however, a number of studies have shown that when a flow void at the carotid bifurcation was present on 2D TOF MRA this generally was associated with a stenosis of 70 % or greater, thus indicating the potential need for carotid endarterectomy. Furthermore, with careful evaluation of the MRA with multiple different projections, in nearly all cases, the patency of the distal internal carotid artery could be established by identification of flow within the ICA beyond the flow void.-

Evaluation of carotid stenosis using 3D TOF MRA technique shows better correlation with catheter angiography [25]. Thus, several studies have shown that the sensitivity and specificity for quantification of stenosis with 3D TOF is in the range of 90% or better when compared with carotid catheter angiography [26, 27]. This prompted recommendation for utilizing both techniques for complete neck MRA evaluation. The 2D TOF MRA is utilized for full neck coverage of the vascular anatomy and the 3D TOF MRA yields a limited FOV or a "targeted" evaluation of the carotid artery bifurcation that also provides a more accurate determination of the percent carotid stenosis.

Contrast enhanced MRA is now the most commonly utilized technique for cervical vessel evaluation due to its speed, its high detail of the neck vasculature combined with relatively lower incidence of artifacts such as from minor patient motion. The contrast enhanced technique also shows good visualization of carotid stenosis that does not appear to have the problem with a flow void at relatively high degrees of stenosis that is associated with the 2D TOF technique. Nevertheless, a recent report by Townsend et al. comparing CE MRA with 3D TOF MRA suggests that contrast enhanced MRA overestimates the degree of stenosis in approximately 40% of cases compared with 3D TOF MRA [28]. They noted, however, that the degree of overestimation was greatest in vessels with less than 70% stenosis and was less critical in vessels with greater than 70% stenosis (in contrast to the experience documented with 2D TOF). Based on this, the authors recommended using 3D TOF MRA as a supplement to CE MRA to most accurately determine the degree of carotid stenosis. It should be noted, however, that they did not have catheter angiography correlation in the cases they reported. A number of other authors have noted a high degree of correlation between determination of degree of stenosis with contrast enhanced MRA versus DSA [29-34]. There may be several reasons for this discrepancy in results. The first is that Townsend compared contrast enhanced MRA with 3D TOF MRA and had no direct correlation with DSA. They did employ phantom study measurements but this may also be limited by the fact that it is not truly physiologic. Since neither 3D MRA or CE MRA is 100% percent accurate, inherent discrepancies in each of these two techniques might, in combination, overestimate projected inaccuracy of CE MRA relative to the "gold standard" of carotid angiography. Secondly, there are a number of variables in CE MRA technique used among the various studies including the type of MR scanner

used, the specific pulse sequence, the timing of the contrast bolus and the rate of injection that might also alter results of these comparisons. Finally, it has been shown that, in addition to looking at the discrepancies between cross sectional stenosis, it is also important to realize that stenosis grading with catheter angiography is based on two or three different projections while MRA utilizes multiple different projections together with cross sectional views of the vessel to determine maximum stenosis. Neidercorn et al. demonstrated that when similar projections were compared between catheter angiography and 3D TOF MRA the correlation was much better than when minimum stenosis alone was graded which tended to show an overestimation of stenosis on the MRA that averaged about 7.5 percent compared with DSA [35].

Doppler ultrasound has for many years been a major diagnostic technique for evaluation of carotid stenosis. The technique is noninvasive, rapid and relatively low cost and is reasonably sensitive and accurate in the evaluation of the degree of carotid bifurcation stenosis. It has several limitations, however. The technique does not provide anatomical detail of the vessels within the neck. It has a limited area of coverage and thus cannot see tandem lesions or even isolated lesions within the distal internal carotid artery near the skull base. Thus, while doppler ultrasound is valuable in screening patients with carotid vessel disease, its limitations require complementary studies to provide information in instances where doppler ultrasound has major limitations. Early in the 1990's it was recognized that MRA provided good complementary information that increased the diagnostic accuracy of noninvasive carotid vascular evaluation. Anderson et al. have shown that this combination misses very little significant disease and provides a good noninvasive technique for screening as well as for surgical decision making [36]. Improvements in MRA, especially with evolution of modern contrast enhanced MRA, have further strengthened the robustness of this approach. The degree of stenosis is well evaluated with doppler ultrasound as well as with contrast enhanced MRA [37] (Fig. 17a, b). In addition, recent papers have shown that the use of contrast enhanced MRA not only provides detection of tandem vascular lesions proximal or distal to the carotid bifurcation but also improves the diagnostic confidence level in interpretation of the degree of stenosis and the presence of high grade stenosis versus total carotid occlusion at the carotid bifurcation [38].

In addition to carotid artery atherosclerotic disease, CE MRA is also well suited to evaluate vertebral artery disease (Fig. 18a, b). Segmented stenosis within a vertebral artery is easily demonstrated and diagnosed. However, because vertebral arteries in the neck may be asymmetric in size as

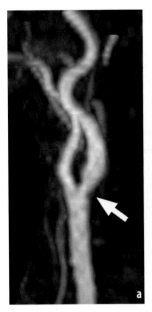
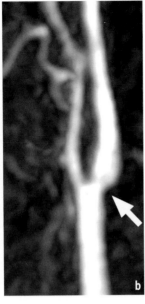

Fig. 17a, b. MRA is very sensitive for showing mild degrees of stenosis at the common carotid artery bifurcation using different techniques. **a** 2D TOF MRA of carotid bifurcation shows mild narrowing at origin of internal carotid artery (*arrow*). **b** CE MRA of carotid bifurcation in a different patient shows a similar mild degree of stenosis at the internal carotid artery origin (*arrow*). Note that in both of these cases the degree of stenosis is compared with the distal ICA according to the NASCET method

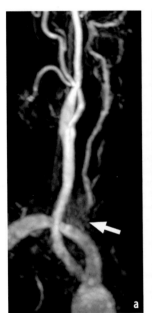
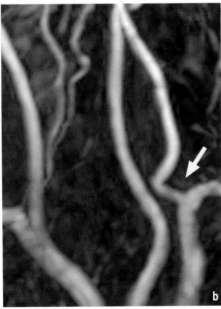

Fig. 18a, b. Right vertebral artery origin stenosis. **a** Severe stenosis of the RVA is demonstrated in this rotated MIP view of CE MRA. Note the presence of a pseudo occlusion (*arrow*) due to high velocity-related signal loss through the stenotic RVA. **b** Another rotational view from the same MRA shows normal origin of LVA (*arrow*)

already discussed, it is important to distinguish a hypoplastic vertebral artery that represents a normal variant from a small vertebral artery secondary to proximal stenosis and reduced flow. This is readily distinguished by observation of the proximal vertebral arteries and the vertebral artery origins. In the case of a diseased vertebral artery with reduced flow there will be a change in caliber at the level of stenosis while the primary hypoplastic variant will demonstrate uniform small lumen size that extends to the vertebral artery origin.

Tandem lesions of the carotid vasculature in the proximal common carotid artery or the distal internal carotid artery are well shown on the contrast enhanced MRA. The presence of intraluminal clot, which is generally considered to be an indication for urgent surgical intervention is also demonstrated using MRA techniques (Fig. 19a-c). Ulceration of the carotid vessels can be shown in many cases with MRA. (Fig. 20a-d) However, catheter angiography as well as high resolution MR imaging have both been shown to provide better information about carotid plaque rupture and ulceration [39].

High-resolution carotid plaque imaging in particular is currently an investigational technique

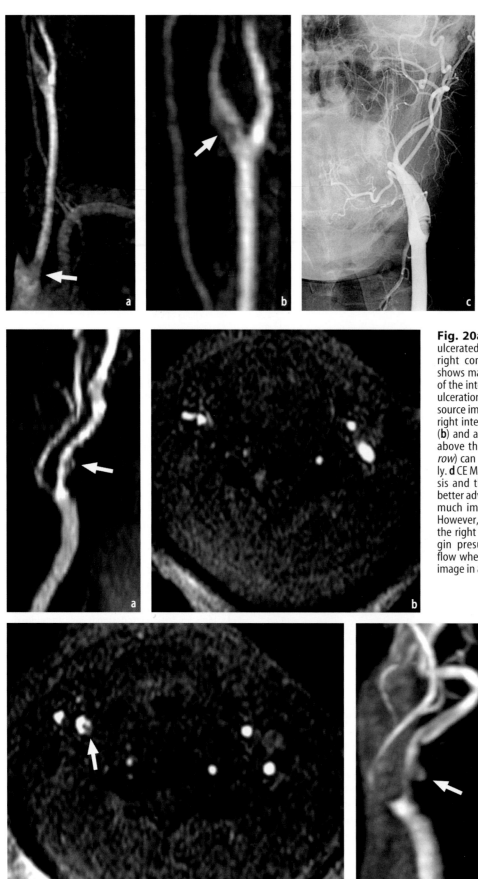

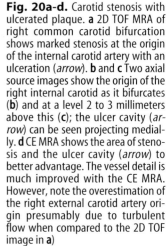

Fig. 19a-c. Intraluminal thrombus in left internal carotid artery bulb. **a** Edited MIP image of the left carotid artery from a CE MRA shows filling defect in the left carotid bulb. Note also the bovine origin of the left common carotid artery (*arrow*).
b Close up view and slightly different projection confirms the intraluminal filling defect (*arrow*).
c Catheter carotid angiogram confirms the presence of intraluminal thrombus, which was subsequently removed surgically

Fig. 20a-d. Carotid stenosis with ulcerated plaque. **a** 2D TOF MRA of right common carotid bifurcation shows marked stenosis at the origin of the internal carotid artery with an ulceration (*arrow*). **b** and **c** Two axial source images show the origin of the right internal carotid as it bifurcates (**b**) and at a level 2 to 3 millimeters above this (**c**); the ulcer cavity (*arrow*) can be seen projecting medially. **d** CE MRA shows the area of stenosis and the ulcer cavity (*arrow*) to better advantage. The vessel detail is much improved with the CE MRA. However, note the overestimation of the right external carotid artery origin presumably due to turbulent flow when compared to the 2D TOF image in **a**)

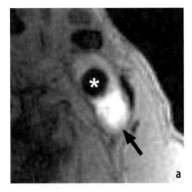

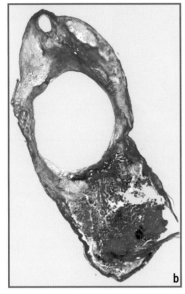

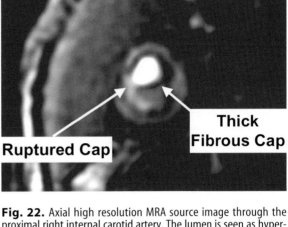

Fig. 22. Axial high resolution MRA source image through the proximal right internal carotid artery. The lumen is seen as hyperintense signal surrounded by a thick, complex atherosclerotic plaque. The dark band surrounding the carotid lumen represents a thick fibrous cap. The lateral portion of the fibrous cap line is absent indicating rupture of the fibrous cap [Case courtesy of Chun Yuan, Ph.D. and Thomas Hatsukami, M.D.]

Fig. 21a, b. a T1-weighted high-resolution axial image obtained just below CCA bifurcation shows flow void in carotid lumen (*asterisk*) together with bright signal from an intraplaque hemorrhage (*arrow*). Intraplaque hemorrhage is best shown on T1 weighted images when intraluminal flow signal is suppressed. **b** Histologic section of endarterectomy specimen of same patient sectioned at same level and orientation as in (**a**) confirms intraplaque hemorrhage (Mallory's Trichrome stain) [Case courtesy of Chun Yuan, Ph.D. and Thomas Hatsukami, M.D.]

being assessed to help better define the vulnerable carotid plaque in comparison to the presumed stable atherosclerotic plaque. Using these techniques high resolution MRI has been shown to reveal intra plaque hemorrhage (Fig. 21a, b) and fibrous cap rupture (Fig. 22) in patients with complex atherosclerotic plaque disease [40]. Detection of intraplaque hemorrhage is a very important finding since it likely distinguishes the biologically active, fragile plaque that is more likely to lead to stroke

from a more stable lesion [41]. Identification of fibrous cap rupture with MRI is another finding associated with an unstable plaque and it has been shown to be highly associated with recent transient ischemic attack or stroke [39]. In the future these techniques may become a major tool in the diagnosis and surgical decision making for evaluating patients with atherosclerotic cerebrovascular disease.

Arterial Dissection

Arterial dissection involves intimal disruption or tearing of the intima with subsequent dissection of blood into the arterial vessel wall. This intramural hemorrhage may result in luminal narrowing or total occlusion of the vessel lumen [42]. Vessel dissection can be divided into two major categories. The first is traumatic in origin usually following blunt injury to the head and neck or injury from chiropractic manipulation. The second major category is that of spontaneous vessel dissection and occurs without predisposing trauma. In the second type of dissection there is usually underlying disease involving the vessel wall that predisposes these patients to dissection. Such predisposing factors include hypertension, fibromuscular dysplasia, genetic diseases such as Marfan syndrome with cystic medial necrosis (Fig. 23), Ehlers Danlos syndrome, alpha-1 anti-trypsin deficiency, or other etiologies including drug abuse with sympathomimetics and infection [2, 43, 44]. Dissection of the carotid or vertebral arteries has a high association with ischemic injuries of the brain either due to vessel occlusion at the dissection site or to embolization. Early recognition of a vessel dissection is important to initiate treatment, often directed to the use anticoagulants or antiplatelet therapy in an attempt to prevent or minimize cerebral ischemic complications [43]. In some cases, invasive treatment may be indicated with either trapping of the dissected segment of the vessel (therapeutic occlusion of the vessel proximal and distal to the level of dissection) or with stenting of the dissected vessel segment to prevent severe luminal stenosis or occlusion. Posttraumatic dissection may not be amenable to anticoagulant therapy if there are accompanying brain contusions or systemic injuries that may result in hemorrhage.

Traumatic carotid dissection most often occurs at the level of C1 – C2 just inferior to the skull base. It is due to a hyperextension and rotation injury that leads to shearing injury of the vessel wall as it is pulled across and stretched over the interior arch of C1. This type of injury is often associated with mandibular fractures (Fig. 24a-c).

Spontaneous carotid artery dissection often is accompanied by a Horners syndrome with ipsilateral ptosis and miosis. Dissection of the carotid or vertebral arteries is often accompanied by neck pain and ipsilateral headache. Chiropractic manipulation more often results in vertebral artery dissection and is less commonly responsible for carotid artery dissection [45].

The diagnosis of vessel dissection is best made with the combination of MRI and MRA. The MRA findings include vessel lumen narrowing that usually occurs over a relatively long segment compared with atherosclerotic disease. The vessel wall

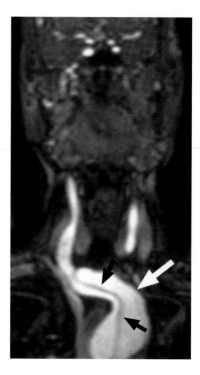

Fig. 23. Dissection of the aortic arch with extension into the right innominate artery in a patient with Marfan's Syndrome. Note the prominent dilatation of the innominate artery (white arrow) and the intimal flap that extends from the aorta into the innominate artery (*black arrows*)

is thickened due to the presence of intramural hematoma and in some cases aneurysmal dilatation due to false aneurysm formation in the area of dissection may be seen rather than luminal narrowing. The MRI findings are generally best shown on T1-weighted images with fat saturation. In the case of acute dissection, intramural hematoma can be seen as high intensity (Fig. 24c) or intermediate signal intensity (Fig. 25) depending on the age of the hematoma within the vessel wall. This finding is highly specific for vessel dissection [46, 47].

MRI and MRA have been shown to be more sensitive for carotid vessel dissection then for vertebral artery dissection (Fig. 26a-c). The sensitivity for carotid artery dissection using a combination of MRI and MRA [43, 48-50] is very high and comparable with carotid catheter angiography. The sensitivity for detection of vertebral artery dissection has been variable with most reports indicating that it is significantly less sensitive compared with catheter vertebral angiography missing up to 30% of vertebral artery dissections. On the other hand, the specificity of MRI/MRA combination in carotid or vertebral artery dissection was higher when compared with catheter angiography [43]. Thus, although less sensitive MRA is very specific for vertebral artery dissection compared with angiography [48].

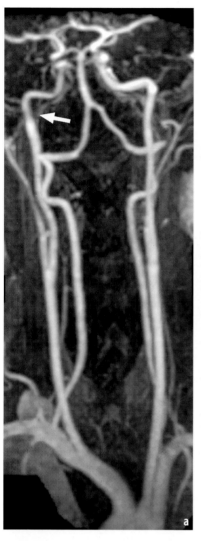

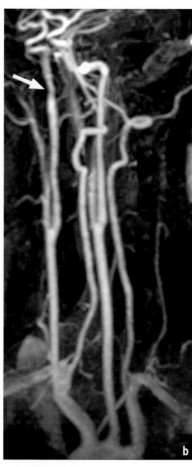

Fig. 24a-c. Acute traumatic dissection of the right internal carotid artery suffered in an automobile accident. **a** Coronal CE MRA shows good filling of all of the neck vessels. Note that there is a subtle, abrupt change in caliber of the distal right internal carotid artery just before it enters the skull base (*arrow*). **b** Rotation of the MRA in a different plane confirms the caliber change (*arrow*). **c** Axial T1-weighted fat saturated image just below the skull base shows hyperintense signal within the wall of the right internal carotid artery indicating intramural hemorrhage from the traumatic dissection (*arrow*). The change in vessel caliber, while highly suggestive of an acute dissection in the appropriate clinical setting, is a non-specific imaging finding. However, the presence of intramural hemorrhage in the wall of the vessel is highly specific for vessel dissection. It is the presence of the intramural hemorrhage that makes MRA more specific than catheter angiography for the diagnosis of vessel dissection

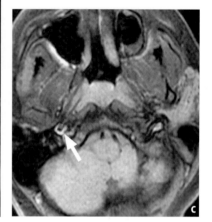

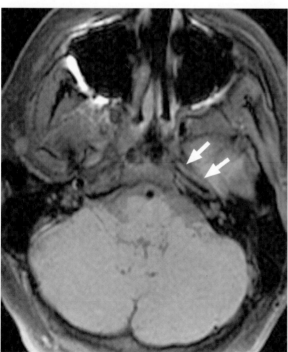

Fig. 25. Axial T1-weighted fat saturated image in a patient with an acute left internal carotid artery dissection that extends into the intrapetrous portion of the internal carotid artery. Note that the wall of the carotid artery is thickened (arrows) but is not hyperintense since this is a very acute carotid dissection that is less than six hours old. It generally takes 24 to 36 hours for the intramural hemorrhage to appear hyperintense on the T1-weighted MR images. Note also the importance of fat saturation so that the thickened wall is visualized without interference from hyperintense perivascular fat

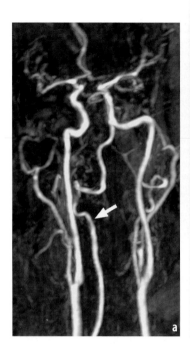
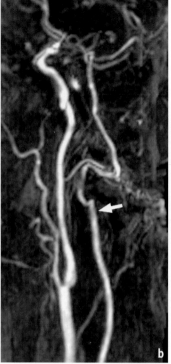
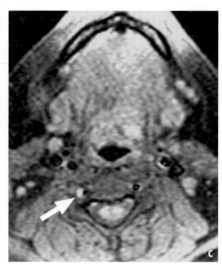

Fig. 26a-c. Right vertebral artery dissection post-chiropractic manipulation. **a** Oblique view of the CE MRA shows only very subtle, minimal narrowing of the right vertebral artery (arrow) beginning just below its turn around the C2 level. **b** Edited view of the right carotid and right vertebral arteries again shows minimal narrowing (*arrow*) which is non-specific and not definite for dissection. **c** Axial T1-weighted fat saturated image at the level of C3 shows hyperintense intramural hematoma partially surrounding the wall of the right vertebral artery (*arrow*). Note that the underlying vessel lumen is not significantly compromised by the dissection, which accounts for the near normal appearance on the MRA

The recommended protocol for diagnosis and detection of suspected cervical neck vessel dissection is axial T1-weighted spin echo images with fat saturation and an inferior saturation pulse to suppress flow through the neck to demonstrate the presence of intramural hemorrhage in combination with contrast enhanced 3D MRA. The fat saturated T1-weighted anatomic images should be obtained prior to the contrast enhanced MRA since the presence of circulating gadolinium may cause perivascular enhancement, which can be confused with intramural hemorrhage.

MRI and MRA are also indicated for follow-up evaluation of patients with known cervical vessel dissection. This is valuable to detect possible pro-

gression of stenosis or occlusion of the dissected vessel. Such progression of disease may indicate the need for invasive therapy such as surgery or stenting to prevent ischemic cerebral complications. In addition, evaluation of response to therapy, which usually consists of anticoagulant, and/or antiplatelet therapy is needed. Signs of possible healing with resolution of intramural hemorrhage and return of the vessel lumen to normal or near normal caliber following treatment will help to determine the end point of anticoagulant therapy [5, 42]. Thus, it is recommended to follow the patient at periodic intervals until complete vessel wall healing is determined.

Head and Neck Tumor Evaluation

Head and neck tumors adjacent to major cervical vessels can be evaluated with MRA. (Fig. 27a-c) The relationship of the mass to the neck vessels and the presence of vessel displacement and/or vessel narrowing can be seen. Assessment is usually directed at determining the presence or absence of vessel wall involvement with tumor prior to attempting surgical resection. Signs of vessel wall involvement with tumor include loss of the normal wall outline and loss of the normal perivascular fat plane that defines the outer border vessel wall. Also narrowing and irregularity of the vessel lumen adjacent to the tumor is another indication of vessel wall involvement. Vascular encasement or vascular wall invasion will usually indicate non-operability of a tumor [3, 51]. In one noteworthy series,

by Yousem, et al, it was determined that involvement of the vessel wall encompassing 270 degrees or more of the vessel circumference was a good indicator of inoperability [52]. Using this criteria the sensitivity of MR imaging for determination of unresectable neck tumor was 100% and specificity was 88%. MRA has proven less useful in determining vascularity of head and neck tumor or for detecting the presence of vascular neoplasms such as paragangliomas compared with contrast-enhanced MRI.

Benign tumors and associated complications can be evaluated by CE MRA. For example, angiomatoid tumors of the head and neck area can be frequently found in children and are easily diagnosed and followed-up with MRA. Moreover, complications such as AV-shunts can be diagnosed and interventional treatment planned (Fig. 28a, b).

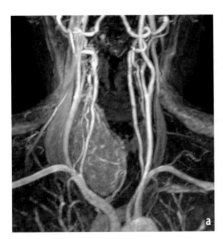
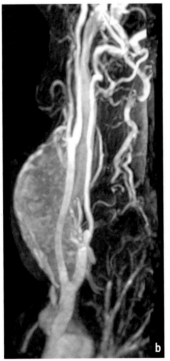
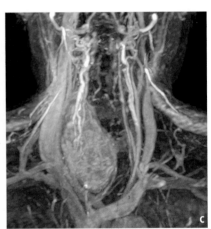

Fig. 27a-c. Time-resolved CE MRA for evaluation of a thyroid tumor at the base of the right neck and extending into the upper mediastinum.
a Coronal view of the arterial phase of the CE MRA shows the mass displacing the proximal portion of the right common carotid artery. The vessels are not narrowed by the mass and the other vessels within the neck appear normal.
b Rotated view of the CE MRA shows that the mass projects anteriorly. Note the degree of hypervascularity with vessels defined along the surface of the tumor as well as small vessels within the tumor.
c Venous phase of the time-resolved MRA shows displacement of the right internal jugular vein but, again, there is no evidence for invasion or narrowing of this vessel. The hypervascular nature of the tumor is again noted

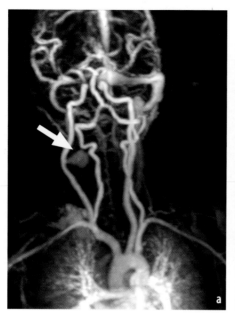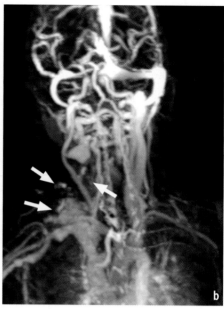

Fig. 28a, b. 12-year old boy with history of a large hemangioma of the right neck extending into the mediastinum. Post surgery and laser therapy a pulsating mass rapidly increasing in size, was observed. **a** Early arterial phase MRA shows aneurysm of the common carotid artery (arrow). Note that some early enhancement of residual hemangioma in the area of the right subclavian artery can also be visualized. **b** In a second acquisition the aneurysm is clearly shown not to connect to the angioma. Note the enhancing residual parts (arrows) of the angioma. Based on MR findings, coiling of the aneurysm was performed leading to its complete occlusion [Image courtesy of Dr. G. Schneider]

Post-Treatment Surveillance

MRA is often used to evaluate patients following treatment for vascular disease. Again, the major area of evaluation is in patients with carotid atherosclerotic disease. Determination of possible restenosis after carotid endarterectomy is an indication for cervical carotid MRA. Techniques for this type of study are identical with those for preoperative carotid vascular evaluation. Images can detect and quantify restenosis and help determine the need for further interventional therapy.

Although still largely investigational, endovascular treatment of carotid stenosis is becoming more accepted in recent years. A number of patients have received treatment with carotid angioplasty without stenting. Evaluation of these patients is also similar to that of patients following carotid endarterectomy. Patients with prior carotid stent placement, however, present added problems. Safety considerations due to possible magnetic attraction of the intravascular stent must be considered. Most stents are not attracted in a magnetic field and therefore are generally safe to image. To be absolutely certain, since most often one is not aware of the exact stent type used, we generally limit MR imaging of post-stented patients for any reason to imaging only after the stent has been in place for a minimum of six weeks. This is to ensure that there is adequate scarring and endotheliazation around the stent, which will help stabilize the

device should there be any magnetic field attraction. In terms of evaluation for possible restenosis, local artifacts due to magnetic susceptibility from the metallic stent material may interfere to varying degrees with evaluation of the vessel lumen. In the case of significant artifact, evaluation for restenosis with MRA is impossible. CTA may then be a better alternative although this too may have difficulty due to interference with the CT visualization of the vessel lumen inside the stent. In these cases, catheter angiography may be the only viable alternative for evaluating vessel lumen status.

Role of MRA vs. CTA

There is considerable overlap in the indications and the utility of MRA versus CTA. Either technique can be utilized for diagnosis and evaluation of atherosclerotic carotid vascular disease, vertebral artery stenosis, posttraumatic and spontaneous vessel dissection and preoperative evaluation for carotid vessel involvement with head and neck tumors.

CTA may be useful in evaluating degree of lumen stenosis similar to that with contrast enhanced MRA. However, when dense calcium deposits are present within an atherosclerotic plaque at the carotid bifurcation this may limit accurate quantitation of vessel lumen stenosis using CTA. For these cases, contrast enhanced MRA may be superior to CTA.

Posttraumatic vessel injury or vessel dissection can also be evaluated with either CTA or MRA. MRA has the advantage of being more specific for traumatic vessel dissection since it detects the presence of intramural hematoma. In the acute situation, however, CTA is more rapidly available in many emergency departments. CTA provides good SNR images of the neck and provides very rapid imaging of the cervical vessels with modern multi-row detector array CT scanners. In addition, there are not the critical safety concerns with CTA. Since many trauma patients may be unable to give a proper history, MR safety considerations may preclude use of MRA in the acute situation.

Future Perspectives

Future advances in MR technology will further improve the accuracy, speed and utility of MRA. Already we are seeing improvements with 3T MR scanners compared with 1.5T MR systems. The 3T MR systems provide higher SNR, which can be used to either shorten the examination time or to increase the potential resolution of the images obtained.

The application of parallel imaging techniques combined with better RF coils and higher SNR with 3T MR scanners promise to shorten the imaging time of the MRA examination. This will result in less chance for degradation of the images due to patient motion. Parallel imaging techniques combined with partial k-space imaging sequences such as TRICKS may also allow acquisition of more rapid dynamic serial imaging studies that can potentially allow physiologic or flow information analogous to that obtained with serial images obtained with catheter angiography studies.

No doubt newer pulse sequences and unique approaches to MRA that have not yet been conceived will be forthcoming. One must remember that clinical use of MR imaging technology has only about a 20-year clinical history. MRA has an even shorter duration of experience. It is probable that MRA, perhaps in conjunction with CTA, will one day replace all of diagnostic catheter angiography. Invasive catheter manipulations will then be reserved only for patients who are candidates for endovascular treatment procedures.

References

1. National Institute of Neurological Disorders and Stroke and Trauma Division. North American Symptomatic Carotid Endarterectomy Trial (NASCET) investigators (1991) Clinical alert: benefit of carotid endarterectomy for patients with high-grade stenosis of the internal carotid artery. Stroke. 22(6):816-87
2. Klufas RA et al (1995) Dissection of the carotid and vertebral arteries: imaging with MR angiography. AJR Am J Roentgenol 164(3):673-67
3. Endres D, Simonson T, Funk G et al (1995) The role of magnetic resonance angiography in head and neck surgery. Laryngoscope 105(10):1069-1076
4. Pisaneschi MJ, Samii M (1995) Applications of MR angiography in head and neck pathology. Otolaryngol Clin North Am. 28(3):543-561
5. Jacobs A et al (1997) MRI- and MRA-guided therapy of carotid and vertebral artery dissections. J Neurol Sci 147(1):27-34
6. Keller PJ et al (1989) MR angiography with two-dimensional acquisition and three-dimensional display. Work in progress. Radiology 173(2):527-532
7. Patel SG et al (2002) Outcome, observer reliability, and patient preferences if CTA, MRA, or Doppler ultrasound were used, individually or together, instead of digital subtraction angiography before carotid endarterectomy. J Neurol Neurosurg Psychiatry 73(1):21-28
8. Riles TS et al (1992) Comparison of magnetic resonance angiography, conventional angiography, and duplex scanning. Stroke 23(3):341-346
9. De Marco JK et al (1994) Prospective evaluation of extracranial carotid stenosis: MR angiography with maximum-intensity projections and multiplanar reformation compared with conventional angiography. AJR Am J Roentgenol 163(5):1205-1212
10. Binaghi S et al (2001) Three-dimensional computed tomography angiography and magnetic resonance angiography of carotid bifurcation stenosis. Eur Neurol 46(1):25-34
11. Morasch MD et al (2002) Cross-sectional magnetic resonance angiography is accurate in predicting degree of carotid stenosis. Ann Vasc Surg 16(3):266-272
12. Sundgren PC et al (2002) Carotid artery stenosis: contrast-enhanced MR angiography with two different scan times compared with digital subtraction angiography. Neuroradiology 44(7):592-599
13. Wutke R et al (2002) High-resolution, contrast-enhanced magnetic resonance angiography with elliptical centric k-space ordering of supra-aortic arteries compared with selective X-ray angiography. Stroke 33(6):1522-1529
14. Wilman AH, Riederer SJ (1997) Performance of an elliptical centric view order for signal enhancement and motion artifact suppression in breath-hold three-dimensional gradient echo imaging. Magn Reson Med 38(5):793-802
15. Korosec FR et al (1996) Time-resolved contrast-enhanced 3D MR angiography. Magn Reson Med 36(3):345-351
16. Kopka L et al (1998) Differences in injection rates on contrast-enhanced breath-hold three-dimensional MR angiography. AJR Am J Roentgenol 170(2):345-348
17. Kim JK, Farb RI, Wright GA (1998) Test bolus examination in the carotid artery at dynamic gadolinium-enhanced MR angiography. Radiology 206(1):283-289
18. Foo TK et al (1997) Automated detection of bolus arrival and initiation of data acquisition in fast, three-dimensional, gadolinium-enhanced MR angiography. Radiology 203(1):275-280

19. Fellner FA et al (2000) Fluoroscopically triggered contrast-enhanced 3D MR DSA and 3D time-of-flight turbo MRA of the carotid arteries: first clinical experiences in correlation with ultrasound, x-ray angiography, and endarterectomy findings. Magn Reson Imaging 18(5):575-585

20. Heiserman JE et al (1994) Neurologic complications of cerebral angiography. AJNR Am J Neuroradiol 15(8):1401-7 discussion 1408-1411

21. Mani RL et al (1978) Complications of catheter cerebral arteriography: analysis of 5,000 procedures. I. Criteria and incidence. AJR Am J Roentgenol 131(5):861-865

22. Kuntz KM et al (1995) Carotid endarterectomy in asymptomatic patients–is contrast angiography necessary? A morbidity analysis. J Vasc Surg 22(6):706-14 discussion 714-716

23. El-Saden SM et al (2001) Imaging of the internal carotid artery: the dilemma of total versus near total occlusion. Radiology 221(2):301-308

24. Nederkoorn PJ et al (2002) Time-of-flight MR angiography of carotid artery stenosis: does a flow void represent severe stenosis? AJNR Am J Neuroradiol 23(10):1779-1784

25. Patel MR et al (1995) Preoperative assessment of the carotid bifurcation. Can magnetic resonance angiography and duplex ultrasonography replace contrast arteriography? Stroke 26(10):1753-1758

26. Nederkoorn PJ, van der Graaf Y, Hunink MG (2003) Duplex ultrasound and magnetic resonance angiography compared with digital subtraction angiography in carotid artery stenosis: a systematic review. Stroke 34(5):1324-1332

27. Scarabino T et al (1998) MR angiography in carotid stenosis: a comparison of three techniques. Eur J Radiol 28(2):117-125

28. Townsend TC et al (2003) Contrast material-enhanced MRA overestimates severity of carotid stenosis, compared with 3D time-of-flight MRA. J Vasc Surg 38(1):36-40

29. Nederkoorn PJ et al (2003) Carotid artery stenosis: accuracy of contrast-enhanced MR angiography for diagnosis. Radiology 228(3):677-682

30. Scarabino T et al (1999) Contrast-enhanced MR angiography (CE MRA) in the study of the carotid stenosis: comparison with digital subtraction angiography (DSA). J Neuroradiol 26(2):87-91

31. Remonda L et al (2002) Contrast-enhanced 3D MR angiography of the carotid artery: comparison with conventional digital subtraction angiography. AJNR Am J Neuroradiol 23(2):213-219

32. Lenhart M et al (2002) Time-resolved contrast-enhanced magnetic resonance angiography of the carotid arteries: diagnostic accuracy and inter-observer variability compared with selective catheter angiography. Invest Radiol 37(10):535-541

33. Huston J et al (2001) Carotid artery: elliptic centric contrast-enhanced MR angiography compared with conventional angiography. Radiology 218(1):138-143

34. Sardanelli F et al (1999) MR angiography of internal carotid arteries: breath-hold Gd-enhanced 3D fast imaging with steady-state precession versus unenhanced 2D and 3D time-of-flight techniques. J Comput Assist Tomogr 23(2):208-215

35. Nederkoorn PJ et al (2002) Overestimation of carotid artery stenosis with magnetic resonance angiography compared with digital subtraction angiography. J Vasc Surg 36(4):806-813

36. Anderson CM et al (1992) Assessment of carotid artery stenosis by MR angiography: comparison with x-ray angiography and color-coded Doppler ultrasound. AJNR Am J Neuroradiol 13(3):989-1003 discussion 1005-1008

37. Turnipseed WD et al (1993) Combined use of duplex imaging and magnetic resonance angiography for evaluation of patients with symptomatic ipsilateral high-grade carotid stenosis. J Vasc Surg 17(5):832-9 discussion 839-840

38. Willig DS et al (1998) Contrast-enhanced 3D MR DSA of the carotid artery bifurcation: preliminary study of comparison with unenhanced 2D and 3D time-of-flight MR angiography. Radiology 208(2):447-451

39. Yuan C et al (2002) Identification of fibrous cap rupture with magnetic resonance imaging is highly associated with recent transient ischemic attack or stroke. Circulation 105(2):181-185

40. Yuan C et al (2001) Carotid atherosclerotic plaque: noninvasive MR characterization and identification of vulnerable lesions. Radiology 221(2):285-299

41. Lusby RJ et al (1982) Carotid plaque hemorrhage. Its role in production of cerebral ischemia. Arch Surg 117(11):1479-1488

42. Leclerc X et al (1999) Preliminary experience using contrast-enhanced MR angiography to assess vertebral artery structure for the follow-up of suspected dissection. AJNR Am J Neuroradiol 20(8):1482-1490

43. Auer A et al (1998) Magnetic resonance angiographic and clinical features of extracranial vertebral artery dissection. J Neurol Neurosurg Psychiatry 64(4):474-481

44. Vila N et al (2003) Levels of alpha1-antitrypsin in plasma and risk of spontaneous cervical artery dissections: a case-control study. Stroke 34(9):E168-169

45. Dziewas R et al (2003) Cervical artery dissection–clinical features, risk factors, therapy and outcome in 126 patients. J Neurol 250(10):1179-1184

46. Mascalchi M et al (1997) MRI and MR angiography of vertebral artery dissection. Neuroradiology 39(5):329-340

47. Ozdoba C, Sturzenegger M, Schroth G (1996) Internal carotid artery dissection: MR imaging features and clinical-radiologic correlation. Radiology 199(1):191-198

48. Levy C et al (1994) Carotid and vertebral artery dissections: three-dimensional time-of-flight MR angiography and MR imaging versus conventional angiography. Radiology 190(1):97-103

49. Stringaris K et al (1996) Three-dimensional time-of-flight MR angiography and MR imaging versus conventional angiography in carotid artery dissections. Int Angiol 15(1):20-25

50. Kirsch E et al (1998) MR angiography in internal carotid artery dissection: improvement of diagnosis by selective demonstration of the intramural haematoma. Neuroradiology 40(11):704-709

51. Colletti PM, Terk MR, Zee CS (1996) Magnetic resonance angiography in neck masses. Comput Med Imaging Graph 20(5):379-388

52. Yousem DM et al (1995) Carotid artery invasion by head and neck masses: prediction with MR imaging. Radiology 195(3):715-720

III.2

Intracranial MR Angiography

Nicoletta Anzalone and Armando Tartaro

Clinical Indications/Background

Clinical indications for noninvasive vascular diagnostic modalities have increased in the last ten years due to rapid developments in technology and subsequent improvements of spatial resolution. Improvements in imaging of intracranial vessels have occurred in large part due the possibility to acquire larger volumes. Major advantages of MRA over CTA for the study of intracranial circulation are that it is less invasive, is not entirely dependent on the need for contrast media, and permits better separation of arteries from veins.

Prior to the advent of noninvasive vascular techniques, digital subtraction angiography was the primary imaging modality for the diagnosis of intracranial vessel pathology, even though its indications were largely restricted to the exclusion of vascular malformations in the presence of intracranial hemorrhage, to the study of tumour circulation and to the evaluation of venous thrombosis. On the other hand, its applicability for the exclusion of arterial vessel thrombosis was limited, since there was no effective treatment for acute stroke. The demonstrable efficacy of intravenous thrombolysis and, to a lesser extent intrarterial thrombolysis, has increased the need of a more complete evaluation of patient with acute stroke.

Possibly the major advantage of MRA for evaluation of the intracranial circulation is the possibility to intergrate this with conventional MR studies of the brain. In this regard recent sophisticated techniques such as diffusion and perfusion MR imaging, in conjunction with MRA, now permit a considerably more precise diagnosis of vascular lesions.

The recent diffusion of Stroke Unit departments for treatment of acute stroke has increased the need for a more precise and fast diagnosis of cerebral infarction and the evidence that MR can reveal the presence of tissue at risk, the so called "ischenmic penumbra", has further elevated the importance of MRA as a diagnostic technique in the intracranial vasculature. MRA in this setting permits a rapid demonstration of the occluded vessel thereby facilitating rapid decision-making concerning the most appropriate treatment.

Integration of MR imaging and MRA has been shown to be particularly useful for the evaluation of major sinus venous thrombosis and intracranial carotid dissection, two indications for which conventional angiography is less frequently employed.

Although conventional angiography is still considered the gold standard technique for pretreatment evaluation of intracranial vascular malformations, MRA has progressively gained ground for both diagnosis and follow-up of cerebral malformations, especially of cerebral aneurysms.

Normal Anatomy

The cerebral blood supply is provided by four arteries: the two internal carotid arteries and the two vertebral arteries. The internal carotid artery (ICA) originates from the bifurcation of the common carotid artery and penetrates the skull base through the jugular foramen. The vertebral artery enters the cranium by way of the occipital foramen and, unlike other arteries which dichotomize, they join to form the larger basilar artery.

Schematically, the intracranial arterial system is divided into an anterior portion which consists of the carotid circulation (Fig. 1), and a posterior portion which consists of the vertebro-basilar circulation (Fig. 2). Both vascular territories anastomose by way of the circle of Willis located at the base of the brain (Fig. 3). Three sets of arteries originate from the circle of Willis: the anterior, middle and posterior cerebral arteries. These arteries provide the blood supply to the cerebral hemispheres, while the brainstem and the cerebel-

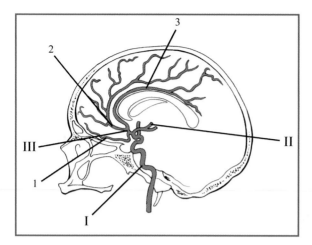

Fig. 1. Schematic representation of the internal carotid artery, its bifurcation and the anterior cerebral artery with its cortical branches

I Internal carotid artery (ICA)	1 Medial frontobasal artery
II Middle cerebral artery (MCA)	2 Callosomarginal artery
III Anterior cerebral artery (ACA)	3 Pericallosal artery

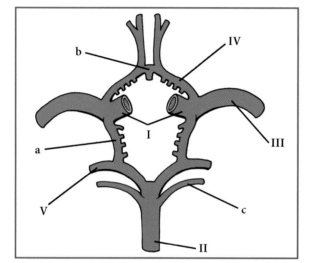

Fig. 3. Schematic representation of the complete circle of Willis

I Internal carotid artery (ICA)
II Basilary artery (BA)
III Middle cerebral artery (MCA)
IV Anterior cerebral artery (ACA)
V Posterior cerebral artery (PCA)

a Posterior communicating artery (PCoA)
b Anterior communicating artery (ACA)
c Superior cerebral artery

lum are supplied exclusively by branches of the vertebro-basilar circulation.

Internal Carotid Artery

After emerging from the petrosal portion of the temporal bone, the intracranial tract of the ICA passes anteriorly to the petrous apex and runs along the sides of the sella, within the cavernous si-

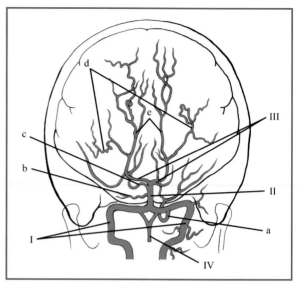

Fig. 2. Schematic representation of the vertebro-basilar circulation from the vertebral arteries to the distal branches of the posterior cerebral arteries

I Vertebral artery (VA)	a Inferior posterior cerebellar artery
II Basilary artery (BA)	b Inferior anterior cerebellar artery
III Posterior cerebral artery (PCA)	c Superior cerebellar artery
	d Temporooccipital arteries
IV Anterior spinal artery	e Medial occipital arteries

nus. This segment is also called the carotid siphon due to its double curved path within the cavernous sinus. After emerging from the cavernous sinus, the ICA lies within the subarachnoid space. Important branches originating from the ICA at this point include the meningohypophyseal trunk, the inferolateral trunk, and the ophthalmic arteries (OA). Within the supra-cavernous segment, the ICA has a vertical orientation and enters the subarachnoid space adjacent to the anterior clinoid process. The branches which originate at this point include the posterior communicating artery (PCoA) and the anterior choroidal artery (AChA). Only the PCoA and OA are generally well represented on MRA images (Fig. 4a, b) (Table 1) [1-3].

The OA originates from the anterio-medial surface of the ICA while the PCoA and the AChA originate from the posterior surface. The PCoA runs immediately above the III cranial nerve and merges with the posterior cerebral artery (PCA). The AChA is the last vessel which originates from the ICA and is not always seen on MRA (Figs. 5-6) [4-7]. The ICA terminates by dividing into two arteries: the middle cerebral artery (MCA) and the anterior cerebral artery (ACA).

Persistence of fetal carotid-vertebrobasilar anastomoses, such as the trigeminal artery which directly connects the intracavernous ICA with the basilar artery, is the most common form of anatomical variation of the ICA (Fig. 7).

Each ACA is subdivided into two tracts: the pre-

Table 1. Path and branches which originate from the internal carotid artery

Segment	Path	Collateral branches	MRA visibility
Cervical	Vascular space, parapharyngeal space	None	–
Intrapetrous	Carotid canal	Carotico-tympanic artery, vidian and periostea arteries	No
Cavernous			
C5	Petrous apex at the posterior bend	Meningohypophyseal trunk	No
C4	Petrous apex at the anterior bend	Inferolateral trunk	No
C3	Intradural segment	McConnel's capsular artery	No
C3-C2	Mostly intradural	Ophthalmic artery	Fair
Supra-cavernous C2-C1	Within the subarachnoid space medial to the anterior clinoid process and under the optic nerve	Superior hypophyseal artery	No
C1	Vertical segment which divides in a T to form the anterior and middle cerebral arteries	Posterior communicating artery	Good
		Anterior choroidal artery	Rarely

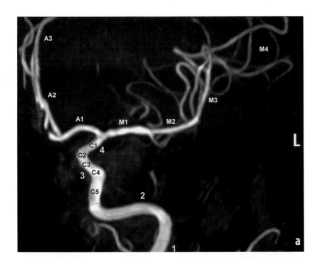

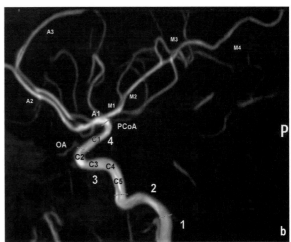

Fig. 4. (a-b). 3D TOF MRA of a normal internal carotid artery, and the anterior and middle cerebral arteries in anterior (**a**) and lateral view (**b**) (see Table 1)

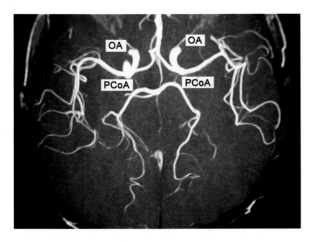

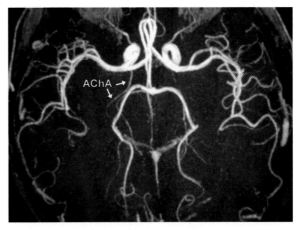

Fig. 5. 3D TOF MRA (*axial view*). Both ophthalmic arteries and posterior communicating arteries are well defined

Fig. 6. 3D TOF MRA (*axial view*). Demonstration of the origin and normal course of the right anterior choroidal artery

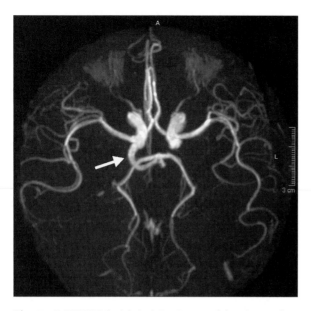

Fig. 7. 3D TOF MRA (*axial view*). Persistence of the trigeminal artery (*arrow*) with direct connection of the right cavernous internal carotid artery to the basilar artery

communicating A1 tract from which originate the lenticular-striat arteries and, sometimes, Heubner's artery, and the A2 tract, which bifurcates into the frontal-polar and orbital-frontal arteries (Fig. 8a). The ACA divides into the marginal callosum and the pericallosum arteries at the level of the bend of the corpus callosum (Fig. 8b). The most frequent anatomical variants of the ACA are the "azygos" ACA (Fig. 8c) and the triple pericallosal artery (Fig. 8d). The anterior communicating artery (ACoA) forms an anastomosis between the two ACAs. Fenestrations and duplications of the ACA are rare anatomical anomalies which may be associated with small aneurysms of the ACoA [8, 9].

The MCA is divided into four segments (Fig. 9): the horizontal or sphenoidal segment (M1) from which originate the perforating lenticulostrate arteries which are not visible on MRA, the insular segment (M2), the opercular segment (M3) and the M4 segments which are outside of the sylvian fissure and supply the frontal and parietal convexity. Anatomical variants of the MCA are uncommon. The most frequent are duplications, fenestrations, or accessory arteries (Fig. 10) [10].

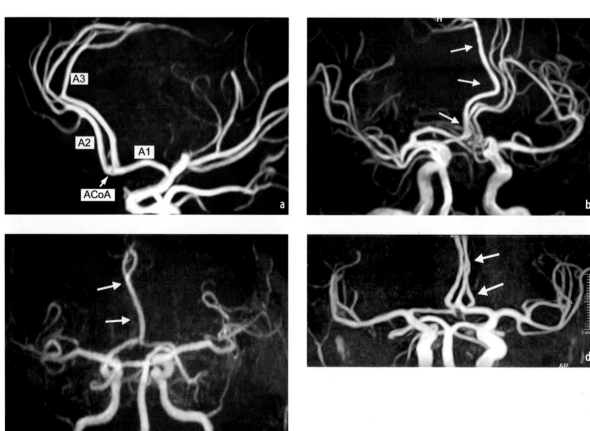

Fig. 8a-d. 3D TOF MRA of the anterior circulation. Representation of the anterior cerebral artery (**a**), callosal artery (**b**), azygos artery (**c**) and triple pericallosal artery (**d**)

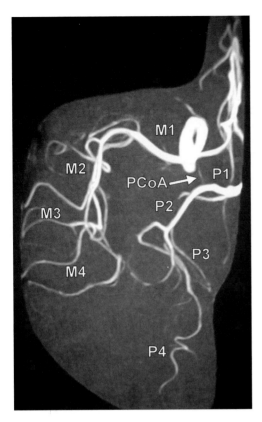

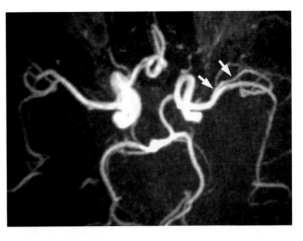

Fig. 10. 3D TOF MRA (*axial view*). Duplication (*arrows*) of the left middle cerebral artery

Fig. 9. 3D TOF MRA (*axial view*). Normal representation of the middle and posterior cerebral arteries with their different segments

Vertebro-Basilar System

The vertebro-basilar circulation comprises the vertebral, basilar, and posterior cerebral (PCA) arteries (Fig. 11). The posterior inferior cerebellar artery (PICA) usually originates before the vertebral arteries merge to form the basilar artery. This artery is usually visible on MRA images (Fig. 12). Conversely, the other branches (meningeal, spinal and bulbar) are seldom visible. Asymmetrical variations of the vertebral arteries are common: most frequently, one of the vertebral arteries is either absent, hypoplastic or ends directly in the PICA, resulting in the basilar artery originating directly from the contralateral vertebral artery.

The basilar artery runs within the pre-pontine cistern and terminates by dividing into two at the PCA. The two anterior-inferior cerebellar arteries (AICA) and the two superior cerebellar arteries (SCA) originate from the caudal tract of the basilar artery. Both AICA and SCA are often visible on MRA images (Fig. 13) [11]. Anatomical variants of the basilar artery are uncommon. The most frequent anomaly is fenestration of the proximal segment (Fig. 14) [12].

The PCA is divided into four segments (Fig. 9): the pre-communicating segment (P1), the per-

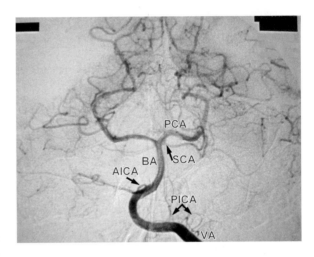

Fig. 11. Selective angiogram of the left vertebral artery with opacification of the basilar artery, cerebellar arteries and posterior cerebral arteries

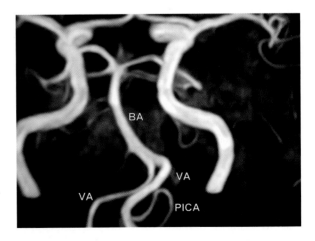

Fig. 12. 3D TOF MRA (*coronal view*). Normal representation of the posterior circulation and of the normal left posterior inferior cerebellar artery (PICA) originating from the left vertebral artery

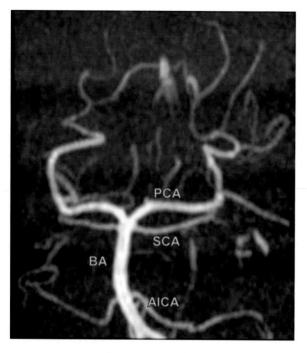

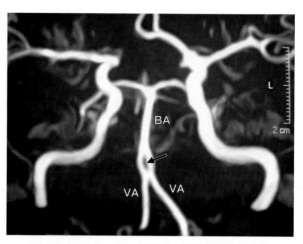

Fig. 14. 3D TOF MRA (*coronal view*). Fenestration (*arrow*) of the proximal segment of the basilar artery

Fig. 13. 3D TOF MRA (*coronal view*). Normal representation of the posterior circulation and of both anterior inferior cerebellar arteries (AICA) and the superior cerebellar arteries (SCA)

Table 2. Vertebro-basilar system and branches

Segment	Path	Collateral branches	MRA visibility
Vertebral arteries	Medullary cistern	PICA	Good
Basilar artery	Prepontine cistern	AICA, SCA	Good
		Perforators	No
PCA	Perimesencephalic cistern	Posterior choroidal	No
		Lenticulostriate	No
		Parieto-occipital	Good
		Calcarine	Good

imesencephalic segment (P2) from which originates the lenticulostriate and posterior choroidal (PChA) arteries which are not detectable on MRA, segment (P3) which runs behind the quadrigeminal lamina and which divides into two branches which are visible on MRA images, and the parieto-occipital and calcarine arteries, and the most distal branches (P4) (Table 2).

The Circle of Willis

The circle of Willis is the most important system of anastomosis between the carotid and vertebro-basilar systems; it also connects the circulation of the right and left hemispheres thereby providing a possible mechanism for hemodynamic compensation in cases of severe stenosis or occlusion of the

ICA and/or basilar artery. In its complete or "balanced" form which occurs in 20% of cases, the circle of Willis is composed of the two ICAs, the two A1 tracts of the ACA, the ACoA, the two PCoAs and the two P1 segments of the PCA (Fig. 15).

The circle of Willis presents with a wide range of anatomical variants due either to hypoplasia or agenesis of one or more components (Fig. 16). The most frequent sites of hypoplasia or agenesis are the PCoA (34%) and the A1 tract (25%) with "fetal" origin of the PCA from the ICA. Hypoplasia or absence of the P1 segment is also relatively common (17%) (Fig. 17a-b) [3-6].

Anastomosis between the intracranial and extracranial arterial circulation is provided by the OA and leptomeningeal arteries. In pathological

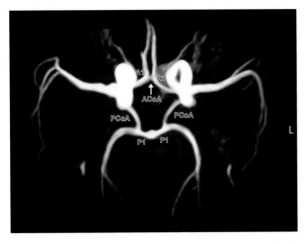

Fig. 15. 3D TOF MRA (*axial view*). Normal complete circle of Willis

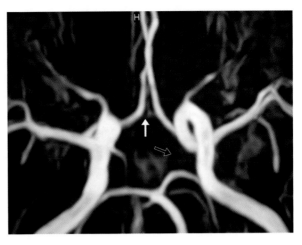

Fig. 16. 3D TOF MRA (*axial view*). Normal variant of the circle of Willis. Agenesis of the anterior communicating artery (*white arrow*) and the left posterior communicating artery (*black arrow*)

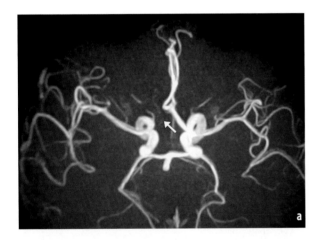

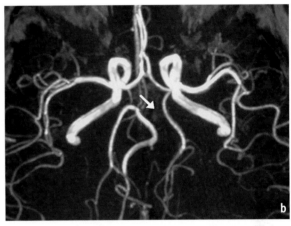

Fig. 17a-b. 3D TOF MRA (*axial view*). Normal variant of the circle of Willis. Agenesis of the right A1 segment of the anterior cerebral artery (**a**) (*arrow*) and of the left P1 segment of the posterior cerebral artery with "fetal" origin from the internal carotid siphon (**b**) (*arrow*)

conditions in which the ICA is obstructed, these anastomoses permit the spontaneous revascularization of the cerebral arteries [13]. While the leptomeningeal arteries are seldom visible on MRA images, revascularization of the intracranial ICA by way of the OA can be observed due to the hypertrophy of this vessel.

Cerebral Venous Anatomy

The venous system is composed of dural sinuses, diploic veins, meningeal veins, and superficial and deep cerebral veins. Schematically, the blood is drained from the brain to the deep venous system (centripetal flow) and to the superficial venous system (centrifugal flow). Both these systems drain into the dural venous sinuses which also col-

lect blood from the diploic and meningeal veins. This is the most important venous drainage pathway of the brain [14, 15], (Fig.18a-b).

The dural sinuses are: the superior sagittal sinus (SSS) that runs along the midline within the superior insertion of the falx cerebri and terminates in the confluence of sinuses indicated as torcular herophili (Fig. 19a-b) [16]; the inferior sagittal sinus (ISS) that originates at the rostral margin of the corpus callosum and runs within a dural fold in the inferior margin of the falx cerebri following the superior profile of the corpus callosum; and the transverse sinuses (TS) contained within the tentorium of each side and run along the insertion with the internal surface of the occipital bone (Fig. 20a-b). The two TS systems continue caudally with the sigmoid sinus and then finish in the jugular vein. The right TS is generally larger than the

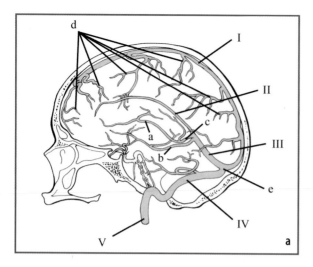

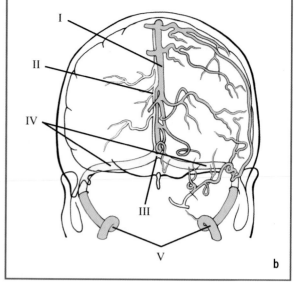

Fig. 18a-b. Schematic representation of the cerebral venous drainage system in the lateral (**a**) and coronal (**b**) views

a lateral view

I	Superior sagittal sinus (SSS)	a	Internal cerebral vein (ICV)
II	Inferior sagittal sinus (ISS)	b	Basal vein (BV)
III	Sagittal sinus (SS)	c	Vein of Galen (VG)
IV	Transverse sinus (TS)	d	Superior cerebral veins
V	Sigmoid sinus	e	Sinus confluence (SC)

b coronal view

I Superior sagittal sinus (SSS)
II Inferior sagittal sinus (ISS)
III Sinus confluence (SC)
IV Transverse sinus (TS)
V Sigmoid sinus

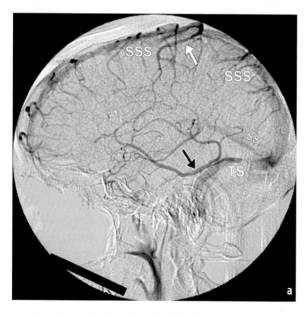

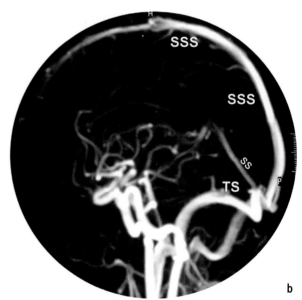

Fig. 19a-b. Cerebral angiography (**a**) in the venous phase and corresponding 3D PC MRA (**b**) of the principal intracranial dural sinuses: Superior Sagittal Sinus (SSS) (*white arrow*), Straight Sinus (SS) and Transverse Sinus (TS) (*black arrow*)

left but a wide range of anatomical variants may be encountered [17].

The cavernous sinus is located in the anterior portion of the cranial base on both sides of the sphenoid body, within the dural space which constitutes the walls of the various canals within which the siphon runs, perpendicular to the III, IV, $V_{1,2}$ and VI cranial nerves. The cavernous sinus receives blood from the orbit by way of the superior ophthalmic vein and from the anterior portion of

the sfeno-parietal sinus [2]. The superior petrosal sinus and the inferior petrosal sinus flow into the lateral and medial portions, respectively, of the posterior portion of the cavernous sinus (Fig. 21). The superior petrosal sinus provides a connection between the cavernous sinus and the TS. The inferior venous sinus provides a connection between the inferior petrosal sinus and the ipsilateral sigmoid sinus.

The superficial veins of the brain which flow

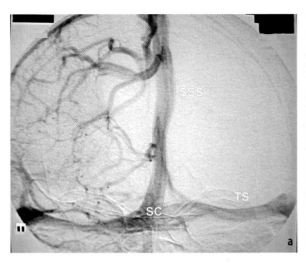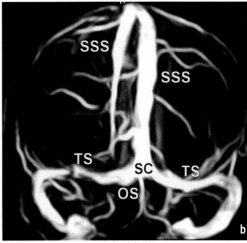

Fig. 20a-b. Cerebral angiography (**a**) in the venous phase and corresponding 3D PC MRA (**b**) of the principal intracranial dural sinuses and of the Sinus Confluence (SC)

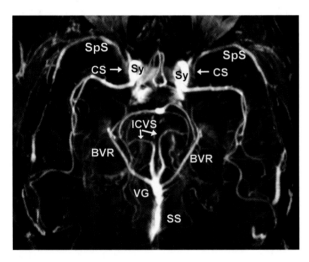

Fig. 21. 3D PC MRA of the deep venous system: Vein of Galen (VG), Basilar vein of Rosenthal (BVR), Internal cerebral vein (ICV), Straight sinus (SS); the sphenoparietal sinus (SpS) and the cavernous sinus (CS) are also shown

Table 3. Affluences of major dural sinuses and veins

Venous sinus	Affluent veins (venous inflow from)	MRA visibility
Superior Sagittal Sinus	Superficial veins of the brain	Good
	Vein of Trolard	Fair
Transverse sinus	Vein of Labbe	Good
	Superficial middle cerebral vein	Good
	Emissary veins	Seldom
Vein of Galen	Internal cerebral vein	Good
	Basilar vein of Rosenthal	Good
Straight sinus	Vein of Galen	Good
	Inferior sagittal sinus	Fair
Cavernous sinus	Superior ophthalmic vein	Good
	Sphenoparietal sinus	Good
	Superior petrosal sinus	Fair
	Inferior petrosal sinus	Fair
	Clival venous plexus	Seldom

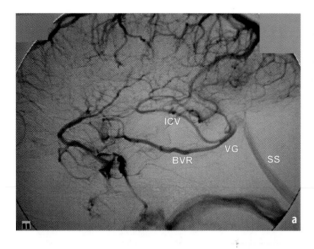

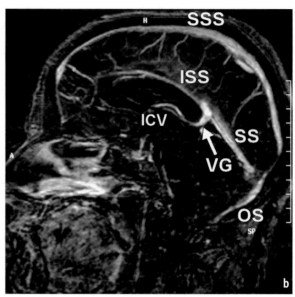

Fig. 22a-b. Cerebral angiography (**a**) in the venous phase and 2D PC MRA (**b**) of the deep and superficial cerebral venous system

into the SSS and the TS constitute the superficial venous system (Table 3). The deep venous system consists of the subependimal, terminal, anterior caudate, and the septal veins which merge into the internal cerebral vein (ICV). These veins run within the superior portion of the III ventricle and after reaching the basilar vein of Rosenthal, flow into the vein of Galen (VoG) (Fig. 22a-b).

Techniques

Intracranial Arterial System

Currently, the arterial circulation is most often studied using 3D time-of-flight (TOF) MRA. This non-invasive technique allows the visualization of the major intracranial arteries and peripheral branches in a relatively short time and generally does not require the use of contrast agent [18]. The principal advantages of the technique are that the overall acquisition time is shorter than those of phase contrast (PC) techniques, a single slice thickness of 1 mm or less can be obtained, a matrix of 512x512 can be acquired within a reasonable time, and, finally, the arteries can be imaged selectively due to the elevated saturation of the veins [19]. Its major limitation, however, is that the distal arterial branches are often less optimally visualized on MIP reconstructions due to the progressive saturation of these vessels during image acquisition [19]. Furthermore, intracranial arteries are often tourtuos and course predominantly within the imaging volume, thereby experiencing repetitive RF pulses and saturation effects. Saturation effects can sometimes be reduced on 3D TOF MRA by optimizing the scan parameters (TR, FA, TE, acquisition volume and scan plane) for preservation of arterial signal or by reducing background noise.

Numerous refinements have been implemented during the last ten years in order to improve the 3D TOF technique. Early developments included the Multiple Overlapping Thin Slab Acquisition (MOTSA) sequence which combines the advantages of both 2D and 3D TOF acquisitions while reducing saturation effects [20, 21]. Among the benefits of MOTSA sequences are that they permit evaluation of the cerebral arterial vessels from the intrapetrous segment of the ICA and the origin of the PICA from the vertebral arteries to the distal branches of the middle, anterior and posterior cerebral arteries. However, a disadvantage of MOTSA is that the acquisition time increases proportionally with the number of slabs required to cover the anatomic region of interest. A subsequent improvement on 3D MOTSA was achieved with the development of the Sliding-INterleaved kY (SLINKY) acquisition sequence which equalizes flow-related signal intensity across the entire slab dimension and thereby eliminates slab boundary artifact (SBA), also called "Venetian" blind artifact [22].

Since the flip angle (FA) also influences the degree of saturation, there is always an optimal value for this variable which is correlated with the blood flow velocity. In the intracranial circulation the ideal FA depends on the segment to be imaged since the blood flow velocity varies greatly from the carotid siphon to the proximal portion of the cerebral arteries and the most distal branches. To overcome this problem, a technique known as Tilted Optimized Non-saturating Excitation (TONE) was introduced in 1995 and is now routinely used in 3D TOF intracranial MRA [23, 24]. A further im-

Table 4. Suggested parameters for 3D TOF MRA of intracranial arteries

3D TOF MRA	
Coil	Head
Patient Positioning	Supine – head first
Saturation band	Superior
Sequences	3D TOF GRE (FISP, GRASS, FFE)
Adjunctive techniques	MOTSA, TONE, MTC
Sequence orientation	axial – bi-commissural line
TR, TE, flip angle	20-25 ms, 2-5 ms (flow comp), 20°-30°
Matrix	256 x 512, phase direction LR
FOV, slab, slice thick	220 x 250 mm^2, 80 mm, 0.75 -1.2 mm (no gap) (contiguous)
Voxel size	0.8 x 0.5 x 0.75 -1.2 mm^3
Acquisition time	6-8 minutes
Landmarks for slab position	Use scouts to cover anatomy
Image subtraction	No
Evaluation of images	Source, MIP (optional SD or VRT)

provement of the SNR between mobile and stationary spins is attainable by applying Magnetization Transfer Contrast (MTC) to 3D TOF MRA sequences of the intracranial circulation [25]. The typical parameters employed for 3D TOF MRA of the intracranial arteries are listed in Table 4.

Despite the technical advantages of 3D TOF MRA, a major limitation is the saturation of slow spins in the more distal arterial branches with consequent reduction of diagnostic accuracy. 2D TOF acquisitions can partly overcome this limitation, but these sequences lack 3D spatial resolution and are thus of little practical value for the visualization of intracranial arteries.

At present there are two possibilities to overcome the limitations of TOF MRA techniques: increased magnetic fields and the uses of contrast agent – enhanced acquisitions.

Creasy et al. [26] were among the first to describe the possibility of increasing the quality of MRA images of the intracranial circulation by combining the 3D TOF MRA technique with the intravenous infusion of a gadolinium contrast agent. Although this and other early studies revealed that visualization of the more distal portions of the intracranial arterial circulation was improved on contrast-enhanced (CE) 3D MRA, the relatively long acquisition times (8 to 10 minutes) of these early studies and rapid distribution of contrast agent led to visualization of both cerebral arteries and veins [27-29]. Additionally, the presence of contrast agent in the capillary-venous compartment was shown to lead to increased signal intensity of the stationary encephalic tissue, particularly of the intracranial structures that lack a blood-brain-barrier (e.g., choroid plexus and pituitary gland) [27, 29]. Because of the superimpo-

sition of arterial and venous structures, as well as non-vascular structures, arterial illustration using these early 3D CE MRA techniques was poor and image interpretation was overly complicated [21, 30]. Therefore, this technique did not replace unenhanced 3D TOF MRA in routine practice despite the advantage of greater sensitivity for peripheral portions of the intracranial arterial vessels.

Recently, with the introduction of stronger gradients and the development of ultrafast sequences (acquisition times of just 20-50 seconds), 3D CE MRA has been reconsidered for the diagnosis of intracranial vascular pathologies [29, 31]. The technique, which requires a rapid intravenous injection of paramagnetic contrast agent, has been shown to be more sensitive and more selective then previous techniques. When scan times are in the order of seconds, an almost exclusive visualization of the intracranial arteries without visualization of the venous vessels can be achieved. These results are possible due to recent developments in K space sampling in which the central portion of K space is the first to be acquired. This reduces the overall acquisition time for arterial vessels where the contrast agent is initially concentrated [32-34].

As in 3D CE MRA of other arterial territories, the underlying principle for 3D CE MRA of the intracranial arterial circulation is the "first pass" T1-shortening effect of circulating contrast agent during the filling of the central portions of K space. However, a fundamental difference between the intracranial arterial circulation and other arterial regions is that the arterial-venous time interval in the brain is extremely short, typically only 4 to 6 seconds [35]. Thus, ultrafast sequences and more rigorous acquisition parameters are required in

Table 5. Suggested parameters for 3D CE MRA of intracranial arteries

3D CE MRA	
Coil	Head
Patient Positioning	Supine – head first
CM dose - flow rate	0.01 mMol (Kg/bw) – 2-4 ml/sec
Bolus Timing	CM dose 2 ml - flow rate 2-4 ml/sec
Saline solution flush	15-20 ml/same flow rate of CM
Sequences	3D GRE T1 weighted (FLASH, SPGR, FFE)
Sequence orientation	axial – bi-commissural plane
TR, TE, flip angle	3-5 ms, 1-2 ms, 30°-40°
Matrix	192 x 256 (512), phase direction LR
FOV, slab, slice thick	220 x 250 mm^2, 60 mm, ~1 mm (no gap)
Voxel size	1.0 x 1.0 x 1.0- 1.5 mm^3
Acquisition time	20-40 sec
Landmarks for slab position	Use scouts to cover anatomy
Dynamic evaluation	4 volumes each lasting ~ 10 sec, without delay
Image subtraction	Yes
Evaluation of images	Source, MIP (optional SD or VRT)

order to obtain diagnostically useful MRA images [28, 29, 31].

As in other vascular territories, there are various examination factors that are critical for optimization of the 3D CE MRA examination. These factors include: optimization of scan parameters, modality of contrast agent injection (timing and quantity), relaxivity of the contrast agent, and post-processing. For most 3D CE MRA examinations of the intracranial arterial circulation, the choice of which parameters to select depends on whether the application requires high contrast and good spatial resolution or "time resolved" acquisitions at lower spatial resolution [34]. Several techniques have been proposed that favor either spatial or temporal resolution.

The 3D CE MRA techniques that favor spatial resolution are similar to the T1 weighted GE sequences and acquisition parameters used for CE MRA of the thoracic aorta and arch vessels. Elliptically centric encoded acquisition must be timed precisely to the arrival of contrast agent in the circle of Willis in order to minimize enhancement of the venous components. Although the overall scan time ranges from 20 to 50 seconds, with elliptical centric phase ordering the center of k-space is filled very efficiently during the initial seconds of the scan enabling the selective visualization of major intracranial arteries without significant venous contamination (Table 5). When a phased array head coil is used, parallel imaging techniques such as SENSE (SENSitivity Encoding [36]) or SMASH (SiMultaneous Acquisition of Spatial Harmonics [37]), permit both a shorter scan time and a high-

er spatial resolution or coverage.

When the TR is short enough and a 192x265 matrix is used, dynamic "time resolved" 3D CE MRA can be performed of most vascular territories with a time resolution of 3-6 seconds for each 3D volume acquisition [31]. However, for intracranial arterial studies this temporal resolution is barely sufficient because of the extremely short interval between the arterial and venous phases. When "time resolved" 3D CE MRA or Time Resolved Imaging of Contrast Kinetics (TRICKS [31]) techniques are used for intracranial imaging, the entire dose of contrast agent must be administered as a rapid bolus during the period between the beginning of the arterial phase and the beginning of the venous phase. Therefore, a preliminary bolus test must be performed to determine the arterial delay, the venous delay, and the resulting time interval even though, due to the rapidity of the intracranial circulation, it is sometimes difficult to separate arteries from veins.

To improve time resolution, a 2D thick-slice MR digital subtraction angiography (2D MR DSA) technique can be used instead of 3D CE MRA. This method combines a series of 2D CE thick slices, each frame lasting 1-2 seconds, with subtraction of pre-contrast images from subsequent contrast-enhanced images to allow greater background tissue suppression (Fig. 23a-g). 2D MR DSA requires one or, when multiple "projections" are necessary, two or more rapid intravenous bolus injections of contrast agent. When multiple injections are needed, image subtraction prevents contamination from previously enhanced vessels (Table 6).

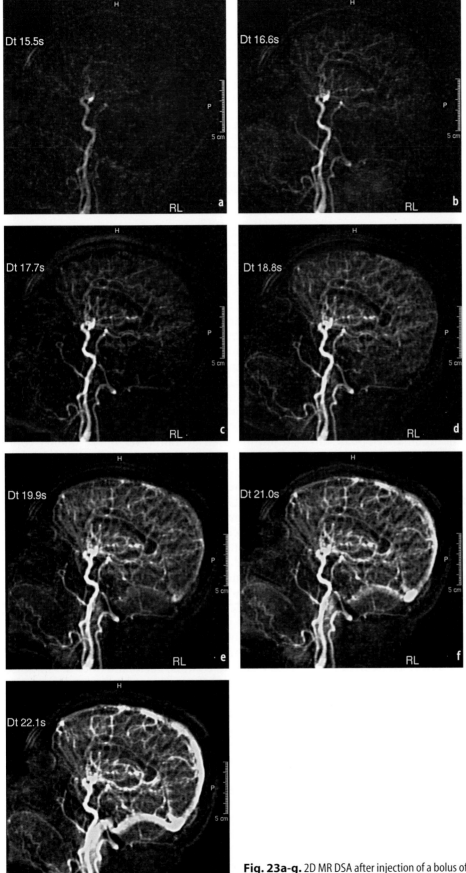

Fig. 23a-g. 2D MR DSA after injection of a bolus of gadolinium contrast agent. Sagittal view of normal cerebral arteriovenous circulation with time resolution of 1.1 seconds

Table 6. Suggested parameters for 2D CE MRA (MR DSA) of intracranial arteries and veins

2D MR DSA	
Coil	Head
Patient Positioning	Supine – head first
CM dose/flow rate	0.1 mMol (Kg/bw) – 4 ml/sec
Bolus Timing	Not required
Saline solution flush	15-20 ml/same flow rate of CM
Sequences	2D GRE T1 weighted (FLASH, SPGR, FFE)
Sequence orientation	sagittal
TR, TE, flip angle	5 ms, 1-2 ms, 40°
Matrix	256 x 256, phase direction AP
FOV, slice thick	220 x 250 mm^2, 60 mm
Acquisition time	1-2 sec for each frame/ 60-30 frames
Landmarks for slab position	Use scouts to cover anatomy
Image subtraction	Yes (automatically subtracted)

Intracranial Venous System

The intracranial venous system is a complex, often asymmetric, system of vessels. MRA was the first non-invasive technique that enabled depiction of the intracranial venous system without using ionizing radiation. Both 2D TOF and 2D-3D PC sequences are available to study the cerebral venous circulation [38].

PC MRA is based on the accumulated phase difference between mobile spins and stationary spins. This characteristic renders PC acquisition more sensitive to slow flow, such as occurs in veins [39]. An appropriate velocity encoding (VENC) (Tables 7 and 8) must be selected based on the velocity of blood within the blood vessel to be imaged [14]. Unlike TOF MRA, PC MRA is not affected by saturation effects. In addition, contrast agents can improve the vascular signal on PC MRA enabling depiction of smaller venous vessels by increasing the signal intensity and hence the spatial resolution achievable [40]. For this reason PC MRA is usually the last sequence acquired during a standard contrast enhanced examination of the brain.

Usually 3D PC MRA is performed in preference to 2D PC MRA for studies of cerebral veins because of the higher spatial resolution and larger coverage achievable. However, 2D PC MRA may also be used to determine blood flow direction and as a pilot study to determine the most appropriate VENC for a definitive 3D PC MRA study. The main disadvantages of 3D PC MRA are the longer acquisition times, which can be overcome in part by the use of parallel imaging technology, and the dependence of the technique on the correct choice of VENC. An inappropriate choice may result in a representation of false stenosis.

2D TOF MRA may also be used to image cerebral veins. With this approach a presaturation band must be collocated below the acquisition to saturate arterial flow and to prevent saturation effects during the TOF acquisition. Usually, a slight oblique coronal plane is chosen to cut perpendicularly the major dural sinuses. As with PC MRA acquisitions, contrast agents have been proposed to increase the signal and to reduce the saturation effect. Unfortunately, 2D TOF MRA has a lower spatial resolution and lower background suppression resulting in an overall lower image quality compared to that achievable with 3D PC MRA [38].

Recently, high resolution 3D fast GE T1 weighted sequences (e.g. MPRAGE, FSPGR, and EPI-FFE) acquired before and during slow administration of gadolinium contrast agent have been proposed. Another suggested protocol involves triggering the sequence with the arrival of contrast agent and fixing a delay of 8-10 seconds to acquire images at the point of maximal venous contrast concentration. The advantages of this technique include a panoramic and consistent visualization of the intracranial venous system. Some protocols propose image subtraction to reduce the signal intensity from arteries which is already very high on acquisitions without contrast agent and does not increase significantly following contrast agent administration. The only inconvenience of this technique is that it doubles the acquisition time, thereby increasing the probability of patient movement and, in consequence, rendering image subtraction futile.

Whichever technique is chosen, the patient should be made as comfortable as possible before initiating the study. For example, ear plugs should be used because the MRA sequences (especially 3D CE MRA sequences) are notably noisier than conventional techniques. When a contrast agent is required, an intravenous line should be connected to

Table 7. Suggested parameters for 3D PC MRA of intracranial circulation

3D PC MRA	
Coil	Head
Patient Positioning	Supine – head first
Saturation band	Inferior
Sequences	3D GRE T1 weighted (FLASH, SPGR, FFE)
VENCs	70-80 cm/sec for arteries; 10-20 cm/sec for veins
Sequence orientation	axial – bi-commissural line
TR, TE, flip angle	80 ms, 10 ms, 20°-30°
Matrix	256 x 256, phase direction LR
FOV, slab, slice thick	200 x 250 mm², 80 mm, 1 -1.5 mm (no gap) (contiguous)
Voxel size	0.8 x 0.9 x 1 -1.5 mm³
Acquisition time	10-12 minutes
Landmarks for slab position	Use scouts to cover anatomy
Image subtraction	Yes (automatically subtracted)
Evaluation of images	Source, MIP (optional SD or VRT)

Table 8. Suggested parameters for 2D PC MRA of intracranial venous system

2D PC MRA	
Coil	Head
Patient Positioning	Supine – head first
Sequences	2D GRE T1 weighted (FLASH, SPGR, FFE)
VENCs	15-20 cm/sec
Sequence orientation	variable
TR, TE, flip angle	80 ms, 10 ms, 20°-30°
Matrix	256 x 256, phase direction LR
FOV, slab, slice thick	200 x 250 mm², 80 mm, 1 -1.5 mm (no gap) (contiguous)
Voxel size	0.8 x 0.9 x 20 mm³
Acquisition time	2-3 minutes
Landmarks for slab position	Use scouts to cover anatomy
Image subtraction	Yes (automatically subtracted)

a power injector prior to initiating the examination in order to avoid repositioning the patient. The patient's head must be securely but comfortably immobilized and the patient should be asked to remain as still as possible during the examination. The field of view should be positioned to include the entire internal portion of the cranium in order to avoid aliasing or back-folding artifacts which significantly reduce SNR.

An important point that must be kept in mind is that MRA is not a substitute for basic brain studies, but is frequently a useful corollary examination.

Clinical Applications

Both TOF MRA and PC MRA have been used for non-invasive studies of cerebral vascular pathologies. New turbo (fast) TOF MRA sequences require at most 5-6 minutes to acquire panoramic images of the entire intracranial arterial district and, therefore, these sequences should be performed routinely to complete standard brain exams. As a general rule, 3D TOF MRA is indicated in all cases where non-invasive and selective studies of specific arterial districts are necessary, while 2D/3D PC or 2D TOF sequences are generally appropriate for selective visualization of the venous sinuses and major central veins.

Both techniques have limitations that reduce their diagnostic accuracy. The saturation phenomena and spin dephasing that occur in TOF MRA when the flow rate is greatly reduced or turbulent, results in an absence of signal on MIP reconstructions and, in consequence, an overestimation of stenosis and an increase in the number of false positives for occlusion. This is a well known problem for the carotid bifurcation, and can be seen in the intracranial circulation when 3D TOF MRA is used.

A decrease in flow velocity is also seen within

cerebral aneurysms, especially in larger lesions in which flow separation and resulting spin saturation of slower blood leads to an underestimation of the size of the aneurysm. In smaller aneurysms this phenomenon may lead to the lesion not being seen. For the most part, these diagnostic pitfalls can be avoided when 3D CE MRA is used since saturation phenomena are no longer a problem. As a consequence, diagnostic accuracy is improved [34].

In cases of recent thrombosis, the presence of methemoglobin (a paramagnetic substance which, like gadolinium, is hyperintense on TOF images) in the coagulum may lead to an underestimation of cerebral artery occlusion which can result in false negative diagnoses.

The limitations of PC MRA are as well known as those of 3D TOF MRA. The possibility to visualize a specific venous or arterial vessel with PC MRA depends upon the VENC sampled for the specific blood vessel. The VENC values under normal conditions have, for the most part, already been determined and each of the producers of MR instruments provides pre-set sequences for the major arterial and venous districts. In pathological situations, however, the arterial and/or venous flow rates are modified and therefore the pre-determined VENC values lead to either an overestimation or an underestimation of vessel patency, thereby greatly reducing diagnostic accuracy. The possibility to utilize alternative 3D CE MRA techniques may avoid this diagnostic pitfall.

Both TOF and PC MRA have notably reduced the overall need for conventional digital subtraction angiography (DSA). On the other hand, DSA still has an important role in diagnostic work-up, especially in cases of vascular malformations (for example, arterial-venous malformations and arterial-venous fistulas) where multiphase dynamic images are required. Multiphase dynamic images can also be acquired using the most recent CE MRA techniques. Although the temporal resolution is not always sufficient with these newer CE MRA techniques, preliminary findings are promising [41].

The following sections summarize the state-of-the-art MRA techniques appropriate for various intracranial pathologies.

Cerebro-Vascular Diseases

Despite recent therapeutic and diagnostic advances, stroke remains the third leading cause of death in industrialized countries and, therefore, is an important social and economic concern. The most common cause of stroke is ischemic infarct of one or more intracranial arteries [42-44]. Cerebral ischemia is the result of a critical decrease in blood flow due to vessel stenosis/obstruction or systemic hemodynamic insufficiency. When the cerebral blood flow is reduced by more than 80% (<20 ml/100g/min) for a sufficiently long period of time, irreversible neuronal damage can occur leading to cerebral necrosis [45]. The causes of infarct include arterial thrombosis, cardiogenic or, more frequently, artery-to-artery embolus, reduced blood flow and venous thrombus [42].

MRA has good sensitivity for the detection and evaluation of stenoses of the major intracranial arteries [23, 46-52]. Frequently, the technique is used in conjunction with other techniques to assess the acute phase of stroke and for patient work-up prior to endarterectomy.

3D TOF MRA is often used in the acute phase of stroke (within the first 12 hours after onset) to complete the basic MR exam in order to identify the cause and location of the occluded artery. For example, the identification of an arterial occlusion in a patient presenting with an acute neurological deficit of less than 3-4 hours' duration would tend to indicate ischemia even when the brain MRI is negative. In these cases, 3D TOF MRA, performed in conjunction with perfusion and diffusion studies, permits precise localization and evaluation of the extension of the ischemic areas (Fig. 24a-l). A roadmap of the intracranial arterial vessels previously obtained by means of 3D TOF MRA is necessary in order to correctly detect the arterial input factor (AIF). This factor must be calculated on a patent vessel in order to obtain reliable perfusion parameters: cerebral blood volume (CBV), cerebral blood flow (CBF), and mean transit time (MTT) [53].

3D TOF MRA is routinely used for the preliminary and noninvasive study of the intracranial circulation because it is faster and more accurate than 3D PC MRA. As highlighted above, the major limitation of 3D TOF MRA is signal saturation in the more distal branches of the intracranial arteries which decreases both the sensitivity and specificity of the technique for the detection and characterization of vascular occlusion/stenosis.

The positive predictive value for correctly grading the degree of intracranial stenosis has been shown to be greater for 3D TOF MRA than for 3D PC MRA, due to the high dependance of signal intensity on mean blood flow velocity in the PC MRA acquisition [19]. Various studies have been performed to evaluate the diagnostic accuracy of 3D TOF MRA (Table 9) [19, 48, 49, 54-58]. The results indicate that the major drawback of the technique is its tendency to overestimate the degree of stenosis. Conversely, it has a high negative predictive value and is a completely noninvasive technique meaning that there is no risk of neurological complications in patients with cerebral vascular pathologies. In comparison, there is 1% to

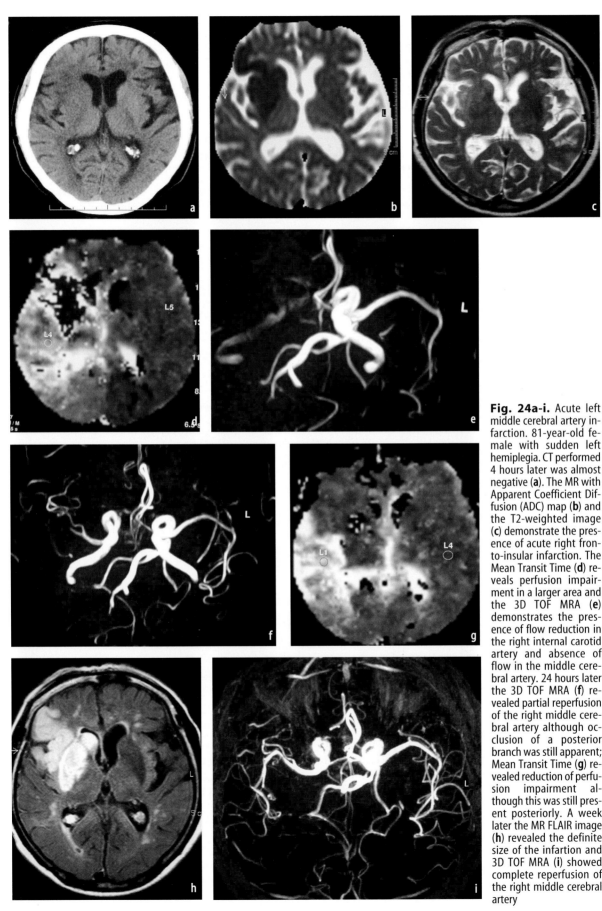

Fig. 24a-i. Acute left middle cerebral artery infarction. 81-year-old female with sudden left hemiplegia. CT performed 4 hours later was almost negative (**a**). The MR with Apparent Coefficient Diffusion (ADC) map (**b**) and the T2-weighted image (**c**) demonstrate the presence of acute right fronto-insular infarction. The Mean Transit Time (**d**) reveals perfusion impairment in a larger area and the 3D TOF MRA (**e**) demonstrates the presence of flow reduction in the right internal carotid artery and absence of flow in the middle cerebral artery. 24 hours later the 3D TOF MRA (**f**) revealed partial reperfusion of the right middle cerebral artery although occlusion of a posterior branch was still apparent; Mean Transit Time (**g**) revealed reduction of perfusion impairment although this was still present posteriorly. A week later the MR FLAIR image (**h**) revealed the definite size of the infarction and 3D TOF MRA (**i**) showed complete reperfusion of the right middle cerebral artery

Table 9. Accuracy of MRA versus DSA for diagnostic imaging of stenosis of the intracranial arterial vessels

Author	MRA Technique	# Pts	Arteries	Sensitivity	Specificity
Heiserman, 1992 [48]	3D TOF	29	stenosis	61%	
			occlusion	100%	
			normal	97%	
			occlusion	100%	
Korogi, 1994 [49]	2DFT and 3DFT TOF MRA	133	Internal carotid artery	85.1%	95.6%
			Middle cerebral artery	88.3%	96.8%
Wentz, 1994 [11]	T1 and T2 weighted SE MRA	284	Intracranial cerebro-basilar system	Normal 100%	100%
					100%
				Stenotic 76%	
Stock, 1995 [54]	MTS VFAE MRA	50		86%	86%
Korogi, 1997 [50]	MIP alone	103	stenosis	78%	
			occlusion	80%	
	3D FT TOF with MIP		stenosis	100%	
			occlusion	100%	
Oelerich, 1998 [19]	3D TOF MRA	18		87%	91%
	PC MRA			63%	92%
Hirai, 2002 [55]	3D TOF MRA MIP and MPR	498	92%	91%	
Mallouhi, 2002 [57]	VR-TOF MIP-TOF VR-CE MIP-CE	82		100%	
Nederkoorn, 2003 [58]	MRA	62	Occlusion	98%	100%
			Overall	95%	90%

MTS VFAE – magnetic transfer suppression and variable flip angle excitation
FT – Fourier transform

3% incidence of complications with DSA [55, 59].

Paramagnetic contrast agents can be used to overcome saturation phenomena and thereby improve the visualization of the more distal portions of the cerebral arteries. As early as 1995 it was reported that CE MRA permitted the visualization of an occlusion of the ICA or MCA in an additional 17% of patients compared to nonenhanced MRA [60].

In patients with severe or pre-occlusive stenosis of the carotid bifurcation, the markedly re-duced blood flow determines a signal saturation of the intracranial district of the ICA which often involves the ipsilateral MCA. The result is that these vessels are either not seen on 3D TOF MRA or are visualized with drastic reduction of the signal. This also occurs in response to a dissection of the ICA. If CE MRA is used, these drawbacks are greatly reduced or are completely eliminated. Several studies have compared unenhanced MRA and 3D CE MRA in acute stroke and have demonstrated that contrast agent application leads to improved

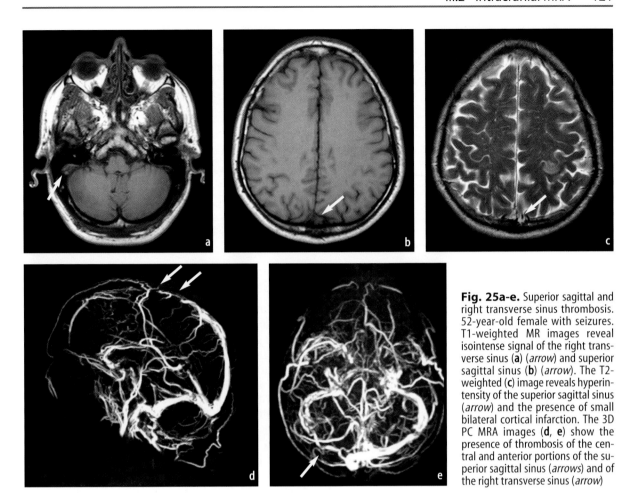

Fig. 25a-e. Superior sagittal and right transverse sinus thrombosis. 52-year-old female with seizures. T1-weighted MR images reveal isointense signal of the right transverse sinus (**a**) (*arrow*) and superior sagittal sinus (**b**) (*arrow*). The T2-weighted (**c**) image reveals hyperintensity of the superior sagittal sinus (*arrow*) and the presence of small bilateral cortical infarction. The 3D PC MRA images (**d**, **e**) show the presence of thrombosis of the central and anterior portions of the superior sagittal sinus (*arrows*) and of the right transverse sinus (*arrow*)

visualization of the remnant patency of the tributary arteries of the ischemic territory [60-62].

Atherosclerosis of the intra- and extracranial vessels is the most common cause of stroke [45]. There is a significant association between stenosis of the intracranial arteries and the risk of stroke [45, 63, 64]. Stenosis of the intracranial arteries is present in 15% of patients with stenosis of neck vessels [65] and in 20% of patients with stroke or transient ischemic attack (TIA) [66]. Therefore, evaluation of the supra-aortic and intracranial arterial segments in patients that undergo work-up for cerebrovascular degenerative disease is very important. MRA is particularly well indicated in these patients while DSA, which is considerably more invasive, should be used only in selected cases.

Turbo or fast CE MRA permits panoramic and high-resolution acquisitions of the arterial vessels of the neck, the carotid arch, and the intracranial circulation with just a single bolus of contrast agent. In order to complete the study of the intracranial circulation, high resolution 3D TOF MRA without contrast agent should be performed and the results compared to the CE MRA acquisi-

tions. Previous studies have shown that unenhanced 3D TOF MRA combined with CTA has a diagnostic accuracy comparable to DSA for determining the degree of stenosis and the presence of occlusions in the intracranial circulation [55].

Venous Vessel Thrombosis

Basic MR combined with MRA has very high sensitivity for the detection of cerebral venous thrombosis. MRA can also be used to monitor the response to thrombolytic therapy. For accurate confirmation of the presence and extension of a venous thrombosis, 3D PC MRA techniques (Fig. 25a-e) are generally preferred over TOF MRA sequences since the latter are frequently unable to distinguish flow from subacute thrombi.

The use of 3D CE MRA and image subtraction minimizes the possibility of false positives due to flow problems. This approach has been proposed as a sensitive technique for evaluation of the dural sinuses, particularly in those regions (transverse sinuses, posterior part of superior sagittal sinus, transverse-sigmoid junction) in which TOF and

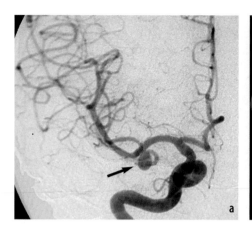 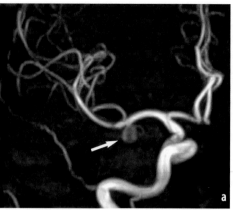

Fig. 26a-b. Small aneurysm (*arrows*) of the right middle cerebral artery bifurcation. (**a**) DSA and (**b**) 3D TOF MRA

PC MRA techniques may be troublesome because of saturation or complex flow. 3D CE MRA enables more complete visualization of venous structures which is most apparent for large dural sinuses [67]. At present this technique seems to be promising, although little has been reported as yet concerning its application in pathological series in comparison with unenhanced techniques.

While unenhanced MRA techniques are capable of distinguishing occlusion and focal stenosis of larger dural sinuses, a diagnostic problem is posed by normal variants or transverse sinus hypoplasia. In these cases improved diagnoses may be achieved with the use of a contrast agent in conjunction with either a PC or TOF MRA technique or preferably a fast 3D CE MRA technique [67].

Another field of possible application in MR venography is in the presurgical evaluation of lesions involving the dural sinuses e.g. meningiomas of the vault. In these cases both 3D PC MRA and fast 3D CE MRA have been proposed.

Intracranial Aneurysms

The term "aneurysm" indicates a dilation of an arterial segment resulting from a defect of the elastic tunica of a blood vessel wall, delimited by just the intima and adventitia.

Asymptomatic (unruptured) cerebral aneurysms are found in 2-8% of autopsies and in 7% of DSA studies [68]. The worst complication for an intracranial aneurysm is a subarachnoid hemorrhage (SAH) which has an annual risk of 1-2% and a mortality rate of 50% [68]. The frequency with which aneurysms rupture should be directly proportional to the dimension of the aneurysm. In other words, the probability of rupture for an aneurysm that is greater than 5 mm in size is greater than that for an aneurysm that is less than 5 mm in size. Nevertheless, even the smallest

aneurysms present a risk of rupture [69]. Symptomatic aneurysms are most frequently seen in the 40 to 60 year-old age range and only 2% are symptomatic in subjects under 20 years of age. The incidence of aneurysms is greater in women than in men by a ratio of 2 to 1, and there is a prevalence of 10% for asymptomatic familial intracranial aneurysms [70]. Intracranial aneurysms may be multiple in 14 to 45% of cases, with multiplicity more frequent among women [71].

An increased prevalence of intracranial aneurysms has been reported for a number of conditions including congenital intracranial vascular malformations, anatomical variations (e.g., persistence of the trigeminal artery, duplication of the MCA and variations of the OA) [72, 73], polycystic renal disease, fibromuscular dysplasia, and Marfan's syndrome [72-75].

Intracranial aneurysms are most often located in the circle of Willis and the trifurcation of the MCA (Fig. 26a-b). One third of all aneurysms are located in the anterior communicating artery and 10% originate in the vertebral-basilar district (Fig. 27a-b) [71].

There are numerous types of aneurysm. Berry (saccular) aneurysms are the result of a defect of the arterial wall which can either be congenital or acquired after continuous local hemodynamic stress. In these aneurysms, the medial elastic tunica terminates in the neck of the aneurismal sac. There is a relatively high frequency of multiplicity for berry aneurysms [71]. Fusiform aneurysms, on the other hand, are localized dilations of an arterial tract caused by arteriosclerosis and are, therefore, more frequent among the elderly. They are typically localized in the basilar artery, vertebral artery or in the supraclinoidal tract of the ICA (Fig. 28a-c). Although they are frequently symptomatic due to compression of the adjacent cranial nerves, these aneurysms rarely rupture. Dissecting aneurysms have a different pathogenesis and can

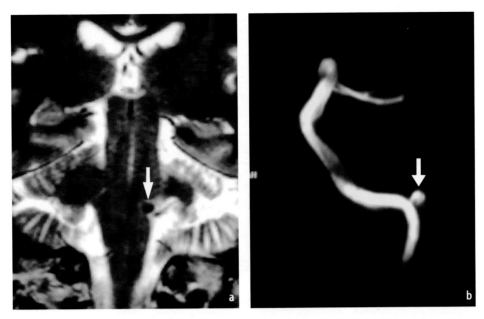

Fig. 27a-b. Small aneurysm (*arrows*) at the origin of the posterior inferior cerebellar artery apparent behind the left middle cerebellar peduncle on the coronal T2-weighted image (**a**) and on the 3D TOF MRA targeted MIP reconstruction (**b**) of the vertebro-basilar circulation [courtesy of Prof. C. Colosimo; University of Chieti]

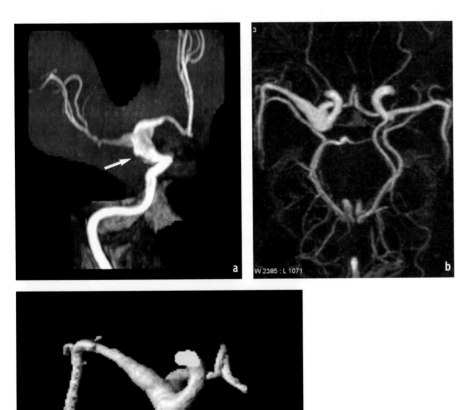

Fig. 28a-c. Fusiform ectasia (*arrow*) of the supraclinoid internal carotid artery with involvment of the middle and anterior cerebral artery. The 3D TOF MRA (**a**) reveals fusiform ectasia of the internal carotid artery and its bifurcation. The CE MRA image (**b**) shows reduced saturation effect and better delineation of the malformation, and allows 3D reconstruction (**c**)

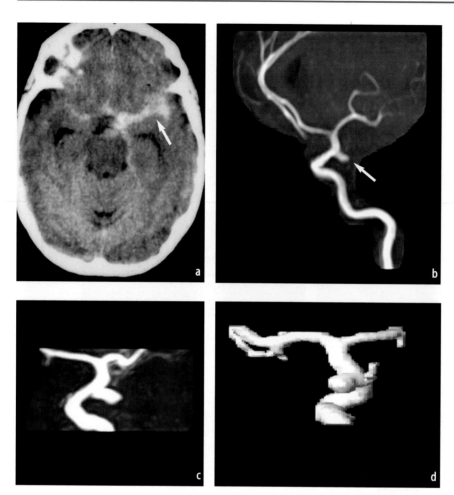

Fig. 29a-d. Acute subarchnoid hemorrhage (*arrow*) at CT (**a**). The 3D TOF MRA image (**b**) reveals a small aneurysm (*arrow*) of the internal carotid artery at the origin of the posterior communicating artery. The CE MRA image (**c**) better delineates the aneurysm morphology and with 3D reconstruction (**d**) the relationship with the posterior communicating artery is apparent

either be spontaneous or occur in response to a direct trauma to the artery. Intracranially, dissecting aneurysms frequently occur near fractures or after a vessel strikes the cerebral falce [76]. Mycotic, infectious or inflammatory aneurysms occur when pathogenic agents attack the intima, for example, in cases of septic emboli which form at a vascular bifurcation, or during propagation of the infection through the vasa-vasorum. Inflammatory processes destroy the adventitia and the muscolaris mucosa. The vessel then dilates as a result of luminal pressure [77, 78].

The particular hemodynamic conditions that are present within an aneurysm are responsible for its growth and rupture. Flow patterns within "berry" aneurysms are characterized by three zones: an inflow zone at the distal margin of the neck and wall of the sac; an outflow zone at the proximal margin of the neck and wall of the sac; and a central slow flow zone where the saturation of moving spins reduces the signal intensity of the aneurysm on 3D TOF MRA acquisitions [79].

3D TOF MRA is currently the non-invasive screening tool of choice for the detection of intracranial aneurysms. The sensitivity of this technique varies from 83% to 97% when the size of the aneurysm is greater than 5 mm, however, for smaller aneurysms the sensitivity decreases markedly [80-85]. The MRA exam must be technically accurate and must favor spatial resolution. Therefore 3D TOF MRA is more sensitive than 3D PC MRA in cases of cerebral aneurysm, especially for lesions less than 5 mm in size [34]. Furthermore, 3D TOF MRA requires markedly less time for the same acquisition volume. However, in cases of SAH, even 3D TOF MRA may require longer acquisition times because the patients are frequently irritable and unstable and hence not totally collaborative. Consequently, the best technique and parameters for each patient are often dictated by the best compromise between acquisition time and spatial resolution (Fig. 29a-d).

The introduction of TOF techniques, such as MOTSA combined with TONE has permitted slice thicknesses to be reduced to 0.75 mm, thereby minimizing saturation effects in the smaller arterial vessels. The scan times of 3D TOF MRA can be reduced by a further 40% by utilizing a section-interpolation technique [83].

3D TOF MRA should be performed within the

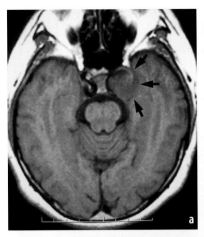

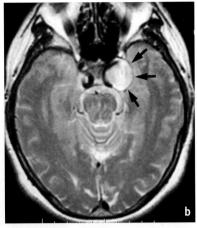

Fig. 30a-d. Axial T1-weighted (**a**) and T2-weighted (**b**) SE images reveal a partially thrombosed left intracavernous ICA aneurysm (*black arrows*). Spin saturation phenomena in the patent portion of the aneurysm results in an underestimation of the size of the residual aneurysm on the 3D TOF MRA image (**c**). MIP reconstruction underestimated the size of the residual aneurysm. The oblique DSA angiogram (**d**) acquired in the early arterial phase shows the real size of the partially thrombosed aneurysm (*black arrow*)

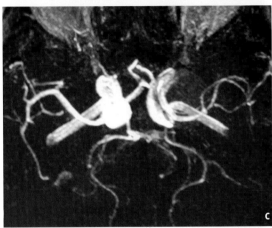

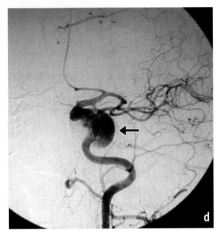

first three days of a SAH. After this time the formation of methemoglobin hampers the detection of smaller blood vessels and reduces the likelihood of seeing a small aneurysm. An alternative to MRA in patients with an acute SAH is CTA which has a sensitivity of approximately 83% for the detection of aneurysms as small as 3 mm. Unfortunately, CTA requires the patient to be exposed to at least 100 ml of iodinated contrast medium and to a considerable amount of radiation. Furthermore, the postprocessing required to obtain satisfactory images that isolate the arterial circulation is elaborate and time consuming, especially for the skull base [81].

Intra-aneurysmal flow dynamics imply that the amount of spin saturation is proportional to the size of the aneurysm, resulting in an underestimation of aneurysm size when 3D TOF MRA is used (Fig 30a-d). 3D PC MRA is affected by this phenomenon to a lesser extent. In the case of a partially thrombozed aneurysm, 3D PC MRA can demonstrate the residual lumen in which blood flow is still present. This may not be possible with 3D TOF MRA if methemaglobin is present in the thrombus as it will appear hyperintense and thus indistin-

guishable from the residual lumen.

For the study of large and giant aneurysms 3D CE MRA is frequently the technique of choice since it can depict the vessel lumen in a similar manner to that of CTA and DSA, even despite the lower spatial resolution of the 3D CE MRA technique. An advantage of 3D CE MRA is that MIP reconstructions are able to depict an aneurysm from numerous angles, permitting accurate visualization of the neck and of the relationship with the parent vessel (Fig. 31a-e). This is particularly useful for pre-treatment evaluation of the malformation when rotational angiography is not available. Another advantage of 3D CE MRA is that it is able to distinguish between possible thrombi and residual lumen: the signal intensity of the thrombus is always lower than that of the circulating blood in which contrast agent is present [34].

Studies comparing 3D CE MRA and 3D TOF MRA for the detection of intracranial aneurysms have indicated that the former technique is more sensitive. For example, sensitivity and specificity values of 100% and 94%, respectively, have been reported for 3D CE MRA [34]. The very short acquisition time makes this technique more feasible

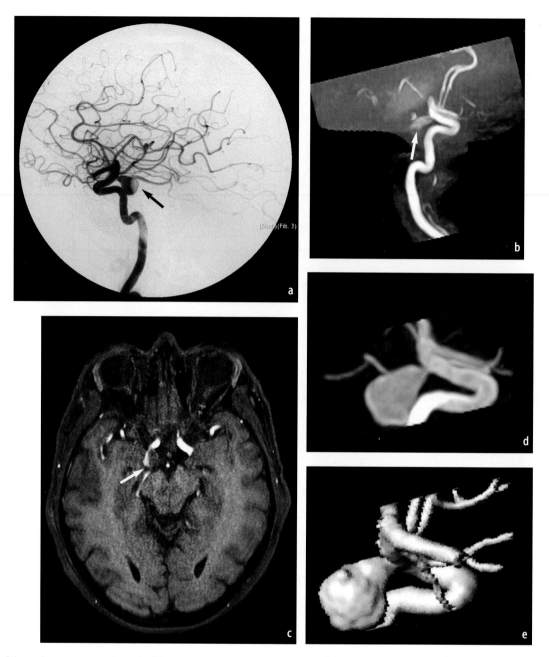

Fig. 31a-e. Large aneurysm (*arrow*) of the right internal carotid artery at the origin of the posterior cerebral artery evident at DSA (**a**). 3D TOF MRA (**b**) shows the dilatation (*arrow*) but underestimates its size due to saturation. This is clearly apparent on the axial source image (*arrow* in **c**). CE MRA (**d**) better delineates the malformation and permits 3D reconstruction (**e**), which clearly depicts the lesion and reveals its relationship to the origin of the posterior communicating artery

for use in emergency conditions such as in cases of SAH. Preliminary studies suggest that 3D CE MRA is comparable to DSA and superior to 3D TOF MRA for the demonstration of "berry-like" aneurysms (Table 10) [54, 80-96]. Nevertheless, 3D CE MRA has not yet been accepted as a routine diagnostic modality in patients with SAH, since the achievable sensitivity does not yet compare with that of DSA. On the other hand, it is frequently used as a screening modality in at-risk patients or

when the presence of aneurysm is suspected from CT or other MR examinations. Whichever technique is employed, the field of view must be positioned to cover the intracranial arterial circulation from the origin of PICA at the vertebral arteries to the pericallosal arteries, both of which are possible sites of aneurysms.

The inferior spatial resolution of 3D CE MRA compared to DSA remains, for now, the major disadvantage of this technique. However, the use of

Table 10. Accuracy of MRA versus DSA for diagnostic imaging of aneurysms of the intracranial arterial vessels

Author	MRA Technique	# Pts	Sensitivity	Specificity
Ross, 1990 [92]	cine volume gradient-echo	28	Cine only 67% Cine+partitions+spin-echo 86%	
Stock, 1995 [54]	MTS VFAE MRA	50	83%	98%
Kadota, 1997 [90]	Conventional MRA	41	< 5mm 0% ≥ 5mm 100%	
	Magnetization transfer contrast and TONE MRA		< 5mm 71% ≥5mm 100%	
Strotzer, 1998 [95]	3D FISP 2D FLASH 3D TONE	40	93% 90% 97%	92% 85% 94%
Metens, 2000 [34]	3D CE T1w MRA MT TONE PC	32	100% 96% 70%	94% 100% 100%
Mallouhi, 2003 [96]	VR-TOF MIP-TOF VR-CE MIP-CE	82	90.7% 83.7% 86% 86%	
Okahara, 2002 [89][1]	3D TOF MRA	82	Neuroradiologists 79% Experienced neurosurgeons 75% Resident radiologists 63%	

[1] lower for smaller aneurysms (<3 mm in maximum diameter) for multiple aneurysms and/or for aneurysms located in the ICA and ACA

larger matrix sizes and isotropic voxel acquisition may improve results.

An accepted application of MRA is in the follow up of coiled aneurysms. Several studies have demonstrated the feasibility and sensitivity of 3D TOF MRA for the detection of aneurysm recanalization [97, 98]. Major disadvantages of this technique however are the relatively low spatial resolution and the presence in nearly 10% of cases of susceptibility artifacts related to the coils. Recently,

MRA techniques with very short TR and TE values have been shown to reduce the number of susceptibility artifacts [99]. Moreover, the use of 3D CE MRA with elliptic centric acquisition, seems to have better sensitivity compared to 3D TOF MRA for the demonstration of aneurysm patency (Fig. 32a-e).

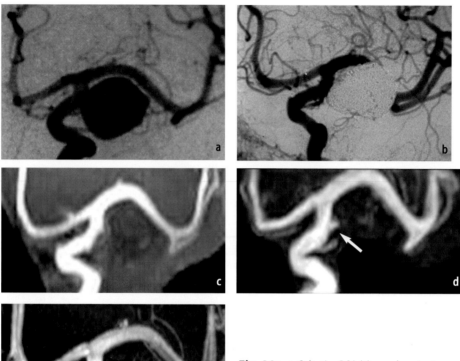

Fig. 32a-e. Selective DSA (**a**) reveals a giant aneurysm of the left internal carotid artery. The selective DSA acquired post-treatment (**b**) suggests complete occlusion of the aneurysm. Almost complete occlusion is similarly suggested by the 3D TOF MRA (**c**). Conversely, the CE MRA image (**d**) reveals the presence of a little residual flow (*arrow*) at the neck of the aneurysm. The corresponding 3D TOF MRA (e) acquired at 3T confirms the observation made in (**d**) of only incomplete occlusion of the aneurysm (*arrow*)

Vascular Malformations

The term vascular malformation is a generic term describing various congenital lesions that can be differentiated using McCormick's classification [100]:
1. Pial (parenchymal), dural or mixed arterial-venous malformations (AVM)
2. Venous angioma
3. Cavernous angioma
4. Capillary telangiectasia

Arterial-Venous Malformations (AVM)

AVM are congenital abnormalities of vascular development and differentiation. Pial AVM have variable dimensions and can occur anywhere in the brain or spine. They are composed of complex accumulations of vascular canals which have incomplete vascular walls that permit direct communication between the arterial and venous compartments, thereby by-passing the capillary-venous districts. The principle characteristic of pial AVM is the presence of a nidus consisting of numerous afferent and efferent vascular canals (afferent and ef-

ferent feeders). The size of the nidus is used to classify the AVM and to determine the appropriate course of treatment: small (<3 cm), medium (between 3 and 6 cm), and large (> 6 cm) [101]. For example, in most cases, radiotherapy is only successful if the nidus has a diameter of less than 3 cm.

The cerebral tissue that surrounds an AVM is generally involved and can demonstrate gliosis, calcifications, and hemosiderin deposits. These alterations can explain the frequent occurance of epilepsy or neurological deficit in patients with pial AVM. The annual probability of bleeding or other neurological complications in patients with AVM varies from 2 to 4% [102].

Dural AVM represent 15% of all AVM and are diagnosed predominantly in adults. They can be distinguished as dural arterial-venous malformations (DAVM) and dural arterial-venous fistulas (DAVF).

DAVM consist of a network of ectasic arterial and venous vessels contained within a venous sinus. They are for the most part acquired, often due to the progressive dilation of arterial-venous micro-fistulas that re-canalize a thrombus of a venous sinus. The transverse and sigmoid sinuses, and to a lesser extent the cavernous sinus, are most

Table 11. Accuracy of MRA versus DSA for diagnostic imaging of vascular malformations of the intracranial arterial vessels

Author	MRA Technique	# Pts	Vessels	Sensitivity	Specificity
Stock, 1995 [54]	MTS VFAE MRA	50		100%	100%
Mallouhi, 2002 [57]	CE MRA	82		100%	
	TOF MRA			64%	
Noguchi, 2004 [108]	3D TOF	15	Intracranial dural fistulas	100%[1]	100%
				76%[2]	86%

[1] multiple high-intensity curvilinear or nodular structures adjacent to the sinus wall
[2] high-intensity areas in the venous sinus

frequently involved. Conversely, the sagittal sinus is rarely involved. DAVM have a tendency to increase in size due to the hemodynamic alterations that they induce in the venous districts.

DAVF are often single and consist of a vessel (rarely more than one) that directly connects an artery with a vein or, more frequently, with a venous sinus, often at a high flow rate.

The symptoms associated with DAVM and DAVF depend upon the site involved and are usually linked to compression of the cranial nerves or to venous hypertension (as occurs when an AVM is located within the cavernous sinus).

In most cases both conventional MRI and MRA permit the diagnosis and characterization of AVM. In pial AVM, conventional MR can show the presence of abnormal vessels and associated parenchymal alterations, such as gliosis or the lack of hemosiderin in chronic bleeding. T2-weighted MR images in particular are able to demonstrate the presence of flow-void in high flow vessels. MRA is able to complement conventional MR by clearly showing the presence of a nidus which characterizes pial or parenchymal AVM. Conventional MR is less useful in identifying DAVF however especially of the posterior cranial fossa. Carotid-cavernous fistulas can be seen directly or due to the presence of indirect signs such as dilation of the superior ophthalmic vein and enlargement of the cavernous sinus (Fig. 33a-e).

The MRA technique most often used is 3D TOF, however, 2D/3D PC MRA with and without contrast agent is also used to characterize flow in abnormal vessels [103-107]. The accuracy values of MRA reported in the literature for the detection of AVM are shown in Table 11 [94, 96, 108] (Fig. 34a-e).

Unfortunately, information concerning the hemodynamics of AVM is often lacking with MRA. For example, despite the panoramic visualization achievable on MRA, accurate definition of the afferent and efferent vessels of the nidus is often poor. This is partly due to the low spatial resolution compared to DSA. The lack of temporal reso-

lution is another important limitation of MRA since hemodynamic data are essential for correct pre-treatment evaluation of AVM and other developmental abnormalities (DVA). To overcome these limitations, various authors have investigated the use of CE MRA [41, 109] and CE MR DSA techniques [86] for the characterization of AVM. The introduction of ultra fast sequences has permitted a dynamic or time resolved approach which permits differentiation of the efferent from the afferent vessels.

Among the advantages of the newer 2D CE MR DSA techniques is a temporal resolution of 1-2 sec which has proven satisfactory for studies of the intracranial arterial-venous circulation [86]. Although 3D CE MRA has also been used to study the vascular architecture of AVM, the longer acquisition times, although still less than a minute, are generally insufficient to permit satisfactory differentiation of the afferent vessels from the efferent vessels [41].

Although DSA is still the most accurate technique for the identification and characterization of AVM, it is impractical and dangerous to use routinely to monitor the progression of the pathology. In these cases 3D TOF MRA [110] and, more recently, CE MRA have proven to be valid alternatives for the planning and follow-up of radiosurgery.

Venous Angioma

Venous malformations (venous angioma) consist of deep small estasic venous vessels with a radial pattern which feed an elastic transcortical vein or, more rarely, a subependimal vein (Fig. 35a-c). They are not vascular malformations but anatomical variations or DVA [111]. DVA are most frequently seen in the frontal or cerebellar semioval centers. Since bleeding is comparatively rare, the cerebral tissue surrounding these malformations is normal. A slight probability of bleeding is present for the

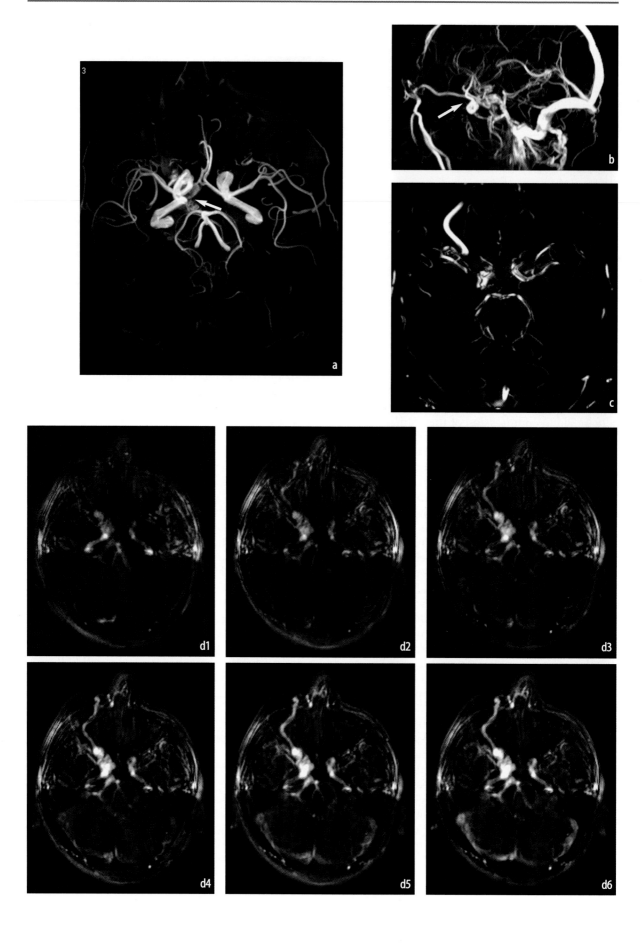

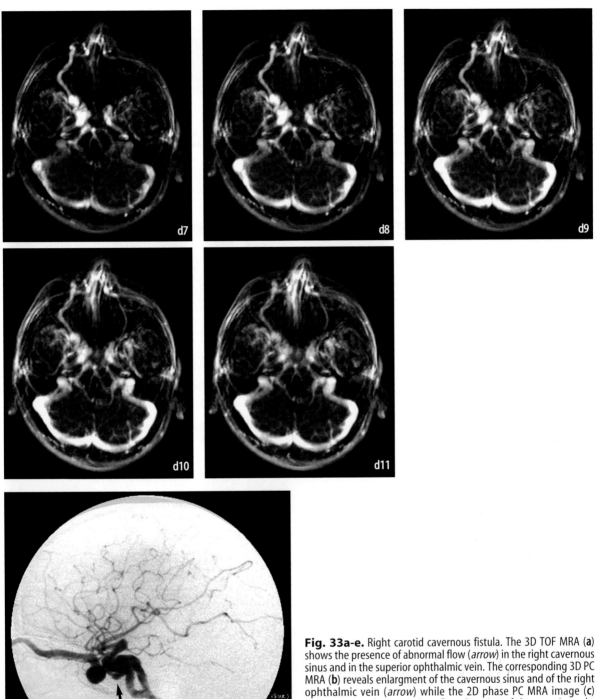

Fig. 33a-e. Right carotid cavernous fistula. The 3D TOF MRA (**a**) shows the presence of abnormal flow (*arrow*) in the right cavernous sinus and in the superior ophthalmic vein. The corresponding 3D PC MRA (**b**) reveals enlargment of the cavernous sinus and of the right ophthalmic vein (*arrow*) while the 2D phase PC MRA image (**c**) demonstrates the anomalous flow direction of the superior ophthalmic vein. The time-resolved CE MRA dynamic series (**d**) acquired in the axial plane with a temporal resolution of 1.2 seconds, reveals early enhancement of the enlarged cavernous sinus and of the ophthalmic vein. Selective DSA (**e**) of the right internal carotid artery confirms the presence of the direct fistula (*arrow*)

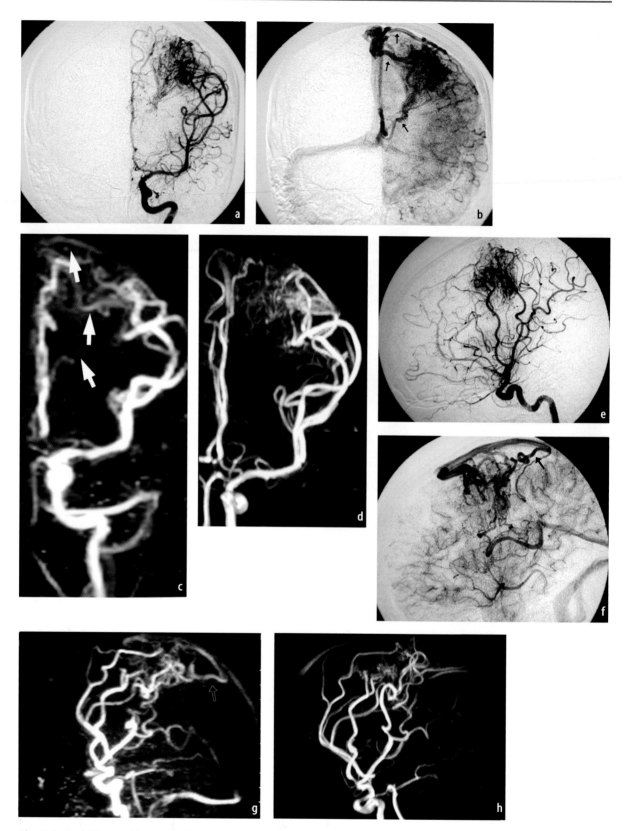

Fig. 34a-h. A 32-year-old woman with arterio-venous malformation (AVM). The frontal DSA angiograms (**a**, **b**) acquired in the arterial and early venous phases reveal a pial (parenchymal) AVM with multiple feeding vessels and large cortical nidus (a) and large cortical draining veins (*black arrows* in **b**). The 2D PC MRA image (**c**) shows the cortical draining veins (*white arrows*), while the nidus and arterial feeders are better shown on the 3D TOF MRA image (**d**). Lateral DSA angiograms (**e**, **f**) acquired in the arterial and early venous phases reval the nidus, and the arterial and venous (*black arrow* in **f**) feeders. The 2D PC MRA lateral view image (**g**) shows one of the large venous feeders (*black arrow*). However, this is not seen on 3D TOF MRA (**h**)

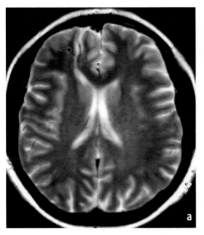 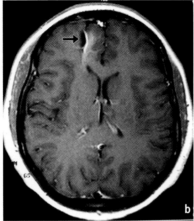 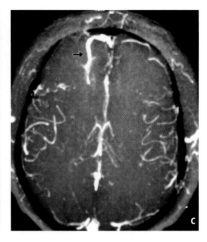

Fig. 35a-b. Right frontal venous angioma. The anomaly is clearly apparent on the T2-weighted (**a**) and contrast-enhanced T1-weighted (**b**) images as a linear vascular structure characterized by flow void and enhancement (*arrows*). The 3D TOF MRA image (**c**) acquired after injection of contrast agent reveals enhancement of the abnormal drainage due to slow flow

mixed form which is associated with venous and cavernous angiomas [112].

Most DVA are asymptomatic and are typically incidental findings. DVA are rarely visible on 3D TOF MRA because the flow within the vessels is very slow with characteristics similar to those of venous vessels. 3D PC MRA acquired with VENC values that range from 10-20 cm/sec are capable of revealing DVA, although the best techniques for identifying DVA are 2D and 3D CE MRA. Both are capable of visualizing the typical characteristics of DVA which include small deep veins flowing to the Medusa head (Caput medusa).

Cavernous Angioma

Cavernous angiomas are vascular malformations which can be seen not only in the brain and spine but also in the vertebra, liver and spleen. Cavernous angiomas are predominantly localized in the cerebral hemispheres but can also be seen in the cerebral trunk and the cerebellum. The presence of hemosiderin at the periphery of an angioma reflects the possibility that red blood cells are deposited outside the incomplete blood vessel for reasons other than bleeding. The probability of bleeding for cavernous angioma, seen on MRI as a breaking of the hemosiderin shell, is very low [113]. Cavernous angiomas are mostly asymptomatic but may induce neurological symptoms due to compression of cerebral structures. Epilepsy is the most common symptom when the lesion involves the cerebral cortex. Multiple cavernous angiomas with a positive family history are consid-

ered hereditary with an autosomal dominant characteristic [114].

The typical appearance of cavernous angiomas on MR include a hyperintense nucleus on T1- and T2-weighted images which reflects the presence of methemoglobin, and a hypointense delimiting ring on T2-weighted images (above all on T2w GRE images) due to the presence of hemosiderin. The most sensitive MR imaging sequence for multiple angiomas is T2w GRE, which should always be included in the scan protocol.

Cavernous angiomas were historically referred to as cryptic angiomas because they were not visible with cerebral angiography. Usually cerebral angiography is not requested except in cases in which a mixed form is suspected. For the same reason, MRA is not typically employed in cases of cavernous angioma. In the case of 3D TOF MRA, the acquisition may be affected by the short T1 of the methaemoglobin component of the malformation.

Capillary Telangectasia

Capillary telangectasia is defined as a mass of dilated capillaries which have an incomplete vascular wall often surrounded by normal cerebral tissue and frequently located in the pons [115]. Gliosis or hemosiderin may be present in the area surrounding the lesion. Patients with capillary telangectasia are usually asymptomatic and diagnosis is typically incidental on contrast enhanced MR examinations. Most capillary telangectasia are too small to be detected by MRA and in most cases by cerebral angiography too.

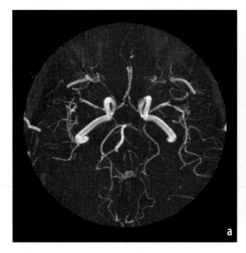
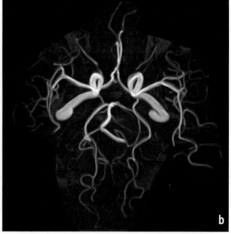

Fig. 36a-b. 3D TOF MRA of the intracranial arteries at 1.5T (**a**) and 3T (**b**). An overall higher signal of all intracranial arteries with better visualization of cortical branches is evident at 3T

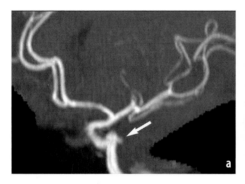
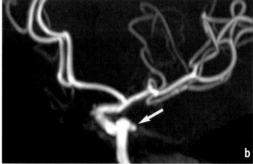

Fig. 37a-b. 3D TOF MRA at 1.5T (**a**) shows the presence of a very small aneurysm of the cavernous ICA (*arrow*). However, better depiction of the aneurysm (*arrow*) is achieved on 3D TOF MRA at 3T (**b**) due to improvements in signal and spatial resolution

Future Perspectives: Intracranial MRA at 3 Tesla

As discussed above the major limitations of MRA at present relate to the relatively low spatial and temporal resolution compared to DSA. Improvents in these areas are essential if MRA is to compete successfully for the evaluation of vascular malformations and other vascular pathologies.

An area which will undoubtedly see rapid progress is in MR imaging at higher magnetic field strengths. It is well established that imaging at higher field strength results in greater SNR, increased vessel-tissue contrast and increased tissue T1 relaxation time. All of these aspects are important for MRA since higher resolution can be obtained, without any loss in signal.

Although little has yet been reported in the lit-erature, preliminary reports have revealed a higher sensitivity of unenhanced 3D TOF MRA at 3T compared to unenhanced 3D TOF MRA at 1.5T for the visualization of small branches of the middle, posterior and anterior cerebral arteries [116] (Fig. 36a-b). More interestingly, a higher sensitivity of 3D TOF MRA at 3T has been reported for the depiction of cerebral aneurysms when compared to DSA [117] (Fig. 37a-b).

Although published data on the application of 3D CE MRA at 3T are not yet available, initial indications suggest the improved suppression of background tissue at higher field strength will markedly benefit the clinical applications for 3D CE MRA of the intracranial vasculature.

Thank you to A. Iadanza and L. Serra for help with the acquisition of images.

References

1. Carriero A, Delle Monache C, Cuonzo G et al (1990) Angiorafia a Risonanza Magnetica del circolo intracranico. Tecnica-anatomia. Radiol med. 80:588-593

2. Pernicone JR, Potchen EJ (1993) Intracranial vascular anatomy. In Potchen EJ, Haacke EM, Siebert JE et al Magnetic Resonance Angiography, St Louis, Mosby

3. Stock WK, Wetzel S, Kirsch E et al (1996) Anatomic evaluation of the circle of Willis: MR Angiography versus Intraarterial Digital Subtraction Angiography. AJNR Am J Neuroradiol 17:1495-1499

4. Katz DA, Marks MP, Napel SA et al (1995) Circle of Willis: evaluation with spiral CT angiography, MR angiography and conventional angiography. Radiology 195:445-449

5. Barboriak DP, Provenzale JM (1997) Pictorial review: magnetic resonance angiography of arterial variants at the Circle of Willis. Clin Radiol 52:429-436

6. Hoksbergen AW, Majoie CB, Hulsmans FJ et al (2003) Assesment of the collateral function of the circle of Willis: three-dimensional time-of-flight MR angiography compared with transcranial color-coded duplex sonograpy. AJNR Am J Neuroradiol 24:456-462

7. Kusunoki K, Oka Y, Saito M et al (1999) Changes in visibility of intracranial arteries on MRA with normal ageig. Neuroradiology 41:813-819

8. Uchino A, Kato A, Takase Y et al (2000) Persistent trigeminal artery variants detecected by MR angiogrphy. Eur Radiol. 10(11):1801-4

9. Friedlander RM, Oglivy CS (1996) Aneurysmal subarachnoid hemorrhage in a patient with bilateral A1 fenestrations associated with an azygos anterior cerebral artery. Case report and literature review. J Neurosurg. Apr; 84(4):681-4

10. Uchino A, Kato A, Takase Y et al (2000) Middle cerebral artery variations detected by magnetic resonance angiography. Eur Radiol. 10:560-563

11. Wentz KU, Rother J, Schwartz A et al (1994) Intracranial vertebrobasilar system: MR angiography. Radiology 190:105-110

12. Goldstein JH, Woodcock R, Do HM et al (1999) Complete duplication or extreme fenestration of the basilar artery. AJNR Am J Neuroradiol. Jan; 20(1):149-50

13. Liebeskind DS (2003) Collateral circulation. Stroke. Sep; 34(9):2279-84. Epub 2003 Jul 24

14. Ayanzen RH, Bird CR, Keller PJ et al (2000) Cerebral MR venography: normal anatomy and potential diagnostic pitfalls. AJNR Am J Neuroradiol 21:74-78

15. Carriero A, Cuonzo G, Iezzi A et al (1992) Venogramma con Risonanza Magnetica del circolo intracranico. Tecnica, anatomia, indicazioni. Rad Med 83:182-191

16. Shane Tubbs R, Jerry Oakes W. (2002) Letter to the Editor. Neuroanatomy, volume 1, p. 14

17. Curè JK, Van Tassel P et al (1994) Normal and variant anatomy of the dural venous sinuses. Semin Ultrasound CT MR 15:499-519

18. Shigematsu Y, Korogi Y, Hirai T et al (1999) 3D TOF turbo MR angiography for intracranial arter-

19. ies: phantom and clinical studies. J Magn Reson Imaging 10:939-944

20. Oelerich M, Lentschig MG, Zunker P et al (1998) Intracranial vascular stenosis and occlusion: comparison of 3D time-to-flight and 3D phase-contrast MR angiography. Neuroradiology 40:567-573

21. Blatter DD, Parker DL, Robinson RO (1991) Cerebral MR angiography with multiple overlapping thin-slab acquisition.I. Quantitative analysis of vessel visibility. Radiology 179:805-811

22. Blatter DD, Parker DL, Ahn SS et al (1992) Cerebral MR Angiography with multiple overlapping thin slab acquisition II. Early clinical experience. Radiology 183:379-389

23. Liu K, Rutt BK (1998) Sliding interleaved kY (SLINKY) acquisition: a novel 3D MRA technique with suppressed slab boundary artifact. J Magn Reson Imaging. Jul-Aug 8(4):903-11

24. Dagirmanjian A, Ross JS, Obuchowski N et al (1995) High resolution, magnetization transfer saturation, variable flip angle, time-of-flight MRA in the detection of intracranial vascular stenoses. J Comput Assist Tomogr. Sep-Oct; 19(5):700-6

25. Nagele T, Klose U, Grodd W et al (1995) Nonlinear excitation profiles for three-dimensional inflow MR angiography. J Magn Reson Imaging. Jul-Aug; 5(4):416-20

26. Catalano C, Pavone P, Laghi A et al (1995) Clementi M, Di Girolamo M, Albertini Petroni G, Passariello R Magnetic resonance angiography of the intracranial circle using magnetization transfer contrast (MTC). Radiol Med. Mar; 89(3):245-9

27. Creasy J, Price R, Presbrery T et al (1990) Gadolinium enhanced MR angiography. Radiology 175:280-283

28. Tartaro A, Severini S, Tonni G et al (1992) Magnetic resonance angiography with gadolinium (Gd-DTPA) versus baseline magnetic resonance angiography in the study of the intracranial circulation. Radiol Med (Torino). 84:536-43

29. Parker DL, Goodrich KC, Alexander AL et al (1998) Optimized visualization of vessel in contrast enhanced intracranial MR angiography. Magn Reson Med 40:873-882

30. Parker DL, Tsuruda JS, Goodrich KC et al (1998) Contrast-enhanced magnetic resonance angiography of cerebral arteries. A review. Invest Radiol 33:560-572

31. Petersen D, Klose U (1997) Indications for contrast medium administration in MR-angiography of cerebral blood vessels. Radiologe 37:508-14

32. Korosec FR, Frayne R, Grist TM et al (1996) Time resolved contrast-enhanced 3D MR angiography. Magn reson. Med 36:345-351

33. Duran M, Schoenberg SO, Yuh WT et al (2002) Cerebral arteriovenus malformations: morphologic evaluation by ultrashort 3D gadolinium-enhanced MR angiography. Eur Radiol 12:2957-2964

34. Suzuki M, Matsui O, Ueda F et al (2002) Contrast-enhanced MR angiography (enhanced 3-D fast gradient echo) for diagnosis of cerebral aneurysms. Neuroradiology 44:17-20

35. Metens T, Rio F, Baleriaux D et al (2000) Intracranial aneurysms: detection with gadolinium-enhanced dynamic three-dimensional MR angiography-initial results. Radiology 216:39-46

35. Klisch J, Strecker R, Hennig J et al (2000) Time-resolved projection MRA: clinical application in intracranial vascular malformations. Neuroradiology 42:104-107

36. Weiger M, Pruessmann KP, Kassner A et al (2000) Contrast-enhanced 3D MRA using SENSE. J Magn Reson Imaging 12:671-677

37. Sodickson DK, McKenzie CA, Li W, Wolff S et al (2000) Contrast-enhanced 3D MR angiography with simultaneous acquisition of spatial harmonics: A pilot study. Radiology 217:284-289

38. Liauw L, van Buchem MA, Slipt A et al (2000) MR angiography of the intracranial venous system. Radiology 214:678-682

39. Walker MF, Souza SP, Domoulin CL (1988) Quantitative flow measurement in phase contrast MR angiography. JCAT 12:304-313

40. Bass JC, Prince MR, Londy FJ et al (1997) Effect of gadolinium on phase-contrast MR angiography of the renal arteries. AJR 168:261-266

41. Suzuki M, Matsui O, Kobayashi K et al (2003) Contrast-enhanced MRA for investigation of cerebral arteriovenus malformations. Neuroradiology 45:231-235

42. Bogousslavsky J, Van Melle G, Regli F et al (1988) The Lausanne stroke registry: analysis of 1000 consecutive patients with first stroke. Stroke 19:1083-1092

43. Caplan LR (1989) Intracranial branch atheromatous disease: a neglected, understudied and underused concept. Neurology 39:1246-1250

44. Chimowitz MI, Kokkinos J, Strong J et al (1995) The warfarin-aspirin symptomatic intracranial disease study. Neurology 45:1488-1493

45. Norrving B, Lowenhielm P (1988) Epidemiology of stroke in Lund-Orup, Sweden 1983-85. Acta Neurol Scand 78:408-413

46. Fujita N, Hirabuki N, Fujii K et al (1994) MR imaging of middle cerebral artery stenosis and occlusion: value of MR angiography. AJNR 15:335-341

47. Furst G, Hofer M, Steinmetz H et al (1996) Intracranial stenoocclusive disease: MR angiography with magnetization transfer and variable flip angle. AJNR 17:1749-1757

48. Heiserman JE, Drayer BP, Keller PJ et al (1992) Intracranial vascular stenosis and occlusion: evaluation with three-dimensional time-of-flight MR angiography. Radiology 185:667-673

49. Korogi Y, Takahasi M, Nakagawa T et al (1994) Intracranial vascular stenosis and occlusion: diagnostic accuracy of three-dimensional, Fourier transform, time-of-flight MR angiography. Radiology 193:187-193

50. Korogi Y, Takahasi M, Nakagawa T et al (1997) Intracranial vascular stenosis and occlusion: MR angiographic findings. AJNR 18:135-143

51. Ley-Pozo J, Reingelstein EB (1990) Noninvasive detection of occlusive disease of the carotid syphon and middle cerebral artery. Ann Neurol 28:640-647

52. Uehara T, Mori E, Tabuchi M et al (1994) Detection of occlusive lesions in intracranial arteries by three-dimensional time-of-flight magnetic resonance angiography. Cerebrovasc Dis 4:365-370

53. Keston P, Murray AD, Jackson A (2003) Cerebral Perfusion imaging using contrast-enhanced MRI. Clinical Radioloy July 505-513

54. Stock KW, Radue EW, Jacob AL et al (1995) Intracranial arteries: prospective blinded comparative study of MR angiography and DSA in 50 patients. Radiology 35:822-829

55. Hirai T, Korogi Y, Ono K et al (2002) Prospective valuation of suspected stenoocclusive disease of the intracranial artery: combined MR angiography and CT angiography compared with digital subtraction angiography. AJNR 23:93-101

56. Masaryk TJ, Modic MT, Ross JS et al (1989) Intracranial circulation: preliminary results with three-dimensional (volume) MR angiography. Radiology 171:793-799

57. Mallouhi A, Chemelli A, Judmaier W et al (2002) Investigation of cerebrovascular disease with MR angiography: comparison of volume rendering and maximum intensity projection algorithms - initial assessment. Neuroradiology. Dec; 44(12):961-7. Epub 2002 Nov 15

58. Nederkoorn PJ, van der Graaf Y, Hunink MGM et al (2003) Duplex ultrasound and magnetic resonance angiography compared with digital subtraction angiography in carotid artery stenosis. Stroke 34:1324

59. Heiserman JE, Dean BL, Hodak JA et al (1994) Neurologic complications of cerebral angiography. AJNR 15:1401-1407

60. Jung HW, Chang KH, Choi DS et al (1995) Contrast-enhanced MR angiography for the diagnosis of intracranial vascular disease: optimal dose of gadopentate dimeglutamine. AJR Am J Roentgenol 165:1251-1255

61. Mathews VP, Ulmer JL, White ML et al (1999) Depiction of intracranial vessels with MRA: utility of magnetization transfer saturation and gadolinium. J Comput Assist Tomogr 23:597-602

62. Yang JJ, Hill MD, Morrish WF et al (2002) Comparison of pre and postcontrast 3D Time-of-Flight MR Angiography for the evaluation f distal intracranial branch occlusions in acute ischemic stroke. AJNR, April 23:557-567

63. Gorelick PB, Caplan LR, Hier DB et al (1984) Racial differences in the distribution of anterior circulation occlusive disease. Neuroradiology 34:54-59

64. Inizitari D, Hachinski VC, Taylor DW et al (1990) Racial differences in the anterior circulation in cerebrovascular disease. How much can be explained by risk factors? Arch Neurol 47:1080-1084

65. Griffths PD, Worthy S, Gholkar A (1996) Incidental intracranial vascular pathology in patients investigated for carotid stenosis. Neuroradiology 38:25-30

66. Wityk RJ, Lehman D, Klang M et al (1996) Race and sex differences in the distribution of cerebral atherosclerosis. Stroke 27:1974-1980

67. Farb RI, Scott JN, Willinsky RA et al (2003) Intracranial venous system: gadolinium-enhanced three-dimensional MR venography with auto-triggered elliptic centric-ordered sequence—initial experience. Radiology. 226:203-109

68. Juvela S, Porrai M, Heiskanen O (1993) Natural History of unruptured intracranial aneurysm: a long term follow-up study. J Neurosurg 79:174-182

69. Schievink WI, Piepgras DG Wirth FP (1992) Ruptured of previously documented small asympto-

matic saccular intracranial aneurysm. J Neurosurg
76:1019-1024

70. Ronkainen A, Hernesnien J, Ryyananen M et al
(1994) A 10% prevalence of asymptomatic familial
intracranial aneurysms: preliminary report on 110
MRA studies in members of 21 Finnish familial intracranial aneurysm families. Neurosurgery 35:9-
19

71. Rinne J, Hernesniemi J, Puranen M et al (1994)
Multiple intracranial aneurysms in a defined population: prospective angiographic and clinical
study. Neurosurgery 35:803-808

72. Takahashi T, Suzuki S, Ohkuma H et al (1994)
Aneurysms at a duplication of middle cerebral artery. AJNR 15:1166-1168

73. Ahmad I, Tominaga T, Suzuki M et al (1994) Primitive trigeminal artery associated with cavernous
aneurysm: case report. Surg Neurol 41:75-79

74. Osborn AG (1994) Intracranial Aneurysms. In Diagnostic Neuroradiology. St Louis: Mosby, 248-283

75. Ruggieri PM, Poulos N, Masaryk TJ, et al (1994)
Occult intracranial aneurysms in polycystic kidney
disease: screening with MRA. Radiology 191:33-39

76. Buckingham MJ, Crone KR, Ball WS et al (1998)
Traumatic intracranial aneurysms in childhood:
two cases and review of the literature. Neurosurgery 22:398-408

77. Barami K, Ko K (1994) Ruptured mycotic
aneurysm as an intraparenchimal hemorrhage and
nonadjacent acute subdural hematoma: case report and review of the literature. Surg Neurol
41:290-293

78. Lawrence-Friedl D, Bauer KM (1992) Bilateral cortical blindness: an unusual presentation of bacterial endocarditis. An Emer Med 21:1502-1504

79. Gobin YP, Counord JL, Flaud P et al (1994) In vitro
study of haemodynamics in a giant saccular
aneurysm model: influence of flow dynamics in
the parent vessel and effects of coil embolisation.
Neuroradiology 36:530-536

80. Grandin CB, Mathurin P, Duprez T et al (1998) Diagnosis of intracranial aneurysms: accuracy of MR
angiography at 0,5 T. AJNR Am J Neuroradiol
19:245-252

81. Harrison MJ, Johnson BA, Gardner GM et al (1997)
Preliminary results on the management of unruptured intracranial aneurysms with magnetic resonance angiography and computed tomography
angiography. Neurosurgery 40:947-955

82. Huston J, Nichols DA, Luetmer PH et al (1994)
Blinded prospective evaluation of sensitivity of
MR angiography to known intracranial
aneurysms: importance of aneurysm size. AJNR
Am J Neuroradiol 15:1607-1614

83. Chung TS, Joo JY, Lee SK et al (1999) Evaluation of
cerebral aneurysms with high-resolution MR angiography using section interpolation technique:
correlation with digital subtraction angiography.
AJNR Am J Neuroradiol 20:229-235

84. Atlas SW, Sheppard L, Goldberg HI et al (1997) Intracranial aneurysms: detection and characterization with MR angiography with use of an advanced
postprocessing technique in a blinded-reader
study. Radiology 203:807-14

85. Brunereau L, Cottier JP, Sonier CB et al (1999)
Prospective evaluation of time-of flight MR an-

giography in the follow-up of intracranial saccular
aneurysms treated with Guglielmi detachable coils.
J Comput Assist Tomogr 23:216-223

86. Mori H, Aoki S, Okubo Tet al (2002) Two dimensional thick-slice MR digital subtraction angiography in the assesment of small to medium-size intracranial arteriovenus malformations. Neuroradiology

87. Korogi Y, Takahashi M, Katada K et al (1999) Intracranial aneurysms: detection with three dimensional CT angiography with volume rendering-
comparison with conventional angiographic and
surgical findings. Radiology 211:497-506

88. Korogi Y, Takahashi, Mabuchi N et al (1994) Intracranial aneurysm: diagnostic accuracy of three-
dimensional Fourier transform, time-of-flight MR
angiography. Radiology 193:181-186

89. Okahara M, Kiyosue H, Yamashita M et al (2002)
Diagnostic accuracy of magnetic resonance angiography for cerebral aneurysms in correlation
with 3D-digital subtraction angiographic images:
a study of 133 aneurysms. Stroke 33:1803-8

90. Kadota T, Hosomi N, Kuroda C et al (1997) [Un-
ruptured intracranial aneurysms: evaluation with
high-resolution MR angiography with magnetic
transfer contrast (MTC) and tilted optimized non-
saturating excitation (TONE)]. Nippon Igaku
Hoshasen Gakkai Zasshi 57:853-9

91. Raaymakers TWM, Buys PC, Verbeeten B Jr et al
(1999) MR Angiography as a screening tool for intracranial aneurysms: feasibility, test characteristics, and interobserver agreement. AJR 1469-1475

92. Ross JS, Masaryk TJ, Modic MT et al (1990) Intracranial aneurysms: evaluation by MR angiography. AJR 11:159-165

93. Jager HR, Ellamushi H, Moore EA et al (2000) Contrast-enhanced MR angiography of intracranial giant aneurysms. AJNR 21:1900-1907

94. Rollen P, Sze G (1998) Small patent cerebral
aneurysms: atypical appearances at 1,5 –T MR imaging. Radiology 208:129-136

95. Strotzer M, Fellner C, Fraunhofer S et al (1998)
Dedicated head-neck coil in MR angiography of
the supra-aortic arteries from the aortic arch to the
circle of Willis. Acta Radiol. 39:249-56

96. Mallouhi A, Felber S, Chemelli A et al (2003) Detection and characterization of intracranial
aneurysms with MR angiography: comparison of
volume-rendering and maximum-intensity-projection algorithms. AJR Am J Roentgenol. Jan;
180(1):55-64

97. Anzalone N, Righi C, Simionato F et al (2000)
Three-dimensional time-of-flight MR angiography
in the evaluation of intracranial aneurysms treated
with Guglielmi detachable coils. AJNR Am J Neuroradiol. 21:746-52

98. Cottier JP, Bleuzen-Couthon A, Gallas S et al
(2003) Intracranial aneurysms treated with
Guglielmi detachable coils: is contrast material
necessary in the follow-up with 3D time-of-flight
MR angiography? AJNR Am J Neuroradiol.
24:1797-1803

99. Yamada N, Hayashi K, Murao K et al (2004) Time-
of-flight MR angiography targeted to coiled intracranial aneurysms is more sensitive to residual
flow than is digital subtraction angiography. AJNR

Am J Neuroradiol. 25:1154-1157

100. McCormick WF (1966) The pathology of vascular ("arteriovenous") malformations. J Neurosurg 24:807-816

101. Spetzer RF, Martin NA (1986) A proposed grading system for arteriovenous malformations. J Neurosurgery 65:476-483

102. Ondra S, Troupp H, Gorge Ed et al (1990) Natural history of symptomatic arteriovenous malformations of the brain: a 24 year followup assessment. J Neurosurg 73:387-391

103. Ducreux D, Trystram D, Oppenheim C et al (2001) Diagnostic imaging of brain arteriovenus malformations. Neurochirurgie 47:190-200

104. Nussel F, Wegmuller H, Huber P (1991) Comparison of magnetic resonance angiography, magnetic resonance imaging and conventional angiography in cerebral arteriovenus malformation. Neuroradiology 33:56-61

105. Tanabe S, Honmou O, Minamida Y et al (2001) Advantages of T2 reversed fast spin-echo image and enhanced three-dimensional surface MR angiography for the diagnosis of cerebral arteriovenus malformations. Prog CI 23:165-175

106. Edelman RR, Wentz KU, Mattle HP et al (1989) Intracerebral arteriovenus malformations: evaluation with selective MR angiography and venography. Radiology 173:831-837

107. Essig M, Engenhart R, Knopp MV et al (1996) Cerebral arteriovenous malformations: improved nidus demarcation by means of dynamic tagging MR-angiography. Magn Reson Imaging 14:227-233

108. Noguchi K, Melhem ER, Kanazawa T (2004) Intracranial dural arteriovenous fistulas: evaluation with combined 3D time-of-flight MR angiography and MR digital subtraction angiography. AJR Am J Roentgenol. 182:183-90

109. Takano K, Utsunomiya H, Ono H et al (1999) Dynamic contrast-enhanced subtraction MR angiography in intracranial vascular abnormalities. Eur Radiol 9:1909-1912

110. Kauczor HU, Engenhart R, Layer G et al (1993) 3D TOF MR angiography of AVMs after radiosurgery. J Comput Assist Tomogr 17:184-190

111. Lasjaunias O, Burrows P, Placet C (1986) Developmental venous anomalies (DVA): the so-called venous angioma, Neurosurg Rev 9:233-244

112. Osterton B, Solymosi L (1993) MRA of cerebral developmental anomalies: its role in differential diagnosis, Neuroradiol 35:97-104

113. Robinson JR, Awad IA, Little JR (1991) Natural history of the cavernous angioma, J Neurosurg 75:709-714

114. Rigamonti D, Hadley MN, Drayer BP et al (1988) Cerebral cavernous malformations: incidence and familial occurence. N Engl J Med 319:343-347

115. Rigamonti D, Johnson PC, Spetzler RF et al (1991) Cavernous malformations and capillary telangectasia: a spectrum within a single pathological entity, Neurosurg 28:60-64

116. Willinek WA, Born M, Simon B et al (2003) Time-of-flight MR angiography: comparison of 3.0-T imaging and 1.5-T imaging-initial experience. Radiology 229:913-920

117. Gibbs GF, Huston J 3rd, Bernstein MA et al (2004) Improved image quality of intracranial aneurysms: 3.0-T versus 1.5-T time-of-flight MR angiography. AJNR Am J Neuroradiol. 25:84-87

SECTION IV

Thorax

IV.1

MR Angiography of the Thoracic Aorta

Günther Schneider

Clinical Indications

Contrast enhanced MRA of the thoracic aorta has long been established as the imaging modality of choice in clinical routine for a variety of pathologic conditions as well as for congenital malformations. In newborns, children and young adults as well as in patients with congenital heart disease the thoracic aorta in most cases is imaged because of a suspected congenital malformation.

Imaging can be performed either to establish the diagnosis or to follow up patients with congenital heart disease. One of the big advantages of contrast enhanced MRA is the possibility to combine non-invasive luminal imaging of the aorta with flow measurements and imaging of extraaortic structures without recourse to ionising radiation or potentially nephrotoxic iodinated contrast media. Further details concerning imaging of pediatric patients are given in chapter VIII.

Concerning elderly patients the thoracic aorta is a frequent focus of arteriosclerotic disease, which can present as either a chronic condition or a life threatening acute condition. For patients with life threatening acute conditions such as aortic trauma or acute aortic dissection, the need for speed, scanner availability and ease of patient management make CT and CTA more favorable diagnostic options for disease evaluation. However, for all other pathologies MRA should at least be considered a viable alternative method if not the imaging modality of choice.

One of the big advantages of contrast enhanced MRA compared with catheter angiography is the possibility to depict the vessel wall and the soft tissue adjacent to a vessel [1]. This can be very useful in patients with acute aortic syndromes in whom intramural hematoma can only be diagnosed by means of cross sectional imaging if the lesion does not have such a large extent (see Fig. 22) [2]. The same holds true for valve pathologies such as congenital bicuspid aortic valve or degenerative-like stenosis or insufficiency of the aortic valve. For this latter condition also the valvular function of the aorta can be imaged with very high accuracy on MRI [3].

Combination of MRA with flow measurements permits quantification of the regurgitation fraction in valve insufficiency as well as estimation of the pressure gradient over a stenosis in conditions affecting the pulmonary and aortic valve and stenotic areas in general.

If evaluation of the thoracic aorta is necessary, cross sectional imaging should be performed in addition to MRA in order to gain as much information as possible about a lesion. In certain cases it may also be important to look at the anatomy of the left ventricle to determine whether aortic insufficiency or stenosis has resulted in dilatation of the left ventricle since this may increase the need for surgery.

Normal Anatomy

The aorta as a complete vessel commences at the upper part of the left ventricle, where it is about 3 cm in diameter. After ascending for a short distance, it arches backward and to the left side, over the root of the left lung. It then descends within the thorax on the left side of the vertebral column, passes into the abdominal cavity through the aortic hiatus in the diaphragm and ends, considerably diminished in size (about 1.75 cm in diameter), opposite the lower border of the fourth lumbar vertebra, by dividing into the right and left common iliac arteries.

Accepted practice is to divide the aorta into three distinct and arbitrary sections: the ascending aorta, the arch of the aorta, and the descending aorta. The descending aorta is then further divided into the thoracic aorta and the abdominal aorta.

The ascending aorta is about 5 cm in length. It commences at the upper part of the base of the left ventricle, on a level with the lower border of the third costal cartilage behind the left half of the sternum; it passes obliquely upward, forward, and to the right, in the direction of the axis of the heart, as high as the upper border of the second right costal cartilage, describing a slight curve in its course, and being situated, about 6 cm behind the posterior surface of the sternum. At its origin three small dilatations called the aortic sinuses are present, opposite the segments of the aortic valve. At the union of the ascending aorta with the aortic arch the caliber of the vessel is increased, owing to a bulging of its right wall. This dilatation is termed the bulb of the aorta, and on transverse section has a somewhat oval shape. The ascending aorta is contained within the pericardium, and is enclosed in a tube of serous pericardium, which is common to this and the pulmonary artery. Thus a rupture of the wall of the ascending aorta, as occurs for example in aortic dissection, may lead to a life threatening hemopericardium, even if the rupture itself is not that dramatic. The only branches of the ascending aorta are the two coronary arteries which supply the heart; they arise near the start of the aorta immediately above the attached margins of the semilunar valves.

The arch of the aorta begins at the level of the upper border of the second sternocostal articulation of the right side. Initially the arch runs upward, backward, and to the left in front of the trachea. It then runs backwards on the left side of the trachea and finally passes downward on the left side of the body of the fourth thoracic vertebra, at the lower border of which it becomes continuous with the descending aorta. It thus forms two curvatures: one with its convexity upward, and the other with its convexity forward and to the left. Its upper border is usually about 2.5 cm below the superior border to the manubrium sterni. Three vessels branch off from the arch of the aorta: the innominate, the left common carotid, and the left subclavian [4].

In the fetal aorta, considerable narrowing of the lumen between the origin of the left subclavian artery and the attachment of the ductus arteriosus leads to formation of the aortic isthmus. Immediately beyond the ductus arteriosus the fetal aorta also presents a fusiform dilation termed the aortic spindle which is the point of junction of the two parts. This is marked in the arch concavity by an indentation or angle. These conditions may persist, to some extent, in the adult, where the average diameter of the spindle exceeds that of the isthmus by roughly 3 mm [5].

The thoracic aorta starts after the arch of the aorta and runs down to the diaphragm whereupon the abdominal aorta begins (Figs. 1, 2). Numerous vessels branch off from the thoracic aorta to supply oxygenated blood to the chest cage and the organs within the chest. Like other sections of the aorta (the ascending aorta, aortic arch and abdominal aorta), the thoracic aorta is an arbitrary anatomic entity.

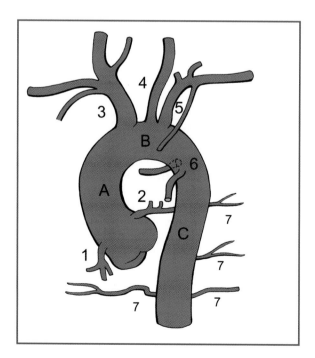

Fig. 1. Normal anatomy of the aorta in the thorax
A Ascending aorta
B Aortic arch
C Descending aorta (thoracic aorta)
1 Right coronary artery
2 Left coronary artery
3 Brachiocephalic trunk
4 Left common carotid artery
5 Left subclavian artery
6 Bronchial arteries
7 Right and left intercostal arteries

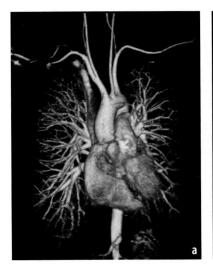
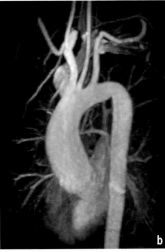

Fig. 2a, b. a Volume rendered CE MRA image of the normal anatomy of the aorta. Note the accurate depiction of the supraaortic vessels (Gd-BOPTA, 0.1 mmol/kg). **b** MIP reconstruction (*lateral view*) of another CE MRA study (Gd-BOPTA, 0.1 mmol/kg)

Patient Preparation

Patients are imaged in the supine position and if possible the arms should be placed above the head to avoid aliasing. In general it is important to cushion the arms carefully if positioned above the head because otherwise the patient may feel uncomfortable or the arms may become numb. This may result in movement of the patient and hence unsatisfactory image quality. If a patient is not able to hold his arms above the head for a sufficient time, cross-sectional imaging (e.g. T1w, T2w, or CINE imaging) can be performed first so that the patient then only has to lift his arms for the duration of the CE MRA examination. A modified imaging strategy may be required for patients who are totally unable to place the arms above the head. Instead of acquiring coronal sections, this may involve positioning the slab for the contrast enhanced MRA scan oblique sagittal to avoid aliasing.

Since it is necessary to perform imaging during breath-hold, the patient should be instructed to do this in slight expiration in order to avoid too great a pressure in the thorax and the possibility of insufficient compactness of the bolus. In order to achieve comparable physiologic conditions, it is important that the patient performs a similar breath-hold for the test bolus examination as for the final CE MRA exam: if the test bolus is done during free breathing and the CE MRA scan during breath-hold significant mistiming may occur.

Since ECG-gating is mandatory for both high resolution cross-sectional dark-blood imaging and CINE imaging of the thorax, either an ECG or a pulse sensor should be attached to the patient prior to the start of the examination.

Technique

A standard body coil generally provides sufficient signal for imaging of the thoracic aorta. However, a phased array torso-coil may significantly increase the signal-to-noise ratio (SNR) resulting in superior image quality and better depiction of smaller vessels. If a phased-array coil is used and the supra-aortic vessels are of clinical interest, then the neck should be included in the evaluation as well. In such cases it is important to fix the phased array-coil adequately in order to prevent movement and malpositioning of the coil in response to repetitive breath-holding of the patient.

Since the anatomy of the thoracic aorta can be variable and complex due to the underlying disease, extensive localizer imaging should be performed prior to positioning the slab for the final contrast enhanced MRA scan. In some cases, for example in patients with extensive kinking of the descending aorta, this may even necessitate positioning the slab sagittal rather than coronal in order to include the whole aorta in the slab.

In patients with sudden onset of thoracic pain for whom ischemic heart disease or acute heart infarct can be excluded, additional dark blood cross-sectional imaging prior to the contrast enhanced study should be performed to detect possible intramural hematoma of the aorta. This condition may sometimes be missed on contrast enhanced T1w images since the hematoma may have a similar high signal to the contrast enhanced lumen [2].

In general breath-holding significantly increases the quality of images. However, if only the descending aorta is of interest even non-breath-hold CE MRA may provide good image quality.

As with all contrast enhanced MRA examinations, it is essential to accurately time the contrast bolus either with an automatic system, interactively by applying MR fluoroscopy or by means of a test bolus. However, automatic triggering systems may not always give optimal results for imaging of the thoracic aorta since the need to perform breath-hold after the arrival of the bolus may result not only in the thoracic aorta being missed, but also in an overlay of venous structures due to early filling of the jugular veins.

At our institution we typically use a test bolus for examinations of the thoracic aorta. The slice level for the test bolus examination is positioned so as to permit visualization of sections of both the ascending aorta and the descending aorta. In this way information is obtained about the delay of filling of the descending versus the ascending aorta. This may be particularly important in cases of coarctation of the aorta or in large aneurysms which may take some time to fill completely. Another clinical scenario in which it may be important to acquire additional information on the dynamics of enhancement is in cases of aortic dissection.

On new state-of-the-art equipment it is now possible to perform two separate MRA studies, the first with a slightly decreased spatial but highly increased temporal resolution and the second with a greatly increased spatial resolution. The first study is aimed at depicting the aorta and obtaining information on dynamics of enhancement and bolus timing, while the second is performed for diagnostic purposes.

As mentioned above, the 3D MRA volume acquisition may be performed in the coronal, sagittal or in an oblique orientation, depending on the anatomy of the patient and his ability to position the arms above the head.

In patients with an enlarged sagittal extension of the aorta, coronal plane imaging requires more sections and thus may be too long to complete in a single breath-hold. In these cases a sagittal acquisition should be performed in order to evaluate the entire thoracic aorta with fewer slices. However, the final choice of whether to perform imaging in the sagittal, coronal or oblique plane depends on the aortic anatomy as displayed on the localizer images.

To ensure complete coverage of the thoracic anatomy an unenhanced scan should be performed first. This scan should later be subtracted from the contrast enhanced scan but should be reviewed prior to the enhanced study in order to establish that all important structures are included and to ensure that no aliasing artifacts are present.

In general, more than one dataset should be acquired after contrast agent injection since a delay of bolus arrival may occur in spite of optimally planned bolus timing. Moreover, additional acquisitions may reveal important additional information concerning venous structures. Typically, the first scan should be timed for optimal enhancement of the thoracic aorta. Thereafter, a deep breath by the patient should be followed by a second breath-hold and the acquisition of a second scan immediately afterwards.

As in imaging of the supra-aortic vessels, injections should be performed into the right arm in order to avoid the T2* effects of residual highly concentrated contrast agent in the venous structures. Injections into the left arm are known to frequently result in artificial depiction of a stenosis of the supra-aortic vessels.

The injection rate should be approximately 3-4 ml/sec if a dose of 0.2 mmol/kg of an extracellular contrast agent is applied. If a weakly protein interacting agent with higher relaxivity (e.g. Gd-BOPTA) is used, a dose of 0.1 mmol/kg is usually sufficient at an injection rate of 2-2.5 ml/sec.

If additional information is required beyond the luminal images derived from CE MRA (e.g. information on anatomic structures), complimentary sequences should be performed, which in the thorax often necessitates ECG- or pulse-gating. Structures outside of the aortic lumen which frequently require further characterization include the vessel wall and the perivascular tissue. The latter may be of particular interest during evaluations of inflammatory changes surrounding the aorta, such as in aortitis [6]. As mentioned above, the same holds true for imaging of intramural hemorrhage which is increasingly of interest due to its recognition as an early form of aortic dissection [7].

Many of the above questions can be answered adequately with conventional ECG-gated unenhanced T1- and T2-weighted SE, TSE or GRE imaging, performed before and in cases of inflammatory changes, immediately after the acquisition of the contrast enhanced MRA. However, additional functional information is often needed, for example, in cases of dilatation of the ascending aorta. In this scenario it is necessary to ascertain whether the dilatation is due to a congenital variation such as a bicuspid aortic valve, or to an acquired disease such as aortic stenosis, aortic insufficiency or a combination of both. In these situations CINE-type imaging can give very good results. The application of CINE phase-contrast imaging additionally permits the absolute quantification of blood flow. This may be applicable for the quantification of regurgitation fraction in aortic valve insufficiency and for the quantification of pressure gradients based on velocity measurements in aortic coarctation [3].

Imaging planes are either perpendicular or along the long axis of the aorta depending on the desired information. Other interesting applications of CINE imaging would be in patients with aortic dissection, in whom diagnosis is unclear based on CE MRA findings due to the tremendous movement of the dissection membrane during the heart cycle and a resulting misregistration of the membrane on CE MRA images. For example, the false lumen may be depicted only during late diastole in some patients and may thus be missed on non ECG-gated contrast enhanced MRA [7].

Anatomic Variations

A number of congenital malformations affect the thoracic aorta. Many of these affect the aortic arch and its branches.

Double Aortic Arch

Double aortic arch is one of the two most common forms of vascular ring. It is a class of congenital anomaly of the aortic arch system in which the trachea and esophagus are completely encircled by connected segments of the aortic arch and its branches. Although various forms of double aortic arch exist, the common defining feature is that both left and right aortic arches are present.

The development of double aortic arch begins early in the course of embryonic morphogenesis. Six pairs of pharyngeal arch arteries develop in conjunction with the branchial pouches. The first through sixth arches appear in a more or less sequential fashion, with left-to-right symmetry, and constitute the primitive vascular supply to the brachiocephalic structures, running from the aortic sac to the paired dorsal aortas. As normal cardiovascular morphogenesis proceeds, patterned regression and persistence of the various arches and right-sided dorsal aorta occur, ultimately resulting in the mature configuration of the thoracic aorta and its branches. The third, fourth, and sixth arches, along with the seventh intersegmental arteries and the left dorsal aorta, are the primary contributors to the normal aortic arch and its major thoracic branches [8].

The segments of the bilateral aortic arch system that normally regress include the distal portion of the sixth arch and the right-sided dorsal aorta. Normally, the left fourth arch becomes the aortic arch, the right fourth arch contributes to the innominate artery, the distal left sixth arch becomes the ductus arteriosus, the proximal sixth arches bilaterally contribute to the proximal branch pulmonary arteries, the left dorsal aorta becomes the descending thoracic aorta, and the dorsal intersegmental arteries bilaterally become the subclavian arteries.

Vascular rings are formed when this process of regression and persistence does not occur normally, and the resulting vascular anatomy completely encircles the trachea and esophagus. Other forms of aortic arch anomaly may occur in which a vascular ring is not present, such as right aortic arch and aberrant left subclavian artery. A double aortic arch is formed when both fourth arches and both dorsal aortas remain present. Various forms of double aortic arch exist. Both arches may be patent, or an atretic (but persistent) segment may exist at one of several locations in either arch. When both arches are patent, the right or left arch may be larger, or they may be similar in size. A cervical arch on either side, variable laterality of the descending thoracic aorta, coarctation of the major arch, and/or discontinuity of the central pulmonary arteries may be present. In more than 75% of patients with double aortic arch, the right arch is dominant [9].

Double aortic arch usually occurs without associated cardiovascular anomalies. Ventricular septal defect and tetralogy of Fallot are probably the most common associated defects, although truncus arteriosus, transposition of the great arteries, pulmonary atresia, and complex univentricular defects sometimes occur in conjunction with a double arch [10].

Right Aortic Arch

A right aortic arch is formed when the right dorsal aorta remains patent and either the left fourth arch or the left dorsal aorta regress abnormally. Two primary forms of vascular ring with a right aortic arch exist, while two other forms are much less common.

In the most frequent form of vascular ring with a right aortic arch, an aberrant origin of the left subclavian artery from a retroesophageal diverticulum (diverticulum of Kommerell) is present, which originates as the last branch of the aortic arch (distal to the right subclavian artery). The ring is completed by a left-sided ductus arteriosus (or its remnant ligamentum arteriosum) passing from the aberrant left subclavian artery to the proximal left pulmonary artery. The retroesophageal diverticulum is distinguished from the aberrant left subclavian artery by its larger caliber. Although the course of the descending thoracic aorta varies, it typically crosses gradually to the left of the vertebral column to pass through the diaphragm in the usual location of the aortic hiatus [11].

In the second major type of vascular ring with a right aortic arch, the brachiocephalic vessels originate from the arch in mirror-image fashion with the left innominate artery the first branch followed by the right common carotid and subclavian arteries. A left-sided ductus arteriosus or ligamentum arteriosum passes between the descending aorta and the proximal left pulmonary artery. In contrast to right aortic arch with aberrant left subclavian artery from a retroesophageal diverticulum, the descending aorta usually crosses to the left side of midline proximally in its course, although in rare cases, it remains to the right of midline until reaching the lower portion of the thorax [11, 12].

Anomalies Involving Aortic Branches

Anomalies concerning the branches of the aortic arch may involve the position and/or the number of primary branches. The branches, instead of arising from the highest part of the arch, may develop from the start of the arch or the upper part of the ascending aorta. Alternatively, the distance between the branches at their origins may be increased or diminished. The most frequent change in this respect is an anomalous proximity of the left carotid toward the innominate artery.

The number of primary branches may be reduced to one, or more commonly two; the left carotid arising from the innominate artery, or (more rarely) the carotid and subclavian arteries of the left side arising from a left innominate artery. In other cases the number of branches may be increased to four, for example, with the right carotid and subclavian arteries arising directly from the aorta while the innominate artery is absent. In most of these latter cases the right subclavian artery is found to arise from the left end of the arch; in other cases it is the second or third branch rather than the first. Another common form in which there are four primary branches is that in which the left vertebral artery arises from the arch of the aorta between the left carotid and subclavian arteries.

Lastly, the number of trunks from the arch may be increased to five; in this instance, the external and internal carotids arise separately from the arch, the common carotid being absent on one or both sides. In a few cases six branches have been found. This condition sees both vertebral arteries arise from the arch [13].

When the aorta arches over to the right side, the three branches have an arrangement which is the reverse of that which is usual; the innominate artery is a left one, and the right carotid and subclavian arteries arise separately. In other cases in which the aorta takes its usual course, the two carotids may be joined in a common trunk. In such cases the subclavians arise separately from the arch, with the right subclavian generally arising from the left end of the arch.

In some instances other arteries derive from the arch of the aorta. Of these the most common

are the bronchial, one or both [11, 12].

Another common developmental abnormality is coarctation of the aorta. It is a relatively common type of congenital heart defect which is often inherited and found mostly in males. Often this defect goes undiagnosed until early adulthood. In over 30% of patients affected by coarctation, a bicuspid aortic valve is also present [14]. Further details about congenital cardiovascular malformations are found in Chapter VIII "MRA in pediatric patients".

Clinical Examples

Developmental Abnormalities

MRI permits an excellent workup of the anatomic and physiologic status particularly as regards congenital cardiovascular malformations of the aorta. Since children or young adults most frequently require evaluation, the lack of ionizing radiation and the excellent safety profile of the applied MR contrast agents are a considerable advantage when compared with other diagnostic modalities. Moreover, since patients with congenital cardiovascular malformations need regular follow-up, it is important to reduce to a minimum the number of examinations that require ionizing radiation.

Aortic Coarctation

Coarctation of the aorta has a male predominance of 4 to 1. Two forms can be distinguished: the localized postductal coarctation (Fig. 3a, b) and the preductal or tubular hypoplasia of the aortic arch.

In the localized form a short discrete narrowing of the aorta close to the ligamentum arteriosum can be found. Although concomitant cardiac anomalies are uncommon in this form of aortic coarctation, there is an association with bicuspid aortic valve in 25-50% of cases. Diagnosis is often made in young adults but sometimes even later in life (Fig. 4). In contrast, in the preductal, infantile form of aortic coarctation a hypoplasia of a longer segment of aortic arch after the origin of the innominate artery is found [14]. This form is often associated with a variety of coexisting cardiac anomalies as described in Chapter VIII "MRA in pediatric patients".

Collateral supplies in aortic coarctation are often easily depicted on CE MRA and may derive from the intercostal and internal mamarian arteries, the scapular arteries, and the lateral thoracic and transverse cervical arteries (Fig. 5a-c). MRI in coarctation not only allows depiction of the involved segment enabling determination of the length and diameter of the aorta, but may also per-

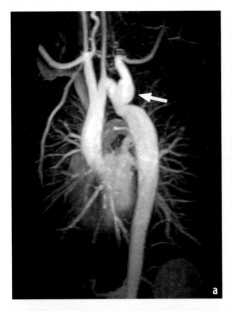

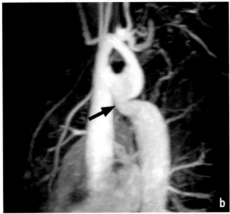

Fig. 3a, b. Localized postductal coarctation in an 18-year old man. Dilatation of the left subclavian artery (*arrow*) and a stenosis of the aorta can be seen in **a**. However, the degree of the stenosis (*arrow*) is much better appreciated on the subvolume MIP image (**b**)

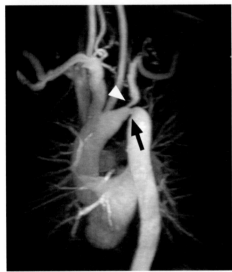

Fig. 4. A 68-year old male patient with hypertension and increasing claudication (Gd-BOPTA, 0.1 mmol/kg). The contrast enhanced MRA study shows coarctation and a high grade stenosis of the aorta distal to the origin of the left subclavian artery (*arrow*) and involving the left subclavian artery (*arrowhead*). This finding is important for surgery since part of the arch has to be reconstructed

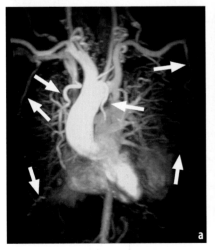
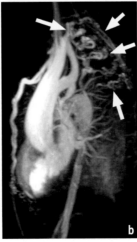
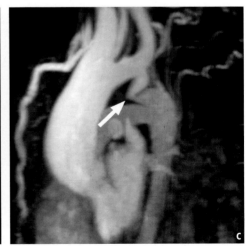

Fig. 5a-c. Depiction of collateral supplies in aortic coarctation in a 17-year old female (Gd-BOPTA, 0.1 mmol/kg). The CE MRA study reveals collaterals from the intercostals, internal mamarian arteries and lateral thoracic arteries (*arrows* in **a**), as well as collaterals from the scapular arteries and transverse cervical arteries (*arrows* in **b**). Note that the degree of stenosis is best displayed on multiplanar reconstructions following the long axis of the aorta (*arrow* in **c**)

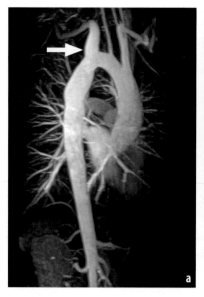

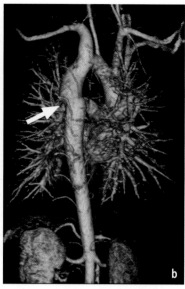

Fig. 6a, b. Follow up study in a patient after surgical repair of aortic coarctation (Gd-BOP-TA, 0.1 mmol/kg). Neither the MIP image (**a**) nor the volume rendered image (**b**) from the CE 3D MRA dataset reveal a residual stenosis although some irregularities of the aortic wall due to patch angioplasty are apparent. Note the persisting dilatation of the left subclavian artery (*arrow* in **a**) and the kinking of the thoracic aorta (*arrow* in **b**)

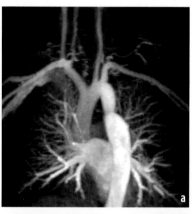

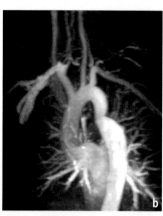

Fig. 7a, d. Pre-intervention (**a**, **b**) and post-intervention (**c**, **d**) evaluations of a patient with aortic coarctation undergoing intraluminal intervention and stent placement. **a** and **b** show coarctation of the thoracic aorta a few centimeters distal to the origin of the subclavian artery. Due to the rather long distance from the subclavian artery stent placement was planned for treatment of the coarctation. On the post-interventional MIP image almost complete signal loss is apparent in the area of the stent (*arrow* in **c**). However, if multiplanar reconstructions are made from the source data the area of the stent can be evaluated on MR images. In this case no hemodynamic relevant residual stenosis is visible (*arrows* in **d**)

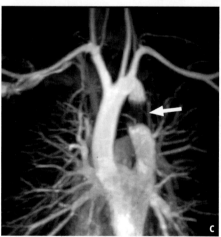

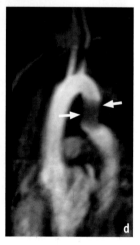

mit estimation of the pressure gradient through evaluation of the maximum flow velocity [15].

Not only diagnosis but also post surgical or post interventional follow-up is of importance (Fig. 6a, b) either to detect residual stenosis of the aorta or to evaluate newly developed stenosis due to scar tissue formation. Furthermore, evaluation of post interventional procedures e.g. dilatation of

the stenosis or stent placement (Fig. 7a-d) is necessary to detect intramural hemorrhage, dissection or aneurysm formation (Fig. 8a-e).

If a diagnosis of coarctation is made, the aortic valve should always be evaluated as well in case a concomitant bicuspid aortic valve is present (see Fig. 18).

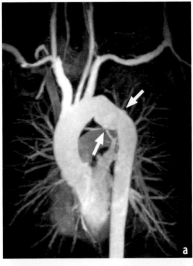
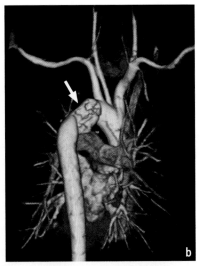
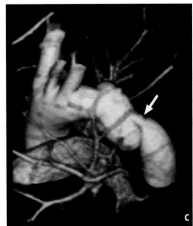

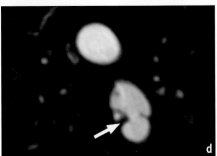
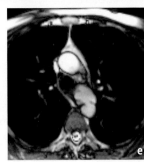

Fig. 8a-e. Aneurysm formation in a patient with recurrent coarctation (Gd-BOPTA, 0.1 mmol/kg). The MIP image (**a**) reveals some irregularities of the aortic wall (*arrows*) in the area of the former coarctation but no signs of a residual stenosis. However, if volume rendering is used for evaluation of the anatomy (**b**, **c**) a tremendously irregular aortic wall and aneurysm formation is demonstrated (*arrow* in **b**) together with a residual stenosis (*arrow* in **c**). The stenosis is confirmed on axial reformations of the CE 3D MRA dataset (*arrow* in **d**) and can be further evaluated by CINE imaging (**e**)

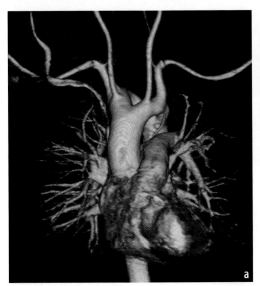
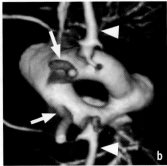

Fig. 9a, b. Incidental finding of a double aortic arch in a 64-year old patient. On conventional thorax x-ray a widening of the upper mediastinum was noted and the patient underwent MRI for further evaluation. The volume rendered images of the CE 3D MRA dataset (Gd-BOPTA, 0.1 mmol/kg) show a complete double aortic arch. This can already be noted on an anterior-to-posterior view (**a**) but is even better displayed if a cranio-caudal view (**b**) is obtained. Note the separate anterior origin of the two common carotid arteries (*arrows*) and the posterior origin of the two subclavian arteries (*arrowheads*)

Arch Anomalies

Anomalies of the aortic arch such as double aortic arch (Fig 9a, b), aberrant right subclavian artery (Fig 10a-c, 11 a-c), right sided aortic arch (Fig 12a, b) and patent ductus arteriosus (Fig 13a-c) are easily and accurately diagnosed on contrast enhanced MRI, as is aortic pseudocoarctation (Fig 14 a, b). In some of these instances patients may be asymptomatic with the diagnosis made due to an incidental finding of, for example, widened upper mediastinum on conventional thorax x-ray.

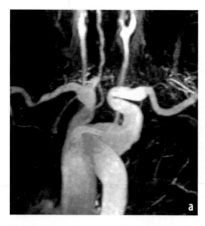
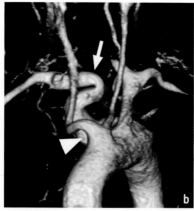
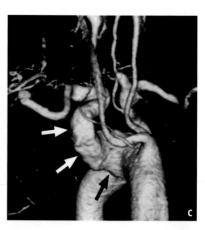

Fig. 10a-c. Aberrant right subclavian artery (Lusoria artery) in a 72-year old male. Whereas the anatomic relationship between the supraaortic vessels is hard to identify on the MIP image (**a**), the volume rendered images in anterior-posterior (**b**) and posterior-anterior (**c**) direction clearly depict an aberrant right subclavian artery (*arrows*) arising as the last vessel from the aortic arch and passing to the opposite site. Note in addition the common trunk of the carotid arteries branching first from the aortic arch (*arrowhead*)

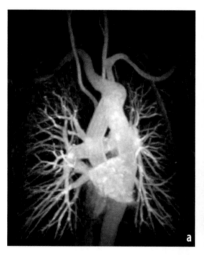
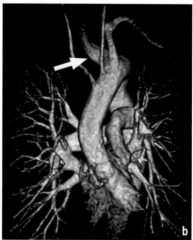
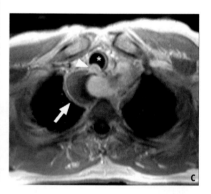

Fig. 11a-c. Aberrant right subclavian artery with development of an aneurysm. Again the relationship between the supraaortic vessels is much better appreciated on the volume rendered image (**b**) than on the standard MIP reconstruction (**a**). As in Fig. 10 an aberrant right subclavian artery (*arrow*) arises as the last vessel from the aortic arch and passes to the opposite site. However in this case a large aneurysm (*arrow*) of the aberrant right subclavian artery with thrombus formation can be noted on the conventional post contrast T1w axial image (**c**). Furthermore note the esophagus (*arrowhead*) and the trachea (*asterisk*) anterior to the aberrant right subclavian artery

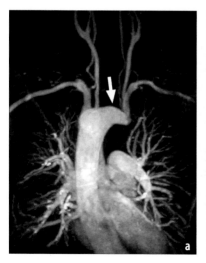
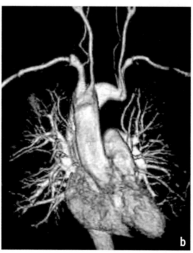

Fig. 12a, b. Right aortic arch giving rise to an aberrant left trunk (Gd-BOPTA, 0.1 mmol/kg). On routine x-ray of the thorax a right descending aorta was noted and the patient was transferred to MRI to further evaluate the vascular structures. The MIP image (**a**) shows the right descending aorta together with a large vessel that passes to the left (*arrow*). The relationship between the vessels is again much better appreciated on the surface rendered image (**b**) which clearly demonstrates that first the right common carotid artery, second the right subclavian artery and last the atypical trunk that gives separate rise to the left common carotid, subclavian and vertebral artery branch from the right aortic arch

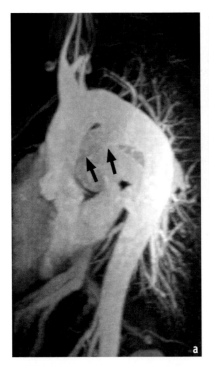

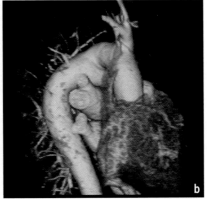

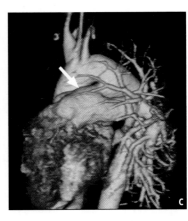

Fig. 13a-c. CE MRA study (Gd-BOPTA, 0.1 mmol/kg) of a patent ductus arteriosus in a 16-year old female patient. A large vessel (*arrows*) connecting the descending aorta with the pulmonary trunk can be identified on the MIP projection (**a**). The volume rendered images (**b**, **c**) identify the site of connection between the patent ductus arteriosus and the pulmonary trunk (*arrow* in **c**) and generally reveal more details of the exact anatomic situation in this complex anatomy

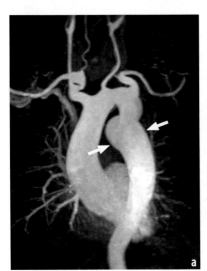

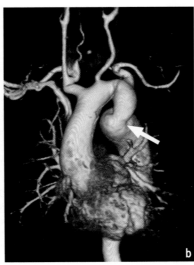

Fig. 14a, b. Aortic pseudocoarctation in a 72-year old male patient. A dilatation of the descending aorta (*arrows* in **a**) can be noted on the MIP reconstruction (**a**) of the 3D CE MRA dataset (Gd-BOPTA, 0.1 mmol/kg). On the volume rendered image (**b**) a slight narrowing of lumen of the aorta (*arrow* in **b**) can be noted with proximal elongation of the vessel which corresponds to aortic pseudocoarctation

Aortic Aneurysm

Aneurysms of the thoracic aorta can be classified according to their shape as either saccular, fusiform or dissecting. The latter are discussed in a separate subchapter. Aneurysms of the thoracic aorta can be distinguished by their location. The most frequent aortic aneurysms are found in the sinus of valsalva, the ascending aorta where they are typically associated with valvular disease, the aortic arch and in the area of the descending aorta. As regards etiology, on rare occasions aortic aneurysms might be congenital. More typically, they are due to atherosclerotic disease, trauma or inflammation.

If the diameter of the aorta is below 4 cm the condition is referred to as aortic ectasia. Conversely, if the diameter exceeds 4 cm the dilatation is generally considered an aneurysm. If an aneurysm of the ascending aorta exceeds a diameter of 5 cm surgical repair has to be considered (Fig. 15a, b), since the risk of rupture is significantly increased. Likewise, aneurysms that are saccular or which develop due to inflammation, as well as aneurysms that increase in diameter by approximately 1 cm over the course of a one year period, should be considered potential surgical candidates since these types of aneurysm have an increased risk of rupture as well [16, 17].

In cases in which the descending aorta is in-

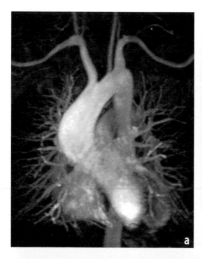
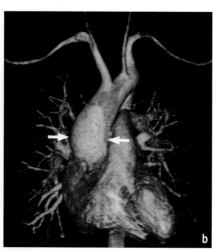

Fig. 15a, b. MIP reconstruction (**a**) and volume rendered image (**b**) of a 3D CE MRA dataset (Gd-BOPTA, 0.1 mmol/kg) of a patient with an aneurysm of the ascending aorta due to aortic valve stenosis. Note the significant dilatation of the ascending aorta (*arrows*) which was measured at 5.2 cm on multiplanar reconstructions perpendicular to the long axis of the aorta. Due to the already large diameter and a progressively increasing diameter of more than 0.5 cm over a one year period surgical reconstruction of the aortic valve and reconstruction of the ascending aorta was performed. Note that the aorta at the level of the origin of the brachiocephalic trunk as well as the trunk itself is not dilated meaning that reconstruction of the arch does not have to be performed

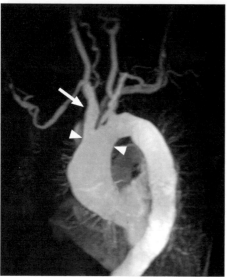

Fig. 16. MIP reconstruction of a 3D CE MRA dataset (Gd-BOPTA, 0.1 mmol/kg) of a patient with aortic aneurysm. In contrast to the case in Fig. 15 in this case the aortic arch also shows dilatation (arrowheads) and the brachiocephalic trunk should at least be described as ectatic (arrow). Note that the supraaortic vessels up to the carotid bifurcation can be evaluated in the same study

volved endoluminal treatment by aortic stent placement may be considered. However, for accurate planning of stent placement and stent size CT imaging should also be considered to allow for exact measurement of the diameters of the aorta above and below the aneurysm as well as to detect extensive calcification [2].

One big advantage of 3D CE MRA is the large field of view (FOV) which with a single contrast agent injection permits evaluation of both the aorta and the relationship of the aneurysm to branching vessels (Fig. 16). Several studies correlating 3D CE MRA with conventional angiography and surgical specimen have shown an almost 100% accuracy for assessing the size and extent of aortic aneurysms and for evaluating their relationship to

aortic branches. To further increase the diagnostic value of CE MRA in patients with aortic aneurysms luminal imaging of the arterial phase of the 3D CE MRA should be combined with cross-sectional imaging either pre or post contrast agent injection (Fig. 17a-c). If post contrast images are acquired they easily allow for differentiation between the patent lumen of an aortic aneurysm and wall thrombosis. Additionally, assessment of inflammation surrounding the aorta, inflammation of the wall and evaluation of surrounding soft tissue is made possible and may provide important additional information [18].

As mentioned above, aneurysms of the ascending aorta are most often caused by valvular disease. Therefore, if an ectasia or aneurysm of the ascending aorta is identified, CINE imaging of the aortic valve and the ascending aorta should be performed to detect congenital malformation of the aortic valve e.g. a bicuspid aortic valve (Fig. 18a-d), or to diagnose stenosis, insufficiency or a combination of both conditions (Fig. 19a, b).

Finally, as discussed previously, MRI allows for quantification of pressure gradients over the aortic valve as well as quantification of the regurgitation fraction in patients with aortic insufficiency.

Aortic Dissection

In contrast to the increased diameter of the aorta in aortic aneurysms the underlying anatomic abnormality in aortic dissection is a spontaneous longitudinal separation of the aortic intima and adventitia. This occurs due to circulating blood gaining access to the media of the aortic wall causing it to split in two. The separation of the intima and the adventitia of the aortic wall results in a dissection membrane which is the typical imaging finding of aortic dissection (Fig. 20a-c). Dissection

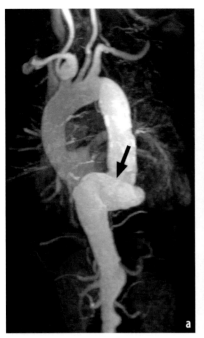
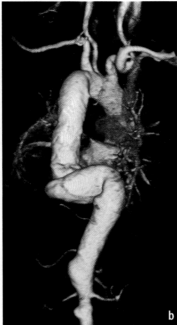
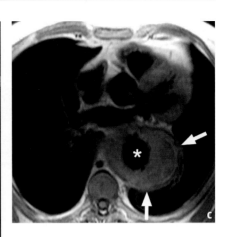

Fig. 17a-c. Kinking and aneurysm formation of the descending aorta in a 74-year old patient. The MIP reconstruction (**a**) of the CE 3D MRA dataset (Gd-BOPTA, 0.1 mmol/kg) shows an elongation of the descending aorta with an almost ascending portion of the aorta (*arrow*) just above the level of the diaphragm. On the volume rendered image (**b**) the anatomy can be appreciated more readily and irregularities of the surface of the aortic lumen can be identified. The unenhanced T1w precontrast image (**c**) clearly identifies a large aneursym of the descending aorta (*arrows*). Partial thrombosis of this aneurysm is apparent and the still perfused part (*asterisk*) demonstrates an almost normal diameter, as indicated by the low signal intensity due to flow void. This case clearly demonstrates the importance of combining CE MRA studies with cross sectional imaging

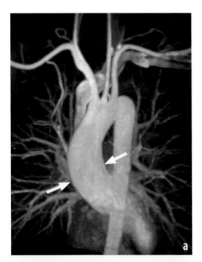
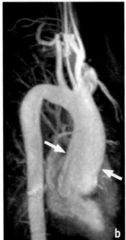
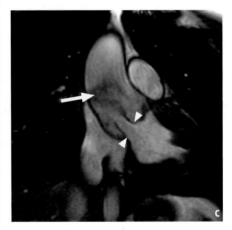

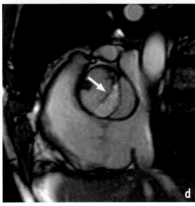

Fig. 18a-d. Aneurysm of the ascending aorta in a 25-year old patient with bicuspid aortic valve. The MIP reconstruction of the 3D CE MRA dataset (Gd-BOPTA, 0.1 mmol/kg) in anterior-posterior (**a**) and lateral (**b**) views shows dilatation of the ascending aorta (*arrows*). Since aortic valve disease is the main reason for aortic aneurysm formation of the ascending aorta in this age group further evaluation of the aortic valve was performed. A True FISP CINE sequence parallel to the axis of the ascending aorta (**c**) shows stenosis (*arrowheads*) and a jet phenomenon (*arrow*) at the aortic valve. A CINE image perpendicular to the aortic root at the level of the aortic valve (**d**) clearly displays the so-called "fish-mouth-appearance" of a bicuspid aortic valve (*arrow*)

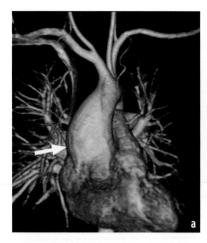

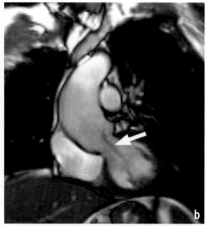

Fig. 19a, b. A volume rendered CE MRA image (Gd-BOPTA, 0.1 mmol/kg) of the thoracic aorta (**a**) shows tremendous dilatation of the ascending aorta (*arrow*) in a 38-year old patient. The corresponding True FISP CINE sequence (**b**) parallel to the axis of the ascending aorta in this case shows a diastolic retrograde jet over the aortic valve (*arrow*) indicating aortic valve insufficiency. This can further be evaluated by phase-contrast GRE images with which a quantification of the regurgitation volume is possible

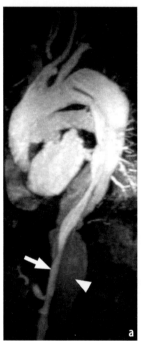

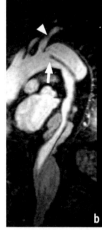

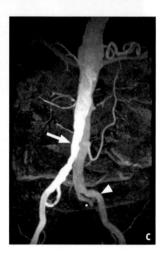

Fig. 20a-c. 3D CE MRA study in a patient with aortic dissection (Gd-BOPTA, 0.1 mmol/kg). The CE MRA study of the thorax (**a, b**) shows dissection of the descending aorta with early filling of the true lumen (*arrow* in **a**) and delayed filling of the false lumen (arrowhead in a). On a multiplanar reconstruction (**b**) following the orientation of the aortic arch the beginning of the dissection (*arrow* in **b**) just distal to the origin of the left subclavian artery (*arrowhead* in **b**) can be identified indicating a Stanford Type B dissection. Further identification of the true (*arrow*) and false (*arrowhead*) lumens is achieved in additional study of the abdomen (**c**). Note that the true lumen ends in the right iliac artery and that the false lumen ends in the left iliac artery

may involve a localized area or the entire circumference of the aorta. Although predisposing underlying diseases include cystic media necrosis, Marfan's syndrome, Ehlers-Danlos syndrome, Turner's syndrome and Behcet disease among others, in the majority of patients no underlying syndrome can be found and the main pathomechanism is systemic hypertension. This is the underlying disease in approximately 60-90% of cases [19].

According to the Stanford Classification, aortic dissections may be categorized as Stanford Type A (70%) and Stanford Type B (20-30%) dissection, with Stanford Type A dissection affecting the ascending aorta +/- the aortic arch and Type B dissection beginning beyond the origin of the left subclavian artery.

In the DeBakey Classification Type I dissection represents a dissection of the ascending aorta and

a portion of the aorta distal to the arch, Type II dissection involves only the ascending aorta, and Type III dissection involves only the descending aorta. In subtype III A of the DeBakey classification the dissection runs down to the level of the diaphragm while in subtype III B the dissection extends below the diaphragm [20].

From the clinical point of view an acute dissection is a dissection that is less than two weeks old while a chronic dissection is one that is more than two weeks old. In the majority of acute Type A dissections, CE MRA or MRI in general does not play an important role since urgent surgery is required as soon as the diagnosis is established. Typically, in the first hours after the onset of a Type A dissection the mortality rate per hour is approximately 8%. In contrast, in chronic Type A dissection MRI and MRA may provide very important clinical information. Similarly, MRA is appropriate for follow up of Type B dissections and for follow up of patients with reconstruction of the ascending aorta following Type A dissection with remaining dissection of the descending aorta [7].

The major questions which should be answered in the setting of aortic dissection are the exact localization and extent of the dissection, the localizations of entries and re-entries, and the involvement of branching vessels. Concerning branching vessels, the supraaortic vessels are of particular interest in Type A dissections while the mesenteric and renal arteries are of interest in Type B dissections. If the involvement of branching vessels cannot be excluded based on the arterial 3D CE MRA dataset, further evaluation with CINE imaging or with contrast enhanced T1w fat suppressed sequences such as VIBE sequences may be helpful.

Simple morphologic criteria can be used to distinguish between the true and the false lumen in aortic dissection. Typically, the true lumen is smaller and if black-blood imaging is performed the faster flowing blood in the true lumen shows complete flow void while the frequently very much slower flow in the larger, false lumen results in an intermediate signal. Occasionally, complete thrombosis of the false lumen occurs (Fig. 21a-c).

It is important to note that other types of dissections or aortic wall anomalies can be distinguished from classical aortic dissection. Examples include intramural hematoma (Fig. 22a-e) which may progress to classical aortic dissection, intimal tear, atherosclerotic ulcer (Fig. 23) and iatrogenic or traumatic dissections.

Atherosclerotic Disease

In atherosclerotic disease not only evaluation of the aorta but also evaluation of the supraaortic vessels is necessary (Fig. 24). Diseases associated with arteriosclerosis are aortic ulcers, kinking of the aorta and aneurysmatic widening of the thoracic aorta as well as stenosis or occlusion with and without elongation of the supraaortic vessels. Anatomy in arteriosclerotic disease of the supraaortic vessels can be complicated and 3D CE MRA generally gives excellent results (Fig. 25a-c).

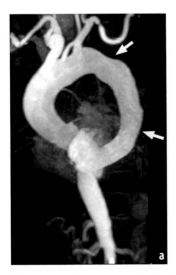 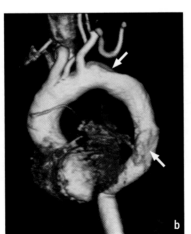 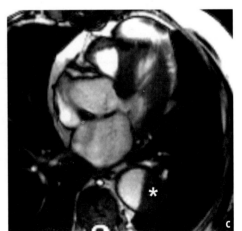

Fig. 21a-c. Complete thrombosis of the false lumen in a patient with Stanford Type B dissection. Whereas only minor wall irregularities (*arrows*) can be noted on the MIP reconstruction (**a**) of the 3D CE MRA dataset (Gd-BOPTA, 0.1 mmol/kg), clear flattening of the perfused aortic lumen in several areas (*arrows*) is apparent on the volume rendered image (**b**). This corresponds to complete thrombosis of the false lumen in Stanford Type B dissection which is clearly demonstrated on a True FISP CINE sequence at the level of the left atrium perpendicular to the axis of the descending aorta (**c**). Note the normal flow signal in the true lumen and the complete thrombosis of the false lumen (*asterisk*)

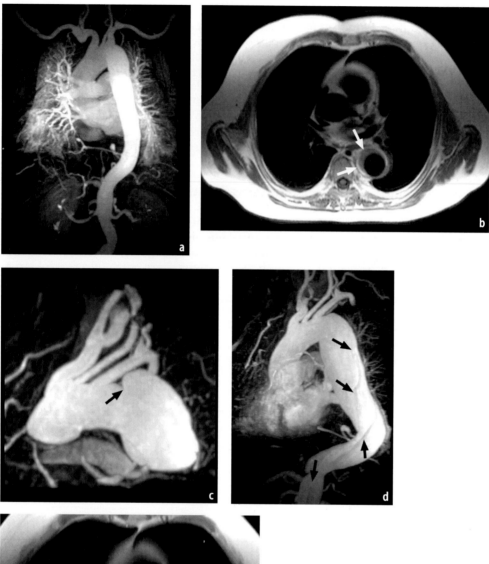

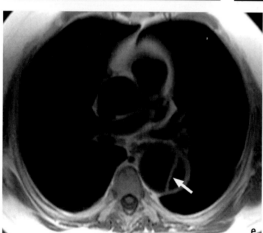

Fig. 22a-e. Intramural hematoma of the descending aorta progressing to a Stanford Type B dissection. The patient first presented with thoracic pain but cardiac infarction was excluded. A MIP reconstruction of a subsequent MRA study (**a**) revealed normal anatomy of the descending aorta. However an intramural hematoma (arrows) of the descending aorta was apparent on axial T1w images of the thorax (**b**). One year later without experiencing another episodes of thoracic pain the patient came back for a follow up study (**c-e**) which revealed Stanford Type B dissection. The MIP reconstruction of the aortic arch (**c**) demonstrates the beginning of the dissection distal to the branching of the left subclavian artery (*arrow*). A complete MIP reconstruction of the thoracic vaculature (**d**) demonstrates the dissection membrane (*arrows*) descending in a spiral course into the abdominal aorta. An axial T1w image (**e**) clearly shows the dissection membrane and no residual high SI of the aortic wall

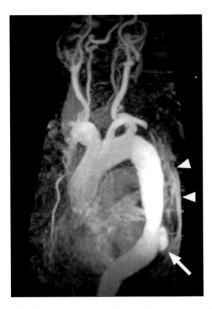

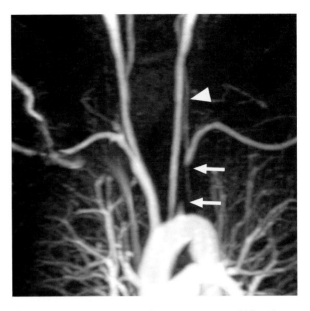

Fig. 23. Arteriosclerotic ulcer in a 74-year old male patient. The contrast enhanced MRA study shows an arteriosclerotic ulcer of the descending aorta (*arrow*). Note in addition the strong enhancement of adjacent lung parenchyma (*arrowheads*) due to atelectasis and inflammation which can be misinterpreted as an inflammatory cause of the aortic ulcer

Fig. 24. Subclavian steal syndrome in a 42-year old female patient. The CE MRA study (Gd-BOPTA, 0.1 mmol/kg) reveals complete occlusion of the left subclavian artery (*arrows*) which is now supplied by the left vertebral artery (*arrowhead*) in which a retrograde flow can be noted

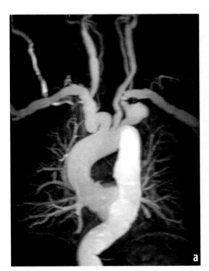

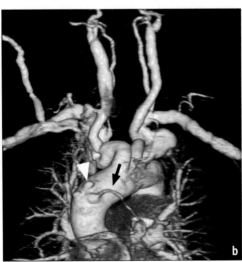

Fig. 25a, b. Arteriosclerosis of the aorta and the supraaortic vessels in a 72-year old male patient. The MIP reconstruction (**a**) of the contrast enhanced MRA study (Gd-BOPTA, 0.1 mmol/kg) reveals elongation and irregular wall formation of the aorta and to an even larger extent of the supraaortic vessels. Again the volume rendered image (**b**) better displays the anatomic situation. Note that both a patent (*arrow*) and an occluded (*arrowhead*) aortocoronary bypass graft are displayed

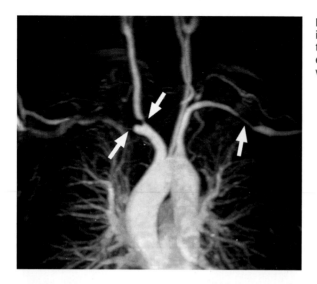

Fig. 26. Contrast enhanced MRA study (Gd-BOPTA, 0.1 mmol/kg) in a 32-year old patient with Takayasu arteritis. Note the occlusion of the right subclavian and vertebral arteries as well as the stenotic areas (*arrows*) of the right common carotid artery and the left subclavian artery

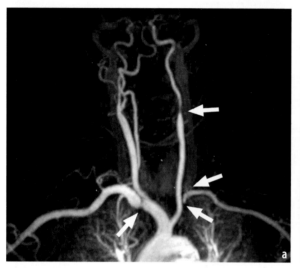

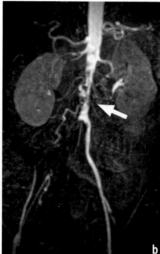

Fig. 27a, b. A patient with advanced Takayasu arteritis. The CE MRA study of the thorax (Gd-BOPTA, 0.1 mmol/kg) shows massive involvement of the supraaortic vessels (*arrows* in **a**). In addition almost complete occlusion of the infrarenal abdominal aorta (*arrow* in **b**) and occlusion of the right common iliac artery can be noted on a CE MRA study of the abdomen

Aortitis

Inflammation of the aorta, also referred to as aortitis, can occur as part of a vascular inflammation syndrome such as Takayasu arteritis (Fig. 26) or as a result of an infectious disease such as syphilitic aortitis. Inflammation may also affect the periaortic tissue, in a similar way to that occurring in Ormond's disease in the abdomen [21]. In such cases the luminal image of arterial phase CE MRA does not depict the surrounding disease. As a result of this and due to the fact that the luminal image does not say anything about the activity of an inflammatory process, T1w fat suppressed post contrast images should be acquired to visualize the enhancement of the involved tissue and to get some information concerning the activity of the disease. In Takayasu arteritis, which is also called pulseless dis-

ease, CE MRA is a very accurate non-invasive method to obtain a complete overview of the arterial status of a patient. As the name pulseless disease suggests, catheter angiography maybe very difficult due to the fact that no peripheral vessel can be catheterized to get access to the aortic lumen [18].

To distinguish between acute active inflammatory processes and more chronic diseases, a combination of T2w and post contrast T1w fat suppressed images is advisable. If high signal intensity is noted on both T2w and post contrast T1w fat suppressed images, this would tend to indicate an active inflammation. Conversely, if a low signal intensity of the involved tissue is noted on T2w images, this would tend to suggest the early stages of fibrosis and hence a more chronic form of disease. If no further enhancement or only slight enhancement is noted on post contrast T1w fat suppressed images, a diagnosis of complete fibrosis without any active inflammation can be made.

Regarding Takayasu arteritis it should be noted that this is the only form of aortitis that can lead to high grade stenosis or occlusion of the aorta (Fig. 27a, b). Therefore, if occlusion of the aorta is found, Takayasu arteritis has to be considered the underlying disease [6].

Pitfalls / Limitations

Due to the sometimes tremendous mobility of the ascending aorta and aortic arch, especially in patients with Marfan's syndrome, it is occasionally possible to observe blurring of the ascending aorta and even depiction of artifacts which might be misinterpreted as aortic dissection.

In cases in which diagnosis of aortic dissection is suspected from contrast enhanced MRA images, conventional ECG-gated cross-sectional images should also be acquired to confirm the diagnosis. Sometimes this can also be accomplished by means of CINE imaging.

Another pitfall in imaging of the thoracic aorta especially in patients with advanced atherosclerotic disease and elongation with increased tortuosity of the thoracic aorta is incomplete coverage of the anatomy. As mentioned above, in some patients elongation and tortousity of the thoracic aorta may be so extreme as to necessitate slab orientation in the sagittal plane in order to completely cover the aorta. In general to avoid this kind of pitfall one should perform extensive localizer imaging before finally positioning the slab for the contrast enhanced 3D MRA study. Similarly, a preliminary unenhanced scan should be reviewed to look for aliasing or incomplete coverage of the thoracic aorta.

Another important issue in imaging of the thoracic aorta is ringing or stripe artifacts. These artifacts in the lumen of the aorta are caused by incorrect timing of the contrast agent bolus. If the contrast agent bolus arrives too late the central parts of k-space are acquired at a time when the maximum Gd concentration has not yet been reached. If a significantly higher Gd concentration in the area of interest is then found during the acquisition of the peripheral parts of k-space, artificial longitudinal dark stripes within the aortic lumen may occur which can simulate the presence of aortic dissection in a similar manner to that found in patients with increased mobility of the ascending aorta and aortic arch.

To avoid or compensate for this kind of artifact a second acquisition of a 3D dataset should be performed immediately after the first, bolus-timed acquisition. If these dark longitudinal lines are only found on the first dataset, a diagnosis of aortic dis-

section can be excluded. Conversely, if these lines also appear on the second dataset, a diagnosis of aortic dissection is likely.

Finally, periaortic inflammation may be misdiagnosed in cases of pneumonia adjacent to the aorta or in cases in which the surrounding lung parenchyma is atelectatic due to dilatation of the aorta. In these cases strong enhancement of the lung tissue is observed which should not be mistaken for inflammation of the aortic wall.

In general to avoid the pitfalls in thoracic 3D CE MRA accurate planning of the examination is necessary and imaging should be performed in conjunction with conventional cross-sectional imaging or CINE imaging. Using this approach in the majority of cases images should be diagnostic and interpretation should be unequivocal.

Accuracy, Review of Literature

Adequate diagnosis of aortic dissection is still a challenge, not because of difficulties in imaging depiction but because of the need to rapidly achieve diagnosis, given that the outcome of patients decreases tremendously with time in cases of acute type A dissection. Furthermore, additional information on the localization and extent of the dissection, on entries and re-entries as well as on the involvement of other vessels or paravascular hemorrhage is needed in order to satisfactorily plan therapeutic strategy.

CT and CTA represent widely available and rapid imaging modalities for the diagnosis of acute aortic dissection. Sensitivity and specificity values between 83% and 94%, and 87% and 100%, respectively, have been achieved with these techniques [20]. With the application of helical CT scans, further improvements in diagnostic accuracy have been achieved especially in type A dissection in which sensitivity was previously below 80% [22, 23]. Unfortunately, CT is disadvantaged by the need for radiation and iodinated contrast material as well as by decreased soft tissue resolution.

In comparison, MR imaging is able to achieve sensitivities and specificities of 95 to 100% for the diagnosis of aortic dissection [7, 19, 20, 24, 25]. Accordingly, this technique represents the imaging modality of choice for both elective examination of suspicious aortic dissection and for follow up studies. Apart from not requiring radiation and potentially nephrotoxic iodinated contrast agents, MR imaging permits a free choice of image orientation and increased soft tissue resolution. Disadvantages, however, are longer examination times, the lack of immediate and widespread availability of scanners and a restriction of monitoring capabilities and patient access due to narrow gantry tubes. However, these limitations will improve with further developments in hardware and software.

Another quick and widely available imaging modality is transesophageal echography (TEE) which permits accurate diagnosis of aortic dissection with a specificity from 63% to 96% and a sensitivity of up to 98% [20, 26, 27]. Clear advantages are the bed-side performance in unstable patients and the possibility to evaluate paravascular hemorrhage, blood flow, dissection membrane and heart with a one-stop-shop approach. Limitations of TEE are the strong dependence on investigator experience, the small field of view and the relative invasiveness of the procedure.

With aortography, which was formerly considered an imaging modality of choice, sensitivities of 86 to 88% and specificities of 75 to 94% have been reached for the diagnosis of aortic dissection [20, 28, 29]. However, due to the invasiveness of the procedure aortagraphy is seldom used as primary diagnostic tool. On the other hand, pre-surgical evaluation of the coronary arteries often requires invasive aorto- and coronarography.

Future Perspectives

With the introduction of parallel imaging the scan times for a high resolution 3D MRA dataset of the thoracic vasculature can be reduced dramatically and thus patients who today are unable to make a sufficient breath-hold may be easily imaged in the future. Furthermore dynamic imaging will be possible facilitating a comprehensive study of the thoracic aorta together with evaluation of the supraaortic vessels. It is likely also that functional as well as morphologic evaluation of the aortic valve will be possible in significantly less than 30 min. Finally, with the introduction of intravascular contrast agents it will become possible to perform both first pass imaging of the aorta and steady state imaging of the coronary arteries thereby permitting a complete non-invasive vascular work-up of patients with atherosclerotic disease.

References

1. Prince MR, Narasimham DL, Jacoby WT et al (1996) Three-dimensional gadolinium-enhanced MR angiography of the thoracic aorta. AJR Am J Roentgenol 166:1387-97
2. Macura KJ, Szarf G, Fishman FK et al (2003) Role of computed tomography and magnetic resonance imaging in assessment of acute aortic syndromes. Semin Ultrasound CT MR 24:232-54
3. Kupfahl C, Honold M, Meinhardt G et al (2004) Evaluation of aortic stenosis by cardiovascular magnetic resonance imaging: comparison with established routine clinical technics. Heart 90:893-901
4. Garcier JM, Petitcolin V, Filaire M et al (2003) Normal diameter of the thoracic aorta in adults: a magnetic resonance imaging study. Surg Radiol Anat. 25:322-9
5. Muster AJ, Idriss RF, Backer CL (2001) The left-sided aortic arch in humans, viewed as the end-result of natural selection during vertebrate evolution. Cardiol Young 11:11-22
6. Choe YH, Kim DK, Koh EM (1999) Takayasu arteritis: diagnosis with MR imaging and MR angiography in acute and chronic active stages. J Magn Reson Imaging. 10:751-7
7. Pereles FS, McCarthy RM, Baskara V et al (2002) Thoracic aortic dissection and aneurysm: evaluation with nonenhanced true FISP MR angiography in less than 4 minutes. Radiology. Apr 223(1):270-4
8. van Son JA, Julsrud PR, Hagler DJ (1994) Imaging strategies for vascular rings. Ann Thorac Surg; Mar 57(3):604-10
9. Chun K, Colombani PM, Dudgeon DL et al (1992) Diagnosis and management of congenital vascular rings: a 22-year experience. Ann Thorac Surg; Apr 53(4):597-602; discussion 602-3
10. Grathwohl KW, Afifi AY, Dillard TA (1999) Vascular rings of the thoracic aorta in adults. Am Surg; Nov 65(11):1077-83
11. Van Dyke CW, White RD (1994) Congenital abnormalities of the thoracic aorta presenting in the adult. J Thorac Imaging 9:230-245
12. Kersting-Sommerhoff BA, Sechtem UP, Fisher MR et al (1987) MR imaging of congenital anomalies of the aortic arch. AJR 149:9-13
13. Billig DM (1973) Congenital anomalies of the thoracic aorta and its branches: pathophysiology, clinical course, and management. Prog Cardiovasc 16:43-67
14. Schulthess GK von, Higashino SM, Higgins SS et al (1986) Coarctation of the aorta. Radiology 158:469-474
15. Stefens JC, Boume MW, Sarkuma H et al (1994) Quantification of collateral blood flow in coarctation of the aorta by velocity encoded cine magnetic resonance imaging. Circulation 90:937-943
16. Benachenhou K, Azarnouch K, Filaire M et al (2004) Evolution of healthy thoracic aortic segment diameter during follow-up of patients with aortic aneurysm or dissection: a magnetic resonance imaging study. Surg Radiol Anat. Oct 29
17. Persson A, Dahlstrom N, Engellau L, Larsson EM et al (2004) Volume rendering compared with maximum intensity projection for magnetic resonance angiography measerements of the abdominal aorta. Acta Radiol 45:453-9
18. Nastri MV, Baptista LP, Baroni RH et al (2004) Gadolinium-enhanced three-dimensional MR angiography of Takayasu arteritis.Radiographics 24:773-86.
19. Hartnell GG (2001) Imaging of aortic aneurysm and dissection: CT and MRI. J Thorac Imaging 16:35-46
20. Khan IA, Nair CK. (2002) Clinical, diagnostic, and management perspectives of aortic dissection. Chest 122:311-328
21. Scheel AK, Meller J, Vosshenrich R et al (2004) Diagnosis and follow up of aortitis in the elderly. Ann Rheum Dis. 63:1507-10
22. Clague J, Magee P, MillsP (1992) Diagnostic dissection in suspected thoracic aortic dissection. Br Heart J 67:428-429
23. Ledbetter S, Stuk JL, Kaufman JA (1999) Helical

(spiral) CT in the evaluation of emergent thoracic aortic syndromes: traumatic aortic rupture, aortic aneurysm, aortic dissection, intramural hematoma, and penetrating atherosclerotic ulcer. Radiol Clin North Am 37:575-589

24. Mathieu D, Keita K, Loisance D et al (1986) Postoperative CT follow-up of aortic dissection. J Comput Assist Tomogr 10:216-8

25. Matsunaga N, Hayashi K, Okada M et al (2003) Magnetic resonance imaging features of aortic diseasees. Top Magn Reson Imaging. 14:253-66

26. Keren A, Kim CB, Hu BS et al (1996) Accuracy of biplane and multiplane transesophageal echocardiography in diagnosis of typical acute aortic dissection and intramural hematoma. J am Coll Cardiol. 28:627-36

27. Vignon P, Gueret P, Vedrinne JM et al (1995) Role of transesophageal echocardiography in the diagnosis and management of traumatic aortic disruption. Circulation 92:2959-6

28. Petasnick JP (1991) Radiologic evaluation of aortic dissection. Radiology 180:297-305

29. Guthaner D, Miller DG (1983) Digital substraction angiography of aortic dissection. AJR Am J Roentgenol 141:157-161

IV.2

MR Angiography of the Pulmonary Vasculature

Jeffrey P. Goldman

Background

Although contrast enhanced x-ray angiography is still considered the diagnostic gold standard for evaluation of pulmonary vascular disease, recent years have seen exciting developments in magnetic resonance angiography (MRA) as a non-invasive diagnostic tool. Today contrast enhanced MR angiography (CE MRA) has moved from the experimental field into clinical practice, thanks in large part to superior resolution deriving from improvements in three dimensional (3D) gradient echo imaging and high performance gradient systems.

Successful MR angiography of the pulmonary vasculature needs to overcome respiratory motion, cardiac pulsation and susceptibility artefacts at air-tissue-interfaces while at the same time resolving small sub-segmental arteries. Non-enhanced techniques have not proven to be reliable and thus are not utilized in clinical routine. With the introduction of 3D CE MRA most of the challenges to successful pulmonary MRA have been overcome. Among the principal challenges to imaging the pulmonary vasculature is that patients with pulmonary vascular disease often have difficulty maintaining an adequate breath-hold. With the advent of novel breath-hold sequences high-resolution imaging of the pulmonary vasculature is now possible and even small vessels can be imaged routinely. Furthermore, new ultrafast sequences can combine both dynamic and morphologic information thereby allowing evaluation of pulmonary perfusion, which further expands the potential indications.

A result of the technical improvements in pulmonary MRA is that extensive clinical experience now exists for a wide variety of pathologies, including pulmonary embolism, pulmonary hypertension, congenital malformations, arteriovenous fistulas and malformations, and the pulmonary vasculature in cases of thoracic tumor. By combining CE MRA with cross-sectional static and dynamic imaging techniques as well as with techniques for flow quantification, it is possible to obtain a comprehensive overview of even complex pathologic processes in one single non-invasive study.

The rapid technical improvements in pulmonary MRA are reflected by the papers published for this indication. For example, in 1997 Meaney et al published a study showing that 3D CE pulmonary MRA had high sensitivity and specificity for the diagnosis of pulmonary embolus when compared to x-ray angiography [1]. In 2001 Goyen et al showed that high resolution 3D MR angiography can be performed of the pulmonary arteries in under 4 seconds [2] and in 2002, Finn et al demonstrated that high resolution 3D MRA can be performed in under a second [3].

This continuing improvement of temporal resolution of MRA allows us to obtain additional functional information on the pulmonary microcirculation. For example, measurements of relative pulmonary perfusion can be calculated by following the passage of an intravenous injection of as little as 5 ml of gadolinium contrast agent through the pulmonary microcirculation (Fig. 1). Studies as far back as 1996 demonstrated that dynamic CE MRI can provide quantitative measurements, which correlate with regional pulmonary blood flow [4-6]. With the improvements and refinements in MRI, MR pulmonary perfusion imaging is now utilized for the evaluation of a wide spectrum of pulmonary vascular disorders [2, 3, 7-10].

Techniques

Coils and Patient Preparation

Imaging can be performed with a phased array torso or body coil. The advantage of using a phased array torso coil is that it provides greater

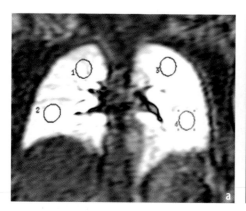 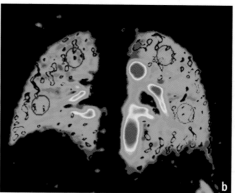

Fig. 1a, b. Pulmonary perfusion study in a normal individual. (**a**) demonstrates a raw data image with overlying regions of interest for measurement of perfusion values. (**b**) represents the corresponding parametric map calculated from the perfusion data in which perfusion values are color coded (red=high perfusion, dark blue=low perfusion)

signal-to-noise ratio (SNR) which can be used to acquire images with higher spatial and temporal resolution. Phased array coils also allow the application of parallel imaging to further increase the spatial and temporal resolution of image acquisition. When pulmonary MRA and pulmonary perfusion are performed in the coronal plane, it is important to have the patient's arms placed over their head in order to reduce or eliminate wrap artifacts. This is especially true if using parallel imaging where wrap can cause extreme artifacts.

Contrast Dosage

Today, there is a tendency to perform more than a single contrast enhanced study during each examination. Often we perform a low dose high temporal resolution functional study followed by a higher dose low temporal but high spatial resolution angiographic study. If more than one contrast-enhanced study is performed within a single examination it is important that the low dose study is performed first so that venous contamination can be minimized. For example in our pulmonary hypertension protocol we first perform an LAO MRA through the aorta to rule out a shunt utilizing 0.025 mmol/kg of contrast agent. Thereafter, we perform a coronal high-resolution pulmonary MRA utilizing 0.15 mmol/kg of contrast agent.

Imaging Protocols

Pulmonary Embolism. We perform a time-resolved pulmonary MRA in 3 seconds utilizing 0.2 mmol/kg of contrast agent at an injection rate of 5 ml/second. Imaging is started 4 seconds after contrast agent administration when breath-holding is initiated. Image acquisition is continued for as long as the patient can maintain a breath-hold. This allows us to obtain both pulmonary MRA and pulmonary perfusion information.

Pulmonary arterial hypertension. We perform a dynamic 3D MRA through the aortic arch in the LAO plane utilizing 0.025 mmol/kg of contrast agent at an injection rate of 5 ml/second. The temporal resolution of each dataset is 0.6 seconds allowing for detection of vascular shunts. We next perform a 3D MRA through the lungs utilizing 0.15 mmol/kg of contrast agent at 5 ml/second. The temporal resolution of this dataset is 3 seconds. This allows us to obtain both perfusion and anatomical information.

Pulmonary arterial vascular malformations (PAVM) or anomalous pulmonary circulation. We perform a dynamic 3D MRA through the lungs in the coronal plane with a temporal resolution of 1 second utilizing 0.1 mmol/kg of contrast agent at an injection rate of 5 ml/second. By obtaining multiple pure arterial phases we can identify small PAVM's. We next perform a 3D MRA through the lungs at a temporal resolution of 3 seconds utilizing 0.1 mmol/kg of contrast agent at an injection rate of 5 ml/second. This allows us to obtain higher spatial resolution images.

To facilitate the accurate planning of interventional therapy, a high resolution study with an acquisition time of up to 20 seconds can be performed. This permits the identification of small feeding vessels.

Normal Anatomy

The pulmonary artery conveys venous blood from the right ventricle to the lungs. It is a short, wide vessel, about 5 cm in length and 3 cm in diameter, arising from the conus arteriosus of the right ventricle. This artery divides into right and left branches under the aortic arch, at approximately the level of the fibrocartilage between the fifth and sixth thoracic vertebrae. The entire pulmonary artery is contained within the pericardium. It is enclosed with the ascending aorta within a visceral

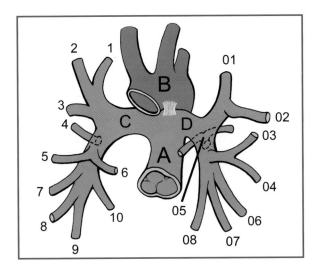

Fig. 2. Normal anatomy of the arterial pulmonary circulation
A Pulmonary artery
B Aortic arch
C Right pulmonary artery
D Left pulmonary artery

Right lung
Segmental arteries supplying:
1   Apical upper lobe segment
2   Posterior upper lobe segment
3   Anterior upper lobe segment
4   Apical superior lower lobe segment
5   Lateral middle lobe segment
6   Medial middle lobe segment
7   Anterior basal lower lobe segment
8   Lateral basal lower lobe segment
9   Posterior basal lower lobe segment
10 Medial basal lower lobe segment

Left lung
Segmental arteries supplying:
01 Apical posterior upper lobe segment
02 Anterior upper lobe segment
03 Superior lingular segment
04 Inferior lingular segment
05 Apical superior lower lobe segment
06 Anterior basal lower lobe segment
07 Lateral basal lower lobe segment
08 Posterior basal lower lobe segment

layer of serous pericardium deriving from the base of the heart. This fibrous layer is gradually lost as the pulmonary artery divides into its right and left branches.

The right branch of the pulmonary artery (right main pulmonary artery), which is longer and larger than the left, runs horizontally to the right, behind the ascending aorta and superior vena cava and in front of the right main bronchus, to the root of the right lung, where it divides into two branches. The lower and larger of these branches goes to the middle and lower lobes while the upper and smaller branch goes to the upper lobe. The left branch of the pulmonary artery (left main pulmonary artery) is slightly shorter and smaller than the right and passes horizontally in front of the descending aorta and left main bronchus to the root of the left lung, where it divides into two branches, one for each lobe of the lung (Fig. 2).

Cranially, the pulmonary artery is connected to the concavity of the aortic arch by the ligamentum arteriosum.

Clinical Indications

Pulmonary Embolism

The clinical presentation of pulmonary embolism (PE) mimics many other common and uncommon diseases. If not quickly and correctly diagnosed PE carries significant morbidity and mortality, especially in the hospitalized patient. The mortality rate for PE is less than 8% when the condition is quickly diagnosed and treated correctly but approximately 30% when untreated [11]. For this reason an accurate screening test for the detection of PE is very important. Strategies for the accurate evaluation of acute and chronic pulmonary embolus have evolved as diagnostic tests have improved.

Acute Pulmonary Embolism

X-ray angiography remains the gold standard but contrast enhanced CTA is rapidly gaining acceptance as the first line test for screening for acute pulmonary embolus. Filling defects within the contrasted lumen of the pulmonary arterial vasculature can identify acute pulmonary embolus on both CE MRA and CTA. Studies have shown similar sensitivity and specificity for detection of pulmonary embolus in the lobar and segmental arteries for both CE MRA and CTA (Fig. 3). However, immediate 24-hour access to MR scanners is not generally available.

Pulmonary perfusion imaging offers additional information to pulmonary angiography (Fig. 4). Several studies have demonstrated the ability of CE MRI to identify perfusion defects in patients with PE. In a study performed by Goldman et al pulmonary perfusion MRI was more sensitive than pulmonary MRA for detection of PE [12]. This was especially true in patients who had difficulty holding their breath.

New techniques for MR ventilation imaging hold great promise for a combined MRI perfusion/ventilation examination. Original studies on ventilation imaging employed hyperpolarized helium [13]. More recent studies have shown promise for ventilation imaging using 100% oxygen [14,15].

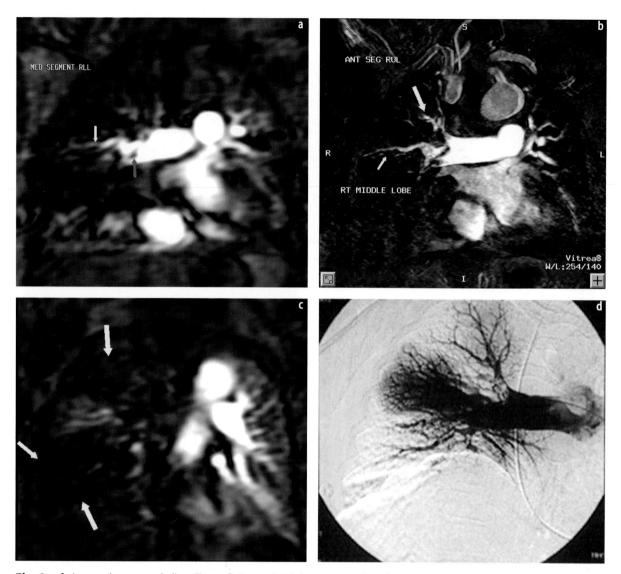

Fig. 3a-d. Acute pulmonary embolism. The perfusion study (**a**) demonstrates thrombus in a right segmental artery which supplies the medial right lower lobe segment (*arrows*). In the corresponding high resolution study (**b**) additional thrombi can be detected (*arrows*). The perfusion study clearly illustrates that large portions of the right lung (**c**) have decreased perfusion (*arrows*). The results of the CE MRA study correlate well with the corresponding catheter angiography (**d**) in the same patient

Chronic Pulmonary Embolism

Signs of chronic pulmonary embolism on pulmonary MRA include vascular webs, wall thickening, distal arterial tapering and multiple distal perfusion defects [16]. We have found pulmonary perfusion imaging especially useful for diagnosis of chronic pulmonary embolism since emboli are often in the distal vasculature where multiple distal perfusion defects are the most conspicuous findings (Fig. 5).

Pulmonary Arterial Hypertension

Pulmonary arterial hypertension (PAH) can arise as a result of congenital heart disease, which caus-

es left-to-right shunting of blood, chronic lung diseases, chronic thromboembolic pulmonary hypertension (CTEPH), and primary pulmonary hypertension (PPH). Usually, the primary condition causes a narrowing of the distal pulmonary arterioles resulting in an increase of pulmonary arterial pressure. PAH is usually diagnosed when the pressure attained is greater than 30 mm Hg by cardiac catheterization.

Although a differential diagnosis between CTEPH and PPH is generally possible on the basis of clinical criteria, chest radiography, echocardiography and V/Q scans alone, further investigation by CPA, CTA, or MRA is frequently required especially in cases in which surgical therapy is considered. One of the advantages of CE MRA as a noninvasive technique is that it can reliably distin-

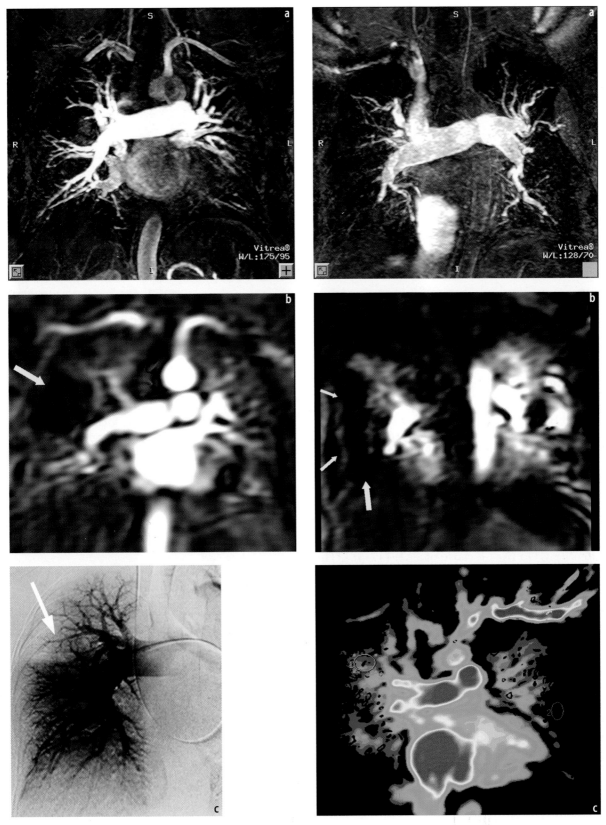

Fig. 4a-c. Acute pulmonary embolism. Whereas acute pulmonary embolism cannot be ruled out on the high resolution CE MRA study (**a**), the perfusion scan (**b**) clearly demonstrates reduced perfusion in the right lung (*arrow*). Again this correlates well with the invasive catheter angiography (*arrow* in **c**)

Fig. 5a-c. Chronic thromboembolic pulmonary hypertension (CTEPH). The high resolution CE MRA study (**a**) shows a decrease in the number of segmental and sub-segmental pulmonary arteries as well as vessel pruning, which is typical of CTEPH. In the perfusion study (**b**) multiple distal perfusion defects are demonstrated (*arrows*). These conspicuous findings of CTEPH are even better depicted on the corresponding parametric map (**c**)

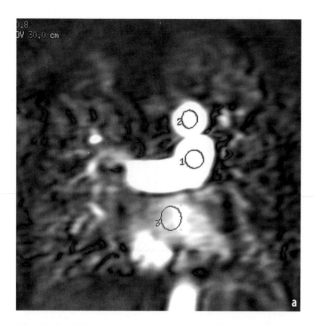
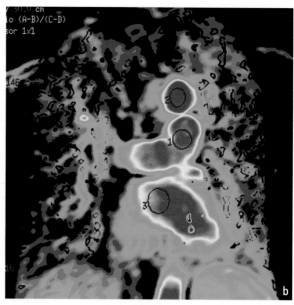

Fig. 6a, b. Primary pulmonary hypertension (PPH). A diffuse distribution of areas demonstrating hypoperfusion rather than distal perfusion defects are shown on a perfusion study (**a**) and the corresponding parametric map (**b**)

guish between characteristic features of CTEPH and PPH. In this regard, patients with CTEPH (Fig. 5) commonly show a decrease in the number of segmental or sub-segmental pulmonary arteries as well as vessel pruning (sensitivity 90±93%). In contrast, patients with PPH (Fig. 6) typically show an abnormal tapering of segmental vessels and the size difference between the proximal and peripheral vessels is often more than twice as great.

CE MRA is a very useful noninvasive test to identify CTEPH as a cause of PAH [17, 18]. The possibility to obtain subsecond temporal resolution permits the direct visualization of right to left shunts [3, 19]. In addition, CE MRA may play a further role in guiding surgeons during thrombendartectomy due to the excellent 3D visualization of the vessel tree.

Pulmonary Arteriovenous Fistulas and Malformations

Direct connections between pulmonary arteries and veins appear predominantly in the peripheral and basal lung zones and can be either congenital or acquired. Congenital and hereditary pulmonary arteriovenous fistulas are typically associated with hereditary hemorrhagic teleangiectasia (Rendu-Osler-Weber disease; Osler's disease), especially if more than one pulmonary arteriovenous malformation (PAVM) is present (Figs. 7, 8). The diagnosis of PAVM in patients with Osler's disease is extremely important since these anatomic right-to-

left shunts may lead to life-threatening cerebral and visceral emboli or abscess formation.

CE MRA may be used for diagnosis, therapy planning and follow up of these patients. Since af-

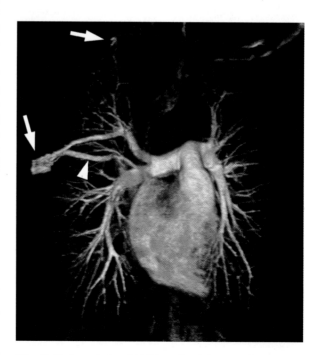

Fig. 7. High resolution CE MRA study of the arterial pulmonary vasculature (Gd-BOPTA, 0.1 mmol/kg) in a patient with proven Osler's disease (Hereditary Hemorrhagic Teleangiectasia = HHT) demonstrating two PAVMs (*arrows*). Note the early filling of the draining vein is clearly depicted for the larger PAVM (*arrowhead*) [Image courtesy of Dr. G. Schneider]

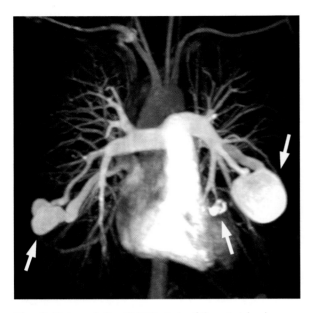

Fig. 8. High resolution CE MRA study of the arterial pulmonary vasculature (Gd-BOPTA, 0.1 mmol/kg) in a patient with multiple, partially giant PAVMs (*arrows*). This is a typical finding in patients with Osler's disease (HHT) [Image courtesy of Dr. G. Schneider]

fected patients are often young and require interventional therapy, radiation dose is an important issue. 3D CE MRA can identify the shunt as a connection between an arterial and venous pulmonary vessel. MIP images provide optimum visualization of the entire sling (Fig. 9). In most instances PAVMs can be demonstrated on 3D CE MRA because both the supplying artery and draining vessels are typically enlarged and there is a form of contrast agent pooling in the dilated vessel segment of the shunt.

The value of pulmonary MRA for both pre and post treatment management of patients with PAVMs has been demonstrated in numerous studies [20]. It has demonstrated 100% sensitivity for the identification of PAVMs greater than 3mm in size, for post embolotherapy assessment of residual aneurysm size, and for the detection of other vascular malformations such as venous aneurysms [21].

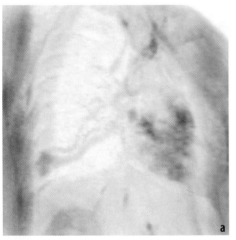
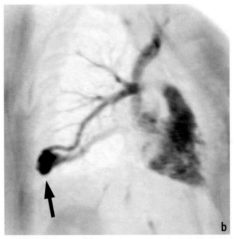
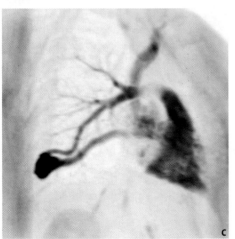
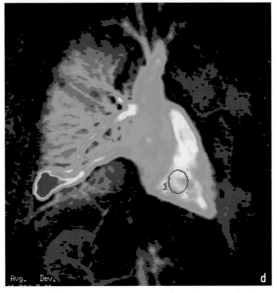

Fig. 9a-d. Pulmonary AV-Malformation evaluated by perfusion imaging. The perfusion images (**a-c**) demonstrate the early arterial enhancement of the PAVM (*arrow*) as well as the early venous drainage. The parametric map (**d**) demonstrates the PAVM as an area of increased pulmonary perfusion

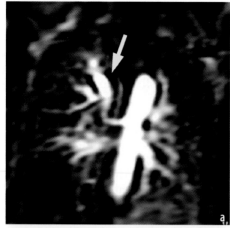
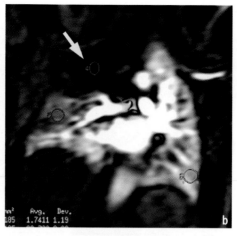
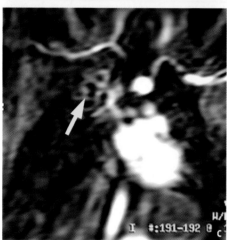

Fig. 10a-c. Perfusion study of aorto-pulmonary shunt. The low resolution MRA shows a direct branch from the aorta to the upper right lobe (*arrow* in **a**). This correlates well with perfusion studies that show lack of perfusion (arrow) of the involved segment in an early phase image (**b**) in which surrounding lung tissue demonstrates normal perfusion. On a later image perfusion of the segment can be demonstrated (*arrow* in **c**) due to systemic arterial perfusion

Anomalous Pulmonary Circulation

Several studies have shown the utility of MRA for the depiction of anomalous pulmonary vasculature [22-30]. Prasad et al showed that 3D CE MRA was accurate for the identification and assessment of patients with major aortopulmonary collaterals (MAPCAs) and partial anomalous pulmonary venous drainage (PAPVD) as compared with echocardiography, cardiac catheterization, or surgical inspection [31]. Goldman et al have shown that rapid pulmonary MRA and perfusion MRI is useful for directly visualizing the path and functional deficits caused by anomalous pulmonary circulation (Fig. 10) [32].

Congenital Heart Disease and Associated Malformations of the Pulmonary Vasculature

Generally, 3D CE MRA is able to identify all forms of vascular anomalies. As congenital abnormalities tend to present early in life, non-invasive assessment without ionising radiation is a major goal in pediatric patients. In pursuing this aim, MRA may and should replace cardiac catheterization or CTA.

In patients with congenital heart disease, MRA for both primary diagnosis and follow up imaging is gaining increasing interest since the very complex anatomy can be imaged both by CE MRA and by cross-sectional static and dynamic imaging techniques in combination. Even flow quantification is possible in one single non-invasive study. This may be of interest for the determination of pressure gradients in cases of, for example, pulmonary valve stenosis (Fig. 11). MR imaging should be performed in close cooperation with cardiologists and thoracic surgeons in order to obtain optimal results. MRI may have a major impact on patient management since post-operative anatomy may not always be displayed completely using catheter angiography approaches.

Intralobar Pulmonary Sequestration

This lesion consists of lung tissue that lacks normal communication with the bronchial tree, shares

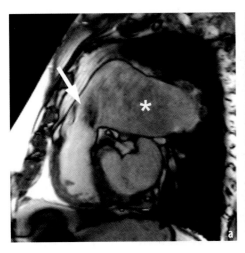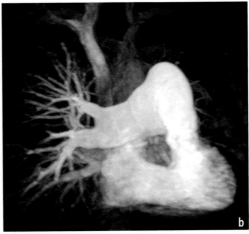

Fig. 11. Congenital stenosis of the pulmonary valve. On a sagittal True FISP image (**a**) a jet phenomenon in the pulmonary artery (arrow) due to stenosis of the pulmonary valve is noted. Note the marked dilatation (*asterisk*) of the pulmonary artery caused by flow turbulence. On the CE MRA study (Gd-BOPTA, 0.1 mmol/kg) (**b**) this dilatation of the pulmonary artery is equally well demonstrated together with an almost normal appearance of the segmental arteries [Images courtesy of Dr. G. Schneider]

the pleura of the parent lobe, and has abnormal blood supply. Sequestration usually occurs in the lower lobes. On plain radiographs, the sequestration appears as a consolidation or mass with or without cavitation. However, the definite clue for non-invasive diagnosis is the presence of systemic arterial blood supply.

CE MRA may non-invasively demonstrate the supplying arterial vessel, which usually originates from the descending aorta as well as the draining vein(s). Hence, surgical planning may be achieved without recourse to invasive X-ray angiography.

Anomalous Venous Return

Anomalies of the pulmonary venous return are typically due to failure of the connection of the primitive pulmonary vein to the left atrium and to the persistence of fetal connections between pulmonary and systemic veins. These abnormalities can result in either complete or partial anomalous venous return and are often combined with other congenital abnormalities (Fig. 12). Typically, the anomalous vein shows a vertical course toward the right cardiophrenic angle, closely paralleling the right atrium. Using 3D CE MRA, the anomalous vein and the location of the drainage can be accurately defined and both surgical planning and post surgical follow-up may be performed non-invasively (Fig. 13). However, physiologic measurements may still require additional catheter angiography.

Pulmonary Vein Thrombosis / Stenosis

Thrombosis of a pulmonary vein with and without accompanying stenosis of the involved vessel has been described as an infrequent complication of lung cancer, pulmonary lobectomy, or in patients post lung transplantation or post surgical correction of anomalous venous return. MR angiography is able to identify a stenosis of a pulmonary vein (Fig. 14) and in cases of thrombosis the thrombus location is depicted as a filling defect of a pulmonary vein and a consequent increase of vessel diameter proximal to the thrombus. Perfusion MRI permits evaluation of the functional effects of a stenosis and an accurate evaluation of perfusion pre and post surgery (Fig. 15). In cases of left atrial myxomas or malignant tumors of the left atrium, the direct extension of the tumor into the proximal veins may lead to hemostasis and thrombosis of larger, more distal veins. In such cases CE MRA allows for a complete non-invasive workup of the patient including evaluation of the heart.

Malignant Tumors of the Pulmonary Arteries and Malignant Tumors Invading the Pulmonary Vasculature

Primary tumors of the pulmonary vasculature are even rarer than cardiac tumors. Sarcomas and lymphomas are the most common primary malignant tumors. Angiosarcomas, in particular, which are typically located in the right heart, are fre-

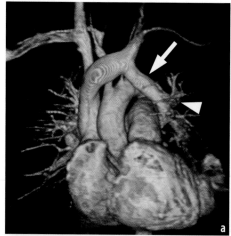
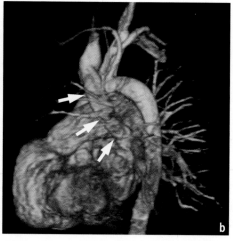
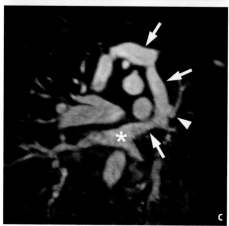

Fig. 12a-c. Partial anomalous venous return together with a persisting upper left caval vein draining into the left atrium. The volume rendered image (**a**) of a 3D CE MRA dataset (Gd-BOPTA, 0.1 mmol/kg) shows a persisting upper left caval vein (*arrow*) into which the upper left pulmonary vein (*arrowhead*) is draining. On a lateral reconstruction (**b**) of the same dataset the extent of the superior caval vein into the region of the left atrium can be followed but the connection to the right or left atrium is not clear. On the curved multiplanar reconstruction of the same dataset (**c**) the left superior caval vein (*arrows*) can be followed continuously to the left atrium (*asterisk*) [Images courtesy of Dr. G. Schneider]

quently found to originate from the wall of the pulmonary arteries. Whereas at CTA they may resemble central pulmonary emboli, MRI allows differentiation between tumor and thrombus in many cases due to contrast enhancement and tumor-like signal behavior.

Secondary infiltration of the pulmonary vasculature in cases of mediastinal tumors and lung tumors (Fig. 16) is another indication for CE MRA especially in patients that do not tolerate iodinated contrast agents.

The combination of CE MRA with multiplanar imaging of the tumor in the coronal and oblique planes may aid in visualizing tumor extension which is relevant for surgical planning.

Pitfalls and Limitations

Among the main pitfalls of pulmonary MRA examinations are artifacts due to motion in patients with poor breath-holding capability and aliasing in patients unable to raise their arms above their heads. In these cases, when a defect is seen in a segmental or sub segmental vessel it becomes difficult to determine if this is due to artifact or a true embolus. Attempts to overcome or minimize limitations due to respiratory artifact include the use of faster imaging protocols. We have found that by obtaining a pure arterial phase scan we can increase our confidence in determining the absence of a vessel. We have also found that perfusion information is very useful in confirming the MRA findings and in many cases is easier to read than the 3D CE MRA examination for evaluation of PE.

Accuracy of the 3D CE MRA Technique as published in the Literature

Few large studies have evaluated the sensitivity and specificity of 3D CE MRA for the evaluation of pulmonary embolus. Comparative evaluation of the accuracy of the technique is especially difficult due to the rapid improvements in technology. Meaney et al performed a first study in 1997 on 23 patients [1]. They performed MRA in the coronal plane utilizing a triple dose of contrast agent and obtained approximate sensitivity and specificity values 87% and 95%, respectively. Gupta et al per-

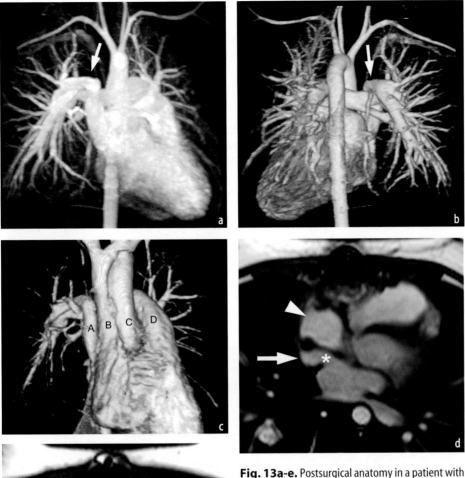

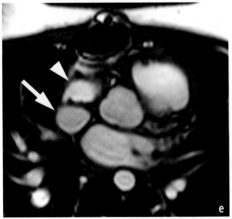

Fig. 13a-e. Postsurgical anatomy in a patient with former right sided anomalous venous return. The MIP image of the 3D CE MRA dataset (Gd-BOPTA, 0.1 mmol/kg) already demonstrates an abnormal configuration of the pulmonary veins on the right. This abnormal configuration is better appreciated on the volume rendered image in posterior to anterior view (**b**) in which the pulmonary vein is shown to override the pulmonary artery (*arrow*). The anterior-posterior projection of a later acquisition (**c**) shows the postoperative anatomy with four vessels side by side: "A" represents the pulmonary vein, "B" represents the superior caval vein, which is now connected to the right atrial appendage, "C" represents the ascending aorta and "D" represents the pulmonary artery. To direct the blood from the pulmonary vein into the left atrium the atrial septum was displaced and an artificial septal defect (*asterisk* in **d**) was created which is best demonstrated on axial true FISP CINE images (**d, e**). These images also show the course of the superior caval vein (*arrowhead*) and the pulmonary vein (*arrow*) [Images courtesy of Dr. G. Schneider]

formed a second study on 46 patients in 1999 and obtained similar sensitivity and specificity values of 85% and 96%, respectively [33]. A larger study on 141 patients was performed by Oudkerk et al in 2002 [10]. They obtained sagittal acquisitions, one through each lung, with high spatial resolution. After reconstructing the images in the coronal and axial planes, they obtained sensitivity and specificity values of 77% and 98% respectively.

Future Perspectives

At present pulmonary MRA and pulmonary perfusion MRI are not in widespread use in routine clinical practice. In large part this is because of the exquisite spatial resolution achievable with contrast enhanced CTA. However, continuing technical developments now allow CE MRA to compete with CTA and even catheter angiography for a variety of

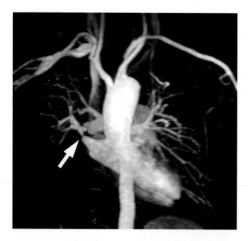

applications. Future development of easy-to-use quantitative pulmonary perfusion analysis tools as well as the possibility to perform pulmonary MRA/perfusion MRI in combination with MRI ventilation imaging may permit a one-stop-shop approach.

The clinical applicability of such a comprehensive examination has already been demonstrated in research studies. Further refinement is underway to permit the transfer of this exciting technology to routine clinical practice.

Fig. 14. Pulmonary vein stenosis in a patient post right middle and lower lobectomy. The postoperative MIP image of a 3D CE MRA dataset (Gd-BOPTA, 0.1 mmol/kg) demonstrates significant stenosis of the upper lobe pulmonary vein (*arrow*) in patient post bilobectomy due to bronchial carcinoma. The stenosis is most likely caused by scar formation since no remaining solid tumor or evidence of recurrent disease could be demonstrated [Image courtesy of Dr. G. Schneider]

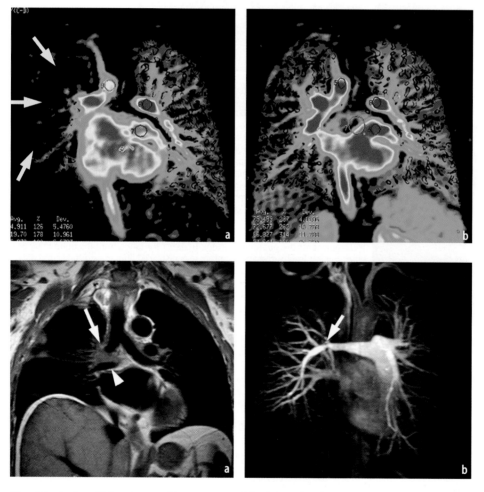

Fig. 15a, b. Evaluation of pulmonary perfusion in pulmonary vein stenosis pre- and post-surgery. Parametric maps before (**a**) and after (**b**) surgery clearly show reduced perfusion of the right lung prior to surgery (*arrows* in **a**). An almost normal parametric map can be demonstrated post surgery (**b**)

Fig. 16a, b. Bronchial carcinoma with encasement of the right main pulmonary artery. **a** The ECG-gated, breath hold coronal T1w image shows a solid tumor (*arrow*) at the right pulmonary hilum infiltrating into the mediastinum with the right main pulmonary artery adjacent to the mass. On a MIP image (**b**) of the corresponding CE MRA study (Gd-BOPTA, 0.1 mmol/kg) a circular stenosis (*arrow*) of the pulmonary artery can be seen which makes the diagnosis of infiltration of the right main pulmonary artery most likely [Images courtesy of Dr. G. Schneider]

References

1. Meaney JF et al (1997), Diagnosis of pulmonary embolism with magnetic resonance angiography. N Engl J Med 336(20):1422-7

2. Goyen M et al (2001) Dynamic 3D MR angiography of the pulmonary arteries in under four seconds. J Magn Reson Imaging 13(3):372-7

3. Finn JP et al (2002) Thorax: low-dose contrast-enhanced three-dimensional MR angiography with subsecond temporal resolution–initial results. Radiology 224(3):896-904

4. Hatabu H et al (1996) Pulmonary perfusion and angiography: evaluation with breath-hold enhanced three-dimensional fast imaging steady-state precession MR imaging with short TR and TE. AJR Am J Roentgenol 167(3):653-5

5. Hatabu H et al (1996) Pulmonary perfusion: qualitative assessment with dynamic contrast-enhanced MRI using ultra-short TE and inversion recovery turbo FLASH. Magn Reson Med 36(4):503-8

6. Uematsu H, Levin DL, Hatabu H (2001) Quantification of pulmonary perfusion with MR imaging: recent advances. Eur J Radiol 37(3):155-63

7. Carr JC et al (2002) Time-resolved three-dimensional pulmonary MR angiography and perfusion imaging with ultrashort repetition time. Acad Radiol 9(12):1407-18

8. Fink C et al (2004) Time-resolved contrast-enhanced three-dimensional pulmonary MR-angiography: 1.0 M gadobutrol vs. 0.5 M gadopentetate dimeglumine. J Magn Reson Imaging 19(2):202-8

9. Ohno Y et al (2004) Dynamic perfusion MRI versus perfusion scintigraphy: prediction of postoperative lung function in patients with lung cancer. AJR Am J Roentgenol 182(1):73-8

10. Oudkerk M et al (2002) Comparison of contrast-enhanced magnetic resonance angiography and conventional pulmonary angiography for the diagnosis of pulmonary embolism: a prospective study. Lancet 359(9318):1643-7

11. Olin JW (2002) Pulmonary embolism. Rev Cardiovasc Med 3 Suppl 2:S68-75

12. Goldman JaC E (2003) Comparison of Pulmonary Perfusion MRI with High Resolution MRA in the Detection of Pulmonary Embolus. RSNA

13. McAdams HP et al (1999) Hyperpolarized 3He-enhanced MR imaging of lung transplant recipients: preliminary results. AJR Am J Roentgenol 173(4): 955-9

14. Mai VM et al (2001) MR ventilation-perfusion imaging of human lung using oxygen-enhanced and arterial spin labeling techniques. J Magn Reson Imaging 14(5)574-9

15. Nakagawa T et al (2001) Pulmonary ventilation-perfusion MR imaging in clinical patients. J Magn Reson Imaging 14(4):419-24

16. Arents DN Jr (2002) Chronic thromboembolic pulmonary hypertension. N Engl J Med 346(11):866

17. Ley S et al (2003) Value of contrast-enhanced MR angiography and helical CT angiography in chronic thromboembolic pulmonary hypertension. Eur Radiol 13(10):2365-71

18. Kruger S et al (2001) Diagnosis of pulmonary arterial hypertension and pulmonary embolism with magnetic resonance angiography. Chest 120(5): 1556-61

19. Wang ZJ et al (2003) Cardiovascular shunts: MR imaging evaluation. Radiographics 23 Spec No:S181-94

20. Goyen M et al (2001) Pulmonary arteriovenous malformation: Characterization with time-resolved ultrafast 3D MR angiography. J Magn Reson Imaging 13(3):458-60

21. Ohno Y et al (2002) Contrast-enhanced MR perfusion imaging and MR angiography: utility for management of pulmonary arteriovenous malformations for embolotherapy. Eur J Radiol 41(2):136-46

22. Balci NC et al (2003) Assessment of the anomalous pulmonary circulation by dynamic contrast-enhanced MR angiography in under four seconds. Magn Reson Imaging 21(1):1-7

23. Choe YH et al (2001) MR imaging of congenital heart diseases in adolescents and adults. Korean J Radiol 2(3):121-31

24. Ferrari VA et al (2003) Images in cardiovascular medicine. Pulmonary venous aneurysms in hereditary hemorrhagic telangiectasia detected by 3-dimensional magnetic resonance angiography. Circulation 108(17):e122-3

25. Gilkeson RC et al (2000) Gadolinium-enhanced magnetic resonance angiography in scimitar syndrome: diagnosis and postoperative evaluation. Tex Heart Inst J 27(3):309-11

26. Puvaneswary M, Leitch J, Chard RB (2003) MRI of partial anomalous pulmonary venous return (scimitar syndrome). Australas Radiol 47(1):92-3

27. Powell AJ et al (2000) Accuracy of MRI evaluation of pulmonary blood supply in patients with complex pulmonary stenosis or atresia. Int J Card Imaging 16(3):169-74

28. Shors SM et al (2003) Heart failure: evaluation of cardiopulmonary transit times with time-resolved MR angiography. Radiology 229(3):743-8

29. Valsangiacomo ER et al (2003) Contrast-enhanced MR angiography of pulmonary venous abnormalities in children. Pediatr Radiol 33(2):92-8

30. Zhang M et al (2001) Contrast enhanced MR angiography in pulmonary sequestration. Chin Med J (Engl) 114(12): 1326-8

31. Prasad SK et al (2004) Role of magnetic resonance angiography in the diagnosis of major aortopulmonary collateral arteries and partial anomalous pulmonary venous drainage. Circulation 109(2): 207-14

32. Goldman JN, J and Poon M (2002) Time Resolved Contrast Enhanced MRA in the Evaluation of Adult Congenital Heart Disease. Proceedings of the ISMRM:165

33. Gupta A et al (1999) Acute pulmonary embolism: diagnosis with MR angiography. Radiology 210(2): 353-9

SECTION V

Coronary Arteries

V
MR Angiography of the Coronary Arteries

Milind Y. Desai and Matthias Stuber

Background

The current gold standard for the diagnosis of coronary artery disease is x-ray coronary angiography. Approximately 1 million cardiac catheterizations are performed each year in the western world. However, x-ray coronary angiography is expensive, invasive, and requires exposure of the patients to ionizing radiation. Moreover, there is a small but finite risk of serious complications to the patient and of operator exposure to radiation. Thus, there exists a strong need for a more cost-effective, non-invasive, and more patient friendly imaging modality. Coronary magnetic resonance angiography (MRA) overcomes a lot of the problems associated with x-ray angiography and has shown great potential for the diagnosis of coronary artery disease (CAD). In addition to being non-invasive, cost effective and patient friendly, it can survey in any image plane and has the ability to achieve high spatial resolution with no exposure to potentially harmful ionizing radiation.

The utility of coronary MRA has been investigated since the late 1980s [1, 2]. Although no coronary stenoses were identified in these early studies, the potential of MR imaging to assess the anatomy of the coronary vessels was demonstrated, and triggered further interest in this field. Simultaneously, it was suggested that coronary artery lumen narrowing is preceded by atherosclerosis and positive arterial remodeling of the vessel wall [3]. Hence, basic and clinical research findings have challenged the notion of flow limiting stenoses and studies have tried to focus away from the vessel lumen and towards the vessel wall. However, using x-ray angiography, the coronary artery vessel wall and hence, the remodeling cannot be visualized. This is where MRI, with its ability to differentiate between coronary lumen and the coronary artery vessel wall, offers great potential.

However, for successful coronary MRA and coronary vessel wall data acquisition, a series of major obstacles has to be overcome. The heart is subject to both intrinsic and extrinsic motion due to its natural periodic contraction and breathing. Both of these motion components exceed the dimensions of the coronary artery, resulting in the need for efficient motion suppression strategies if satisfactory acquisition of coronary MR data is to be achieved in the sub-millimeter range.

Enhanced contrast between the coronary lumen and the surrounding tissue is crucial for successful visualization of both the coronary lumen and the coronary vessel wall. In this chapter, we will discuss the hurdles that need to be overcome in order to acquire adequate coronary images using MRI, the technical details and clinical implications of coronary MRA and the approaches to coronary vessel wall imaging.

Technical Challenges associated with Coronary MRA

Motion Suppression in Coronary MRA

Cardiac Motion

Cardiac Motion, a major obstacle for obtaining adequate coronary MRA images, can be divided into two types: motion related to intrinsic cardiac contraction/relaxation and motion due to superimposed diaphragmatic and chest wall movement during respiration. Since the extent of each motion supercedes the diameter of the coronary artery, blurring artifacts of the coronary lumen occur unless adequate motion suppression techniques are used. To account for intrinsic cardiac motion, ECG gating is absolutely essential. However, considerable ECG signal degradation occurs because of radiofrequency field and gradient-switching noise. To overcome this, a vector ECG approach has been found to be very robust for R-wave detection as compared to alternate gating strategies such as peripheral pulse detection. However, under the influence of a strong static magnetic field, the so called magnetohydrodynamic effect is enhanced and an artifactual voltage overlaid to the T-wave of the ECG results. This artifactual augmentation of the T-wave may frequently mislead the R-wave detection algorithm so that triggering is performed on the T-wave instead of the R-wave. This results in serious artifacts on coronary MRA and coronary vessel wall images. Since this artifact increases with field strength, this presents a major challenge for MRA, particularly at higher field strengths such as 3 Tesla. However, by analyzing the ECG vector in 3D space [4], the true T-wave can be separated from the artifactual T-wave augmentation. Moreover, reliable R-wave detection has recently been shown to be feasible even at higher field strength [5].

Another issue lies with actual coronary artery motion which occurs in a triphasic pattern during the cardiac cycle. Hence, mid-diastolic diastasis has been identified as the preferred time for image acquisition as it also coincides with the interval of rapid coronary filling. This period is inversely related to the heart rate and can be determined using a heart rate dependent formula. However, because of considerable interpatient variation, a recommendation is to determine a patient specific diastasis period which can be achieved by acquiring a cine image perpendicular to the long axis of the proximal/mid right coronary artery (RCA).

Respiratory Motion

The second major impediment to coronary MRA is respiratory motion. Early approaches to suppressing respiratory motion involved the use of breath-hold techniques. Two-dimensional (2D) breath-hold coronary MRA relied on acquiring contiguous images, with the goal of surveying the proximal segments of the coronary arteries during serial breath-holds. More recently, three-dimensional (3D) breath-hold techniques for coronary MRA have also been implemented [6-10]. Breath-hold approaches offer the advantage of rapid imaging and are technically easy to implement in compliant subjects. For coronary MRA techniques that utilize the first-pass enhancement of intravenously injected extracellular contrast agents, breath-holding is a requirement at the present time. However, breath-holding strategies have several limitations. Some patients may have difficulty sustaining adequate breath-holds, particularly when the duration exceeds a few seconds. Additionally, it has been shown that during a sustained breath-hold there is cranial diaphragmatic drift [11], which may be sub-

stantial in many cases (~1cm). Among serial breath-holds, the diaphragmatic and cardiac positions frequently vary by up to 1 cm, resulting in registration errors [6, 12]. Misregistration results in apparent gaps between the segments of the visualized coronary arteries, which could be misinterpreted as signal voids from coronary stenoses. Finally, the use of signal enhancement techniques, such as signal averaging or fold-over suppression is significantly restricted by the duration of the applicable breath-hold duration. Using breath-holding techniques, the spatial resolution of the images is also governed by the patient's ability to hold his/her breath. Thus, while breath-hold strategies are often successful with motivated volunteers, their applicability to the broad range of patients with cardiovascular disease is more limited.

To overcome limitations associated with breath-holding, different methods such as MR navigators [13] have been developed to allow for free-breathing coronary MRA. With vertical positioning of the navigator at the dome of the right hemidiaphragm (lung-liver interface), the diaphragmatic craniocaudal displacement can be monitored. These data can be used to gate coronary MRA acquisitions. The gating process can be either prospective (i.e. before data acquisition) or retrospective (i.e. following data acquisition, but before image reconstruction). Although navigator approaches greatly improve patient comfort and do not require significant subject motivation, their use prolongs the scan duration since coronary MRA data are collected during 50% of the RR intervals on average [14]. To overcome problems associated with narrow gating windows and prolonged scans, coronary MRA with prospective navigator correction has been implemented and has been shown to maintain or improve image quality both for 2D and 3D approaches to coronary MRA [15-17], while scanning time can be shortened. However, it is of utmost importance that the navigator is positioned in close temporal proximity to the imaging part of the sequence [18]. Typical examination times with free-breathing 3D real-time navigator approaches are ~7min.

Currently, inversion-recovery techniques seem to be emerging as the method of choice for contrast-enhanced coronary MRA [19-22]. However, the inversion-pre-pulse precedes the navigator thereby reducing the magnetization at the location of the navigator, which may adversely affect navigator performance. Therefore, countermeasures have been proposed [23] and successfully applied [22].

Spatial Resolution

Even though great progress has been made with regard to motion suppression, MRI hardware, software, scanning protocols and contrast agents, the spatial resolution achievable with MRI is still inferior to that obtainable with x-ray coronary angiography (<300 μm). While an improvement in spatial resolution is always accompanied by a trade-off in terms of signal-to-noise ratio (SNR), this may partly be overcome by the use of high-field systems [5] and contrast agents [22]. However, prior to reducing the voxel size towards the resolution achievable on x-ray angiography, it is important to ensure that the residual intrinsic and extrinsic motion of the coronary arteries is sufficiently constrained [18]. Therefore, current research is focused on optimization of the acquisition interval [24, 25], the utility of k-space reordering techniques with a reduced sensitivity to motion [26, 27], and the use of multiple navigators to account for the complex respiration-induced 3D motion pattern of the heart [28]. These and similar technical developments will be most critical and still remain to be evaluated in a clinical setting.

Coronary Magnetic Resonance Angiography

Contrast-Enhancement in Coronary MRA

Using MRI, the contrast between the coronary blood-pool and the surrounding tissue can be manipulated using the in-flow effect [29] or by the application of MR pre-pulses. Non-exogenous contrast enhancement between the coronary arteries and the surrounding tissue has been obtained by the use of fat-saturation pre-pulses [29], magnetization transfer contrast pre-pulses (MTC) [30] or more recently T2 preparatory pulses (T2Prep) [31, 32] which take advantage of natural T2 differences between blood and the surrounding myocardium. With these techniques, the coronary lumen appears bright while the surrounding myocardium appears with reduced signal intensity. An alternative to bright-blood visualization of the coronary

arteries is black-blood coronary MRA, in which the coronary lumen appears signal attenuated while the surrounding tissue displays with high signal intensity [33].

With the use of MR contrast agents, the T1 relaxation of blood can be shortened, allowing for increased contrast-to-noise ratio (CNR) for coronary MRA [19, 21]. The contrast agents currently available for coronary MRA are the traditional extracellular gadolinium-based contrast agents. However, because extracellular agents quickly extravasate into the extravascular space, their use requires rapid first-pass imaging, thereby necessitating breath-holding [8]. First-pass coronary MRA with extravascular contrast agents is also limited by the need for repeated contrast injections when more than one slab is imaged. With each subsequent injection, the CNR will be lower, as the signal from the extracellular space continuously increases following initial contrast administration.

An attempt to overcome the inherent limitations of extracellular contrast agents has seen the development of newer intravascular agents (the so-called blood-pool agents) based either on gadolinium (e.g. B22956 and MS-325) or iron oxide (e.g. AMI 227 and NC100150) [19-21, 34, 35]. The use of intravascular agents has the advantage of allowing image acquisition over longer time periods after intravenous administration of the contrast agent. Thus, non-breath-hold schemes can be employed, and repeated scans have similar CNR values thereby obviating the need for repeated injections [21]. Figure 1 displays a left coronary arterial system with high contrast acquired with B-22956 (Bracco Imaging S.p.A., Milan, Italy) and a previously described free-breathing navigator-gated and corrected 3D inversion technique [21]. Using this specific intravascular contrast agent, a substantial (50%) enhancement of the SNR was accompanied by a 160% improvement in CNR when compared to a standard non-contrast enhanced technique [22, 36]. Simultaneously, a 20% improvement in vessel sharpness suggested superior vessel

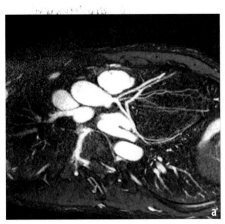 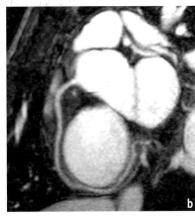

Fig. 1. Left (**a**) and right (**b**) coronary arterial systems acquired with the intravascular contrast agent B-22956 (Bracco Imaging SpA, Milan, Italy) and a free-breathing navigator gated and corrected 3D inversion technique [21]. The images were acquired as part of an international collaboration: IBT ETH Zurich, Switzerland, German Heart Center, Berlin, Germany, Bracco Imaging SpA, Italy, Beth Israel Deaconess Medical Center, MA, USA, Philips Medical Systems, Best, The Netherlands

delineation post contrast [22]. These findings are visually supported by the images displayed in Fig. 1. Similar results were found in a parallel volunteer study using the contrast agent SH L 643A (Schering, Berlin, Germany) [37].

Identification of Coronary Stenosis

Although current breath-hold coronary MRA techniques have relatively limited in-plane spatial resolution, the technique has proven adequate for the identification of proximal coronary stenoses in several clinical series. Gradient-echo techniques depict focal stenoses as signal voids. In one of the earliest patient studies comparing coronary MRA prospectively with x-ray coronary angiography [38], a segmented k-space 2D breath-hold ECG-gated gradient-echo sequence was used. Overall sensitivity and specificity values of the 2D coronary MRA technique for correctly ascertaining whether individual vessels had or did not have significant CAD (50% diameter on conventional contrast angiography) were 90% and 92%, respectively. Subsequent studies [39-43] have reported variable sensitivity and specificity values for the detection of significant CAD. Explanations for this variability in these single center studies include differences in the utilized MR sequences, inadequate patient cooperation with regards to breath-holding, and irregular rhythms, all of which contribute to image degradation. Newer breath-hold [10] and non-breath-hold approaches to 3D coronary MRA have also demonstrated the ability of this technique to detect coronary stenoses. The first international multicenter trial prospectively comparing coronary MRA and the gold standard x-ray coronary angiography using common methodology and identical hardware and software has recently been completed [36]. The major finding of the study was that free-breathing sub-millimeter 3D coronary MRA is able to accurately identify significant proximal and mid coronary disease, while non-significant coronary disease can be excluded with high confidence (Fig. 2). Drawbacks that need to be resolved include a relatively low specificity (false positive readings) while the potential for accurate quantitative *grading* of stenosis has still to be investigated.

Recent Technical Developments

Spiral Coronary MRA

Although early attempts to acquire coronary MRA data in the sub-millimeter range resulted in 2D spiral acquisitions with outstanding image quality [44], this technique has not been widely employed.

An advantage of spiral techniques is that efficient sampling of k-space can be performed with high SNR while minimizing adverse effects due to flow artifacts. An extension of spiral coronary MRA using a 3D acquisition strategy [45, 46], an interleaved segmented approach [46], and real-time navigator technology for free-breathing coronary MRA data acquisition has proven to be a very valuable alternative for high-resolution coronary MRA [47]. An image of a left coronary arterial system acquired with a dual-interleaved free-breathing 3D spiral technique is shown in Figure 3.

Steady-state with free-precession Coronary MRA

With this sequence, high SNR and very high contrast between the ventricular blood-pool and the myocardium can be obtained without the need for exogenous contrast enhancement. The application of SSFP is therefore highly promising for contrast enhancement in 3D coronary MRA, in which the in-flow effect is generally reduced due to relatively thick slab excitations [48]. Presently, more and more cardiac MRI centers are adopting SSFP sequences either in conjunction with a single breath-hold [48] or based on free-breathing with navigators [49]. A first evaluation in an animal model demonstrated that SSFP imaging permits high quality coronary MRA during free breathing with substantial improvements in SNR, CNR and vessel sharpness when compared with standard T2-prepared gradient-echo imaging [49]. Although spiral imaging achieved the highest SNR, SSFP imaging was considered better for image quality and vessel definition. In a small volunteer study to evaluate theoretical considerations concerning the T1-lowering characteristics of contrast agents [50], consistent fat suppression and a 78% increase in blood-myocardial CNR was found post contrast using SSFP.

Black-blood Coronary MRA

Artifacts originating from metallic implants such as clips or sternal wires are accentuated on gradient echo based bright blood coronary MRA. Furthermore, thrombus, vessel wall and various plaque components may appear with high signal intensity on bright blood coronary MRA [51]. As a result, luminal stenosis may be obscured on bright blood images. To overcome this potential drawback, 'black-blood' fast spin-echo coronary MRA techniques have recently been introduced [23, 33]. With these techniques, the coronary lumen appears signal attenuated while the signal of surrounding tissue including epicardial fat and my-

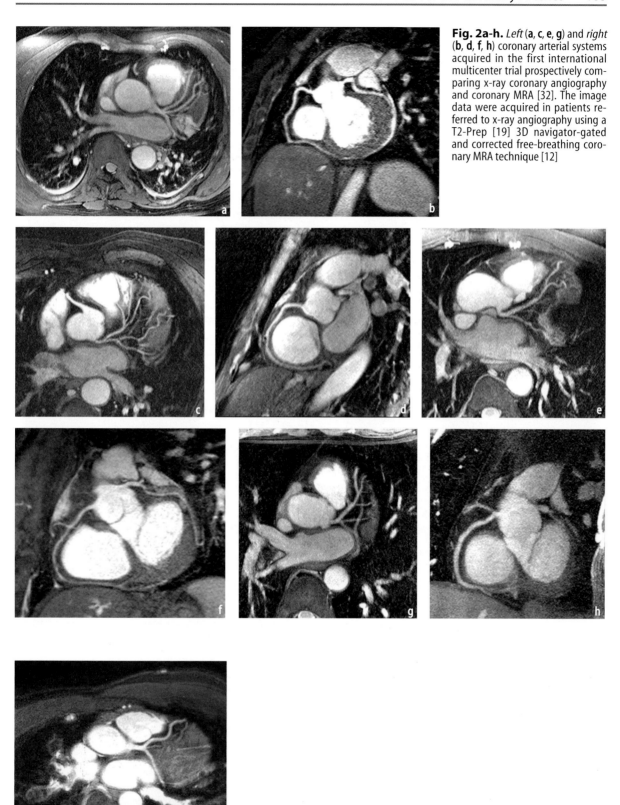

Fig. 2a-h. *Left* (**a, c, e, g**) and *right* (**b, d, f, h**) coronary arterial systems acquired in the first international multicenter trial prospectively comparing x-ray coronary angiography and coronary MRA [32]. The image data were acquired in patients referred to x-ray angiography using a T2-Prep [19] 3D navigator-gated and corrected free-breathing coronary MRA technique [12]

Fig. 3. 3D spiral image of a left coronary arterial system. The image was acquired with real-time navigator technology using a dual-interleaved spiral imaging technique

ocardium appears enhanced. Initial results obtained in patients suggest that artifacts originating from metallic implants can be minimized. However, a principal disadvantage of dual-inversion black-blood coronary MRA is that calcifications appear signal attenuated resulting in the possibility for misinterpretation of calcified stenosis. On the other hand, black-blood coronary MRA has proven very useful for the visualization of the vessel wall as discussed below.

Parallel Imaging for Coronary MRA

An alternative method to compensate for respiratory motion, and thus to allow for free-breathing coronary MR imaging, would be to decrease the acquisition time so that the entire data set is obtained in one cardiac cycle. The development of such rapid strategies is an active field of research in cardiac MRI [52, 53]. Early introductions to parallel imaging for coronary MRA include techniques termed 'SMASH' and 'SENSE'. These parallel imaging approaches are able to reduce the scanning time for cardiac MRI substantially [54] and therefore have great potential. However, a principal

trade-off for reduced acquisition time is a reduced SNR and this has to be evaluated carefully for each individual application. On the other hand, magnets with higher field strengths may overcome some of these limitations while maintaining a suitably short acquisition time.

High Field (3T) Coronary MRA

Currently, the vast majority of research into coronary MRA as well as most technical innovations and clinical applications are performed on 1.5T systems. For many of these applications, limited SNR or lengthy examination times are impediments. The recent availability of high field systems (3T) equipped with dedicated cardiac hardware (real-time spectrometer, parallel receiver technology with high bandwidth, body RF send coil, vector ECG, etc.) and software (SENSE, navigators, interactive interface, SSFP) will permit a major step forward for coronary MRA. Preliminary *in vivo* findings obtained in two healthy adult subjects evaluated on a commercial 3T system (Philips Medical Systems, Best, NL) are displayed in Figure 4. The images were acquired using an ECG trig-

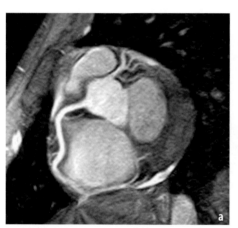
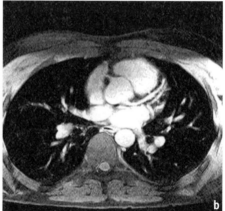

Fig. 4. Preliminary in vivo coronary MRA image acquired at 3T. The 3D image data were obtained during free breathing with a T2-Prep and 2D selective real-time navigator technique. The image of the right coronary system (**a**) was acquired with a 6-element cardiac phased-array surface coil while the image of the left coronary system (**b**) was acquired using a body coil

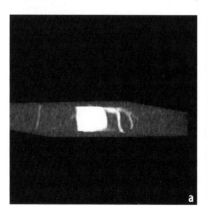
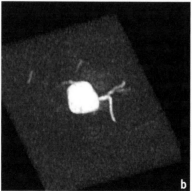
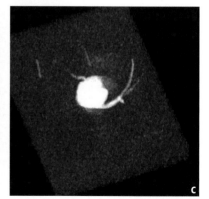

Fig. 5. Arterial spin labeling enables an exclusive and selective 3D visualization of the coronary arterial lumen [42]. The left coronary system (**a, b, c**) is displayed at 3 incremental viewing angles about the left-right axis of the examined healthy adult subject. Signal from the surrounding tissue (chest wall, atria, great cardiac vessels, coronary veins etc.) is entirely suppressed

gered segmented k-space gradient echo technique including T2-Prep and real-time navigator technology for free-breathing data acquisition (0.6 x 0.6 x 3mm voxel size) [5].

Arterial Spin Labeling

Conventional coronary MRA techniques display the coronary blood-pool along with surrounding structures including the chest-wall, myocardium, ventricular and atrial blood-pools, and great cardiac vessels (Figs. 1-4). This representation of the coronary lumen is not directly analogous to the information provided by x-ray coronary angiography, in which the coronary lumen displaced by contrast agent is depicted exclusively. Analogous "luminographic" data may be obtained using MR arterial spin tagging [55]. This technique enables exclusive and selective 3D visualization of the coronary blood-pool without user-assisted segmentation or post-processing (Fig. 5). However, despite its potential, the technique inherently doubles the acquisition time and is sensitive to misregistrations. Consequently, very efficient motion compensation mechanisms are required.

Coronary Vessel Wall Imaging

Coronary Artery Disease and Atherosclerosis

Despite advances in both treatment and prevention, complications of atherosclerotic disease remain the leading cause of morbidity and mortality in the Western World [56]. More than 50% of atherosclerotic deaths can be attributed to coronary heart disease with estimated socioeconomic costs of $112 billion in the year 2002 in the United States alone. While atherosclerosis may progress slowly over years or decades, the occurrence of thrombosis as a consequence of sudden plaque rupture often leads to abrupt life threatening complications. Such acute events may explain why many people who die from coronary artery disease die suddenly without manifestation of typical symptoms. As reported by Glagov et al [3], the initial response to endothelial injury and initial development of atherosclerosis is outward remodeling of the artery, with relative preservation of lumen diameter. Such findings have been confirmed in living patients with invasive [57] and non-invasive techniques [58, 59]. Over 50% of all future myocardial infarctions occur in vascular regions with atherosclerotic thickening but non-critical luminal narrowing [60, 61]. This was confirmed in a prospective study of 4476 elderly subjects for whom carotid wall thickness, assessed non-invasively by high-resolution

B-mode ultrasound, was a stronger predictor of future stroke and myocardial infarction than were conventional coronary atherosclerotic risk factors [62]. The inference was that carotid wall thickening was a marker for diffuse atherosclerosis and thus correlated or predicted concomitant disease in the coronaries. The prognostic value of coronary wall thickness for predicting future events is probably very high. However, this has not yet been demonstrated because ultrasound evaluation of coronary wall thickness can only be performed invasively (intravascular ultrasound) and such studies are precluded in large, prospective, long-term endpoint trials. However, coronary wall disease, as indexed by coronary calcium, can be detected by rapid computed tomography (CT) and this approach has also been useful in predicting future cardiac events [63, 64]. The approach, however, does not directly measure wall thickness and cannot identify or characterize common, non-calcified atherosclerotic plaques. Conventional x-ray angiography is the current gold standard for the detection and treatment of intra-luminal (flow-limiting) coronary artery stenosis, but x-ray "luminography" provides minimal information on the magnitude of underlying atherosclerotic plaque burden. For these reasons, a non-invasive technique capable of measuring coronary wall thickness has great potential not only for the identification of disease at an early stage, but also for the prediction of future events and the evaluation of therapeutic strategies.

Identification of Plaque Components in the Vessel Wall by MRI

Findings from *in vitro* studies demonstrated the ability of MRI to identify various plaque components [65, 66] and T2-weighted sequences have shown promise for the differentiation of plaque components [65, 67]. Serfaty et al. [68] used T2-weighted MR imaging to measure fibrous cap thickness and lipid core volume. Unfortunately, their *ex vivo* study was limited by overestimation of the lipid core. Shinnar et al. [66] suggested the use of two echo times to differentiate the lipid core from fibrocellular areas that contain lipid. However, one limitation of T2-weighted MR imaging is an inherently low SNR. *In vivo* application of these techniques is supported by the strong agreement demonstrated between *in vivo* and *ex vivo* measurements of vessel wall thickness and T2 relaxation of plaque components [69, 70]. Wasserman et al. [71] used gadolinium (Gd) in combination with T1-weighted MRI to describe plaque morphology and demonstrated not only that delayed hyperenhancement preferentially occurs in fibrocellular tissue, but also that SNR is substantially enhanced compared to T2-weighted imaging. Similar results were reported by Yuan et al. [72] who showed that the strongest MRI signal enhancement was observed in fibrocellular tissue and that only modest contrast agent uptake occurred in the lipid core of the carotid vessel wall. A study by Jaffer et al. [73], which included participants who were free of clinically apparent coronary disease, revealed evidence of aortic atherosclerosis in 38% of the women and 41% of the men. Atherosclerotic prevalence was more apparent in the abdominal than in the thoracic aorta. These data demonstrate the ability of MR vessel wall imaging to detect subclinical atherosclerotic disease, and to better risk stratify patients with asymptomatic heart disease. However, it should be noted that all these studies were performed under *ex vivo* conditions, in animal models, or in the carotids or aorta as a surrogate for *in vivo* human coronary arteries, and that a clear correlation between carotid/aortic plaque and coronary events has not been established [73, 74]. Together with the current understanding that luminal disease underestimates plaque burden and that the majority of acute coronary syndromes occur at sites without previously flow-limiting stenoses (<50%) [60, 75], this demonstrates a clear need for an imaging method that allows direct and non-invasive access to the coronary or bypass graft vessel wall. However, coronary vessel lumen, and, especially wall imaging, are among the most challenging tasks for cardiovascular MRI. There are specific technical difficulties that have hampered the transfer of carotid or aortic plaque imaging approaches to the coronary vessel wall. These include the small dimensions (0.5–2mm) of the coronary vessel wall, a very complex geometry, cardiac and respiratory motion, and the proximity of the coronary artery walls to epicardial fat and coronary blood. As discussed above, recent advances in MRI hardware and new imaging software have made it possible to visualize the native coronary artery vessel wall in selected cases [58, 59, 76]. However, limited spatial resolution still hampers further progress and limits the accuracy and sensitivity of quantitative measurements [77]. A major step forward is expected with the availability of higher spatial resolution on 3T MRI systems and by simultaneously taking advantage of vessel wall hyperenhancement after contrast injection.

Measurement of Plaque Regression after Pharmacological Intervention using MRI

Non-invasive MRI has been shown to allow serial monitoring of atherosclerotic plaque size changes in the carotids after lipid-lowering pharmacological interventions [78]. Studies by Corti et al. [79, 80], revealed significant regression of established atherosclerotic carotid and aortic lesions in humans. These studies were performed at baseline and at 6 and 12 months after lipid-lowering therapy. The effects of the treatment on atherosclerotic lesions were measured as changes in lumen area, vessel wall thickness, and vessel wall area, a surrogate for atherosclerotic burden. At 6 months after pharmacological intervention, no changes in lumen area, vessel wall thickness, or vessel wall area were observed. However, at 12 months, significant reductions in vessel wall thickness and vessel wall area, without changes in lumen area, were observed in both aortic and carotid arteries. Unfortunately, the spatial resolution was still not optimal for coronary vessel wall imaging in these studies. In addition to improving spatial resolution, greater sensitivity for the measurement of progression and regression of wall thickness is needed. For this, direct imaging access to the coronary vessel wall is the goal.

Coronary Vessel Wall Imaging using MRI

Imaging of the coronary artery vessel wall is probably the most challenging task in cardiac MRI because of the small dimension and constant motion of the coronary arteries. Simultaneously, the need for high contrast between the coronary lumen blood pool and the surrounding coronary vessel wall is mandatory. However, this is very similar to the challenges faced by coronary MRA in general.

The first successful implementation of coronary vessel wall imaging in humans involved the use of a dual-inversion fast spin echo sequence. Using this method, single slices of the coronary artery wall could be acquired during a prolonged breath-hold period, permitting the demonstration of relative wall thickening in selected cases [59]. Subsequently, and to overcome the limitations associated with breath-holding, this technique was adapted for use with navigators for free-breathing data acquisition [76]. More recently, the free-breathing navigator approach has been combined with 3D spiral imaging in conjunction with a 'local inversion' technique [81]. Using this method, excellent image quality can be obtained because of the high SNR associated with 3D imaging on the one hand and the signal-efficient spiral read-out on the other. This enables larger anatomical coverage with much thinner reconstructed slices than those of the earlier 2D approaches. Therefore, it is now possible to visualize long, contiguous sections of the coronary artery vessel wall as shown in Fig. 6. Additionally, the spiral approach permits data

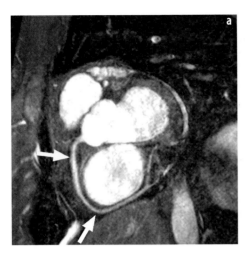

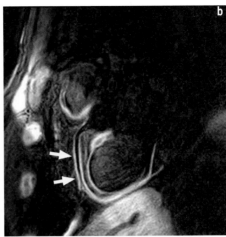

Fig. 6a, b. Coronary vessel wall imaging in a healthy adult subject. The SSFP image (**a**) of a right coronary artery (*arrow*) was used as a scout scan for (**b**) the local-inversion 3D spiral navigator-gated and corrected coronary vessel wall (*arrows* in **b**). A 5-6 cm segment of the coronary vessel wall is clearly seen and high visual contrast between the coronary lumen and the surrounding vessel wall is apparent. The spatial resolution is 0.8x0.8x1 mm and the scanning time during free-breathing is ~12min

acquisition within a short acquisition window of only 50 ms, permitting the effects of intrinsic myocardial motion to be suppressed more effectively while at the same time rendering the technique less susceptible to R-R variability. A disadvantage of the technique is a prolonged scanning time of ~12 min during free breathing with image acquisition during alternate R-R intervals. Preliminary evaluation of this local-inversion 3D spiral technique has been performed in 12 adult subjects comprising 6 clinically healthy subjects and 6 patients with non-significant coronary artery disease (10% to 50% diameter reduction on x-ray angiography). Examinations were performed on a commercial 1.5 Tesla scanner with free-breathing 3D coronary vessel wall imaging performed along the major axis of the right coronary artery with isotropic spatial resolution (1.0x1.0x1.0 mm^3). The proximal vessel wall thickness and luminal diameter were objectively determined with an automated algorithm [32]. The 3D vessel wall scans allowed for visualization of the contiguous proximal right coronary artery in all subjects. The mean vessel wall thickness (1.7 ± 0.3 versus 1.0 ± 0.2 mm) was significantly increased in the patients compared with the healthy subjects (p<0.01). However, the lumen diameter measurement (3.6 ± 0.7 versus 3.4 ± 0.5 mm, p=0.47) was similar in both groups. The findings suggest that free-breathing 3D black-blood coronary MRI may serve as an appropriate non-invasive technique for the identification of increased coronary vessel wall thickness with preservation of lumen size in patients with non-significant coronary artery disease, consistent with "Glagov-type" outward arterial remodeling [3]. This novel approach may have the potential to quantify sub-clinical disease. Future developments will include the use of higher magnetic field strengths, contrast agents for plaque characterization [71, 72], and studies of vessel wall thickness following intervention [82].

Practical Recommendations

Because of the small dimensions and tortuosity of the coronary arteries, high-resolution imaging and sufficient volumetric coverage are essential. However, the need for high resolution and larger volumes results in dramatically lengthened scanning times of contemporary MRI techniques from a few seconds to a few minutes. Unfortunately, imaging of the heart is not practical on this timescale because of breathing and intrinsic myocardial motion. Therefore, ECG triggering, k-space segmentation, short acquisition intervals (Tacq <100ms), and imaging during quiescent periods in the cardiac cycle (typically in late diastole) are recommended, while respiratory artifacts must be suppressed by means of breath-holding or navigator technology. While k-space segmentation, abbreviated acquisition windows, and the use of navigators effectively suppress motion artifacts, a substantial increase in scanning time is inevitable (3-15 min). Breath-holding is an effective method to reduce scanning time, but compromises relating to the acquisition intervals (Tacq >120ms) and spatial resolution have to be made to accommodate practical breath-hold durations of <20 s. As is the case for CTA, improved coronary MRA image quality is achieved at lower heart rates while data collection during arrhythmias must be avoided.

At the present time, clinical multi-center experience only exists for free-breathing navigator approaches. Below are some practical recommendations for performing free-breathing navigator-gated and corrected coronary MRA at 1.5T. For coronary MRA with intravascular contrast agents, the T2-Prep sequence can simply be exchanged for an inversion pulse and a carefully adjusted inversion delay [22]. Parts of the protocols were provided by Marc Kouwenhoven from Philips Medical Systems. For breath-holding, black-blood imaging (coronary vessel wall imaging), and arterial spin label-

Table 1. Scout 3. Free-breathing navigator gated and corrected 3D SSFP

Parameter	Value	Unit	Parameter	Value	Unit
Field of View	270	mm	T2Prep/TE	YES/50	ms
Matrix	128		FatSat	YES	
Slices	35		SENSE	Optional	
Slice Thickness	3.4	mm	Navigator	YES	
Half Scan	YES		Gating Window	7	mm
TR	3.7	ms	Navigator Tracking	YES	
TE	1.9	ms	Tracking Factor	0.6	
Tacq	75	ms	Bandwidth	1086	Hz/Pixel
Alpha	90	Deg	Scan Duration	2-4	min
Spatial Resolution	2.1x2.2x3.4	mm^3			

Table 2. Targeted coronary MRA. High-resolution free-breathing navigator gated and corrected 3D SSFP

Parameter	Value	Unit	Parameter	Value	Unit
Field of View	270	mm	T2Prep/TE	YES/50	ms
Matrix	272		FatSat	YES	
Slices	10		SENSE	NO	
Slice Thickness	3.0	mm	Navigator	YES	
Half Scan	NO		Gating Window	5	mm
TR	5.6	ms	Navigator Tracking	YES	
TE	2.8	ms	Tracking Factor	0.6	
Tacq	73	ms	Bandwidth	543	Hz/Pixel
Alpha	110	Deg	Scan Duration	4-7	min
Spatial Resolution	1.0x1.0x3.0	mm^3			

ing, readers should refer to the literature mentioned in this chapter.

Scout Scanning

For localization of the coronary arteries and for identification of the period of minimal myocardial motion, 3 scout scans are recommended:

Scout 1: A low resolution 2D SSFP scan that covers the chest in 3 orthogonal views (coronal, sagittal, transverse). Multiple (10) 1 cm thick slices per view. The scan is performed during free-breathing.

Scout 2: On a mid-ventricular level (as identified on the first scout), a transverse 2D SSFP cine scan with 40 frames/s is acquired for the visual identification of the diastolic rest period. This scan can either be performed during free-breathing using signal averaging (total duration ~40 sec) or during one breath-hold of ~10 sec.

Scout 3: Transverse 3D SSFP scout scan for localization of the coronary arteries. Image acquisition is performed in late diastole, at the time-point of minimal myocardial motion as identified in Scout 2. The 3D volume of Scout 3 includes the whole heart including the apex and the pulmonary artery as seen on the coronal view of Scout 1. The navigator is localized at the dome of the right hemidiaphragm. Localization of the dome of the right hemidiaphragm is performed on the transverse and coronal views of Scout 1. The end-expiratory gating window for Scout 3 is 7 mm. The scan duration is ~1.5-2 min depending on the heart rate and the respiratory pattern of the patient (Table 1).

For high resolution coronary MRA, 3D volume-targeted SSFP or segmented k-space gradient echo imaging sequences are currently preferred. In the following protocols a compromise between bandwidth for signal-readout and TR was made. Therefore, not all the protocols run with the shortest possible TR values. Shortening of the TR is possible but at the cost of a reduced SNR (Table 2).

Table 3. Targeted coronary MRA. High-resolution free-breathing navigator gated and corrected 3D TFE

Parameter	Value	Unit	Parameter	Value	Unit
Field of View	270	mm	T2Prep/TE	YES/50	ms
Matrix	384		FatSat	YES	
Slices	10		SENSE	NO	
Slice Thickness	3.0	mm	Navigator	YES	
Half Scan	NO		Gating Window	5	mm
TR	7.2	ms	Navigator Tracking	YES	
TE	2.0 (Partial Echo)	ms	Tracking Factor	0.6	
Tacq	71	ms	Bandwidth	135	Hz/Pixel
Alpha	25	Deg	Scan Duration	6-9	min
Spatial Resolution	0.7x1.0x3.0	mm^3			

Table 4. Whole-heart coronary MRA. High-resolution free-breathing navigator gated and corrected 3D SSFP

Parameter	Value	Unit	Parameter	Value	Unit
Field of View	256	mm	T2Prep/TE	YES/50	ms
Matrix	256		FatSat	YES	
Slices	80		SENSE/Factor	YES/2	
Slice Thickness	1.5	mm	Navigator	YES	
Half Scan	NO		Gating Window	7	mm
TR	5.0	ms	Navigator Tracking	YES	
TE	2.5	ms	Tracking Factor	0.6	
Tacq	125	ms	Bandwidth	543	Hz/Pixel
Alpha	90	Deg	Scan Duration	10-15	min
Spatial Resolution	1.0x1.0x1.5	mm^3			

High-Resolution Coronary MRA

For accurate volume-targeting, it is important that the 3D scout scan (Scout 3) and 3D high-resolution coronary MRA are acquired at the same timepoint in the cardiac cycle (identified from the images of Scout 2) and using the same suppression of respiratory motion. For high resolution imaging, the gating window should be reduced to ~5 mm and the localization of the navigator should remain unchanged when compared to Scout 3. Typically, the duration of the acquisition window is also reduced for high resolution coronary MRA (50 – 100 ms). Volume targeting for the right coronary system can be performed using a 3-point planscan tool. Three user-specified points (as viewed on Scout 3) on the proximal RCA, the mid-RCA and the distal RCA define the orientation and location of the center plane of the imaged volume. For the left coronary system, one point on the LM, and one point on the mid-LAD and mid-LCX prescribe a near-transverse view that includes the proximal segments of the left coronary arterial system. The highest (most cranial) point of the left coronary system is not always on the left main. Therefore, it is important to ensure that the prescribed volume encompasses the major proximal segments of the left coronary system. Alternative plane orientations parallel to the LCX and/or the LAD have also been used and long segments of the LCX are often visualized on scans of the RCA. These high resolution volume targeted MRAs provide ideal localizer scans for dual-inversion black-blood coronary vessel wall imaging. In whole-heart coronary MRA as described by Weber and co-workers [83], a transverse volume that encompasses the apex and the pulmonary artery as viewed on Scout 1 is planned. Although the whole-heart scan lasts 10-15 min, near-isotropic resolution is obtained (Tables 3, 4).

Navigator Pitfalls

To maximize navigator performance and efficiency, localization of the navigator at the dome of the right hemidiaphragm is important. Since the 3D shape of the diaphragm is individually dependent, identification of the dome on 2 orthogonal planes is advised. Localization of the navigator with 1/3 above the lung-liver interface and 2/3 below is recommended. Caudal 'drift' of the end-expiratory diaphragmatic position is sometimes observed which may adversely affect the efficiency of the scan. However, this is often related to sleep apnea or a low frequency pattern overlaid to the respiration, and in most cases the end-expiratory diaphragmatic position returns to its original position. On average, the navigator efficiency should approach ~50% which prolongs the nominal scanning time by a factor of 2. Navigator efficiencies below 20% and above 80% are suboptimal meaning that the localization of the navigator may need to be adapted. Stopping and restarting the scan may help in some cases. General patient motion can be minimized by specifically informing the patient that changing the position of the legs (crossed vs. non-crossed) should be avoided during the scan session. Asking the patient to go to the restroom prior to the MR exam helps to minimize general patient motion and improves the respiratory pattern.

Conclusion

MR imaging, because of its non-invasive nature, 3D capabilities, and capacity for soft tissue characterisation, is emerging as a powerful modality for both coronary luminal and vessel wall imaging. With further refinement of the technique and improvements of the spatial resolution on high field MR scanners, there is hope of significantly improving our ability to detect and characterize the tissue and plaque components in the coronary vessel wall. Doing so may have far reaching implications for the management of patients with established coronary heart disease.

References

1. Lieberman JM, Botti RE, Nelson AD (1984) Magnetic resonance imaging of the heart. Radiol Clin North Am 22(4):847-58
2. Paulin S, von Schulthess GK, Fossel E et al (1987) MR imaging of the aortic root and proximal coronary arteries. AJR Am J Roentgenol 148(4):665-70
3. Glagov S, Weisenberg E, Zarins CK et al (1987) Compensatory enlargement of human atherosclerotic coronary arteries. N Engl J Med 316(22):1371-5
4. Fischer SE, Wickline SA, Lorenz CH (1999) Novel real-time R-wave detection algorithm based on the vectorcardiogram for accurate gated magnetic resonance acquisitions. Magn Reson Med 42(2):361-70
5. Stuber M, Botnar RM, Fischer SE et al (2002) Manning, Preliminary report on in vivo coronary MRA at 3 Tesla in humans. Magn Reson Med 48(3):425-9
6. Wang Y, Grimm RC, Rossman PJ et al (1995) Ehman, 3D coronary MR angiography in multiple breath-holds using a respiratory feedback monitor. Magn Reson Med 34(1):11-6
7. Wielopolski PA, van Geuns RJ, de Feyter PJ et al (1998) Breath-hold coronary MR angiography with volume targeted imaging. Radiology 209(1):209-19
8. Goldfarb JW, Edelman RR (1998) Coronary arteries: breath-hold, gadolinium-enhanced, three-dimensional MR angiography. Radiology 206(3):830-4
9. Stuber M, Kissinger KV, Botnar RM et al (1998) Breath-Hold 3D Coronary MRA using Real-Time Navigator Technology. JCMR 1(233-238)
10. van Geuns RJ, Wielopolski PA, de Bruin HG et al (2000) MR coronary angiography with breath-hold targeted volumes: preliminary clinical results. Radiology 217(1):270-7
11. Danias PG, Stuber M, Botnar RM et al (1998) Navigator assessment of breath-hold duration: impact of supplemental oxygen and hyperventilation. AJR Am J Roentgenol 171(2):395-7
12. Liu YL, Riederer SJ, Rossman PJ et al (1993) A monitoring, feedback, and triggering system for reproducible breath- hold MR imaging. Magn Reson Med 30(4):507-11
13. Ehman RL, Felmlee JP (1989) Adaptive technique for high-definition MR imaging of moving structures. Radiology 173(1):255-63
14. Stuber M, Botnar RM, Danias PG et al (1999) Double-oblique free-breathing high resolution three-dimensional coronary magnetic resonance angiography. J Am Coll Cardiol 34(2):524-31
15. McConnell MV, Khasgiwala VC, Savord BJ et al (1997) Prospective adaptive navigator correction for breath-hold MR coronary angiography. Magn Reson Med 37(1):148-52
16. Danias PG, McConnell MV, Khasgiwala VC et al (1997) Prospective navigator correction of image position for coronary MR angiography. Radiology 203(3):733-6
17. Stuber M, Botnar RM, Danias PG et al (1999) Submillimeter three-dimensional coronary MR angiography with real-time navigator correction: comparison of navigator locations. Radiology 212(2):579-587
18. Spuentrup E, Stuber M, Botnar RM et al (2001) The impact of navigator timing parameters and navigator spatial resolution on 3D coronary magnetic resonance angiography. J Magn Reson Imaging 14(3):311-8
19. Hofman MBM, Henson RE, Kovacs SJ et al (1999) Blood pool agent strongly improves 3D magnetic resonance coronary angiography using an inversion pre-pulse. Magn Reson Med 41(2):360-67
20. Li D, Dolan RP, Walovitch RC et al (1998) Three-Dimensional MRI of coronary arteries using an intravascular contrast agent. Magn Reson Med 39: p. 1014-18
21. Stuber M, Botnar RM, Danias PG et al (1999) Contrast agent-enhanced, free-breathing, three-dimensional coronary magnetic resonance angiography. J Magn Reson Imaging 10(5):790-9
22. Huber ME, Paetsch I, Schnackenburg B et al (2003) Performance of a new gadolinium-based intravascular contrast agent in free-breathing inversion-recovery 3D coronary MRA. Magn Reson Med 49(1):115-21

23. Stuber M, Botnar RM , Spuentrup E et al (2001) Three-dimensional high-resolution fast spin-echo coronary magnetic resonance angiography. Magn Reson Med 45(2):206-11

24. Wang Y, Watts R, Mitchell I et al (2001) Coronary MR angiography: selection of acquisition window of minimal cardiac motion with electrocardiography-triggered navigator cardiac motion prescanning–initial results. Radiology 218(2):580-5

25. Kim WY, Stuber M, Kissinger KV et al (2001) Botnar, Impact of bulk cardiac motion on right coronary MR angiography and vessel wall imaging. J Magn Reson Imaging 14(4):383-90

26. Jhooti P, Keegan J, Gatehouse PD et al (1998) Firmin, 3D Coronary Imaging with Phase Reordering for Optimal Scan Efficiency. Proceedings of the International Society for Magnetic Resonance in Medicine 1:318

27. Huber ME, Hengesbach D, Botnar RM et al (2001) Motion artifact reduction and vessel enhancement for free-breathing navigator-gated coronary MRA using 3D k-space reordering. Magn Reson Med 45(4):645-52

28. Manke D, Nehrke K, Bornert P (2003) Novel prospective respiratory motion correction approach for free-breathing coronary MR angiography using a patient-adapted affine motion model. Magn Reson Med 50(1):122-31

29. Edelman RR, Manning WJ, Burstein D et al (1991) Coronary arteries: breath-hold MR angiography. Radiology 181(3):641-3

30. Li D, Paschal CB, Haacke EM et al (1993) Coronary arteries: three-dimensional MR imaging with fat saturation and magnetization transfer contrast. Radiology 187(2):401-6

31. Brittain JH, Hu BS, Wright GA et al (1995) Coronary angiography with magnetization-prepared T2 contrast. Magn Reson Med 33(5):689-96

32. Botnar RM, Stuber M, Danias PG et al (1999) Improved coronary artery definition with T2-weighted, free-breathing, three-dimensional coronary MRA. Circulation 99(24):3139-48

33. Stuber M, Botnar RM, Kissinger KV et al (2001) Free-breathing black-blood coronary MR angiography: initial results. Radiology 219(1):278-83

34. Stillman AE, Wilke N, Jerosch-Herold M (1997) Use of an intravascular T1 contrast agent to improve MR cine myocardial- blood pool definition in man. J Magn Reson Imaging 7(4):765-7

35. Taylor AM, Panting JR, Keegan J et al (1999) Firmin, and D.J. Pennell, Safety and preliminary findings with the intravascular contrast agent NC100150 injection for MR coronary angiography. J Magn Reson Imaging 9(2):220-7

36. Kim WY, Danias PG, Stuber M et al (2001) Coronary magnetic resonance angiography for the detection of coronary stenoses. N Engl J Med 345(26):1863-1869

37. Herborn CU, Barkhausen J, Paetsch I et al (2003) Coronary arteries: contrast-enhanced MR imaging with SH L 643A–experience in 12 volunteers. Radiolo 229(1):217-23

38. Manning WJ, Li W, Edelman RR (1993) A preliminary report comparing magnetic resonance coronary angiography with conventional angiography. N Engl J Med 328(12):828-32

39. Duerinckx AJ, Urman MK (1994) Two-dimensional coronary MR angiography: analysis of initial clinical results. Radiology 193(3):731-8

40. Post JC, van Rossum AC, Hofman MB et al (1996) Three-dimensional respiratory-gated MR angiography of coronary arteries: comparison with conventional coronary angiography. AJR Am J Roentgenol 166(6):1399-404

41. Müller MF, Fleisch M, Kroeker R et al (1997) Proximal coronary artery stenosis: three-dimensional MRI with fat saturation and navigator echo. J Magn Reson Imaging 7(4):644-651

42. Post JC, van Rossum AC, Hofman MB et al (1997) Clinical utility of two-dimensional magnetic resonance angiography in detecting coronary artery disease. Eur Heart J 18(3):426-33

43. Pennell DJ, Bogren HG, Keegan J et al (1996) Assessment of coronary artery stenosis by magnetic resonance imaging. Heart 75(2):127-33

44. Meyer CH, Hu BS, Nishimura DG et al (1992) Fast spiral coronary artery imaging. Magn Reson Med 28(2):202-13

45. Thedens DR, Irarrazaval P, Sachs TS et al (1999) Fast magnetic resonance coronary angiography with a three-dimensional stack of spirals trajectory. Magn Reson Med 41(6):1170-9

46. Bornert P, Aldefeld B, Nehrke K (2001) Improved 3D spiral imaging for coronary MR angiography. Magn Reson Med 45(1):172-5

47. Bornert P, Stuber M, Botnar RM et al (2001) Direct comparison of 3D spiral vs. Cartesian gradient-echo coronary magnetic resonance angiography. Magn Reson Med 46(4):789-94

48. Deshpande VS, Shea SM, Laub G et al (2001) 3D magnetization-prepared true-FISP: a new technique for imaging coronary arteries. Magn Reson Med 46(3):494-502

49. Spuentrup E, Buecker A, Stuber M et al (2003) Navigator-gated coronary magnetic resonance angiography using steady-state-free-precession: comparison to standard t2-prepared gradient-echo and spiral imaging. Invest Radiol 38(5):263-8

50. Deshpande VS, Li D (2003) Contrast-enhanced coronary artery imaging using 3D trueFISP. Magn Reson Med 50(3):570-7

51. Jara H, Yu BC, Caruthers SD et al (1999) Voxel sensitivity function description of flow-induced signal loss in MR imaging: implications for black-blood MR angiography with turbo spin- echo sequences. Magn Reson Med 41(3):575-90

52. Sodickson DK, Manning WJ (1997) Simultaneous acquisition of spatial harmonics (SMASH): fast imaging with radiofrequency coil arrays. Magn Reson Med 38(4):591-603

53. Pruessmann KP, Weiger M, Scheidegger MB et al (1999) SENSE: sensitivity encoding for fast MRI. Magn Reson Med 42(5): 952-62

54. Weiger M, Pruessmann KP, Boesiger P (2000) Cardiac real-time imaging using SENSE. SENSitivity Encoding scheme. Magn Reson Med 43(2):177-84

55. Stuber M, Bornert P, Spuentrup E et al (2002) Selective three-dimensional visualization of the coronary arterial lumen using arterial spin tagging. Magn Reson Med 47(2):322-9

56. AHA, American Heart Association 2002 Heart and Stroke Statistical Update. 2002

57. Nissen SE (2002) Application of intravascular ultrasound to characterize coronary artery disease and assess the progression or regression of atherosclerosis. Am J Cardiol 89(4A): 24B-31B

58. Kim WY, Stuber M, Bornert P et al (2002) Three-dimensional black-blood cardiac magnetic resonance coronary vessel wall imaging detects positive arterial remodeling in patients with nonsignificant coronary artery disease. Circulation 106(3):296-9

59. Fayad ZA, Fuster V, Fallon JT et al (2000) Noninvasive in vivo human coronary artery lumen and wall imaging using black-blood magnetic resonance imaging. Circulation 102(5):506-10

60. Little WC, Constantinescu M, Applegate RJ et al (1988) Can coronary angiography predict the site of a subsequent myocardial infarction in patients with mild-to-moderate coronary artery disease? Circulation 78(5 Pt 1):1157-66

61. Ambrose JA, Fuster V (1997) Can we predict future acute coronary events in patients with stable coronary artery disease? Jama 277(4):343-4

62. O'Leary DH, Polak JF, Kronmal RA et al (1999) Carotid-artery intima and media thickness as a risk factor for myocardial infarction and stroke in older adults. Cardiovascular Health Study Collaborative Research Group. N Engl J Med, 340(1):14-22

63. Detrano RC, Wong ND, Doherty TM et al (1999) Coronary calcium does not accurately predict near-term future coronary events in high-risk adults. Circulation 99(20):2633-8

64. Raggi P, Callister TQ, Cooil B et al (2000) Identification of patients at increased risk of first unheralded acute myocardial infarction by electron-beam computed tomography. Circulation 101(8):850-5

65. Toussaint JF, Southern JF, Fuster V et al (1995) T2-weighted contrast for NMR characterization of human atherosclerosis. Arterioscler Thromb Vasc Biol15(10):1533-42

66. Shinnar M, Fallon JT, Wehrli S et al (1999) The diagnostic accuracy of ex vivo MRI for human atherosclerotic plaque characterization. Arterioscler Thromb Vasc Biol 19(11):2756-61

67. Martin AJ, Gotlieb AI, Henkelman RM (1995) High-resolution MR imaging of human arteries. J Magn Reson Imaging 5(1):93-100

68. Serfaty JM, Chaabane L, Tabib A et al (2001) Atherosclerotic plaques: classification and characterization with T2-weighted high-spatial-resolution MR imaging– an in vitro study. Radiology 219(2):403-10

69. Toussaint JF, LaMuraglia GM, Southern JF et al (1996) Magnetic resonance images lipid, fibrous, calcified, hemorrhagic, and thrombotic components of human atherosclerosis in vivo. Circulation 94(5):932-8

70. Yuan C, Beach KW, Smith LH et al (1998) Measurement of atherosclerotic carotid plaque size in vivo using high resolution magnetic resonance imaging. Circulation 98(24):2666-71

71. Wasserman BA, Smith WI, Trout HH et al (2002) Carotid artery atherosclerosis: in vivo morphologic characterization with gadolinium-enhanced double-oblique MR imaging initial results. Radiology 223(2):566-73

72. Yuan C, Kerwin WS, Ferguson MS et al (2002) Contrast-enhanced high resolution MRI for atherosclerotic carotid artery tissue characterization. J Magn Reson Imaging 15(1):62-7

73. Jaffer FA, O'Donnell CJ, Larson MG et al (2002) Age and sex distribution of subclinical aortic atherosclerosis: a magnetic resonance imaging examination of the Framingham Heart Study. Arterioscler Thromb Vasc Biol 22(5):849-54

74. Fazio GP, Redberg RF, Winslow T et al (1993) Transesophageal echocardiographically detected atherosclerotic aortic plaque is a marker for coronary artery disease. J Am Coll Cardiol 21(1):144-50

75. Falk E, Shah PK, Fuster V (1995) Coronary plaque disruption. Circulation 92(3):657-71

76. Botnar RM, Stuber M, Kissinger KV et al (2000) Noninvasive coronary vessel wall and plaque imaging with magnetic resonance imaging. Circulation 102(21):2582-7

77. Schar M, Kim WY, Stuber M et al (2003) The impact of spatial resolution and respiratory motion on MR imaging of atherosclerotic plaque. J Magn Reson Imaging 17(5):538-44

78. McConnell MV, Aikawa M, Maier SE et al (1999) MRI of rabbit atherosclerosis in response to dietary cholesterol lowering. Arterioscler Thromb Vasc Biol 19(8):1956-9

79. Corti R, Fayad ZA, Fuster V et al (2001) Effects of lipid-lowering by simvastatin on human atherosclerotic lesions: a longitudinal study by high-resolution, noninvasive magnetic resonance imaging. Circulation 104(3):249-52

80. Corti R, Fuster V, Fayad ZA (2002) Lipid lowering by simvastatin induces regression of human atherosclerotic lesions: two years' follow-up by high-resolution noninvasive magnetic resonance imaging. Circulation 106(23):2884-7

81. Botnar RM, Kim WY, Bornert P et al (2001) 3D coronary vessel wall imaging utilizing a local inversion technique with spiral image acquisition. Magn Reson Med 46(5):848-54

82. Nissen SE, Tsunoda T, Tuzcu EM et al (2003) Effect of recombinant ApoA-I Milano on coronary atherosclerosis in patients with acute coronary syndromes: a randomized controlled trial. Jama 290(17):2292-300

83. Weber OM, Martin AJ, Higgins CB (2003) Whole-heart steady-state free precession coronary artery magnetic resonance angiography. Magn Reson Med 50(6):1223-8

Acknowledgments

Part of the work described in this chapter is supported by a Biomedical Engineering Grant from the Whitaker Foundation (RG-02-0745), a grant from the Donald W. Reynolds Foundation and by the National Institutes of Health (HL61912)

Dr. Stuber is compensated as a consultant by Philips Medical Systems NL, and Bracco Diagnostics, Milan, IT, the manufacturers of equipment described in this presentation. The terms of this arrangement have been approved by the Johns Hopkins University in accordance with its conflict of interest policies

SECTION VI

Abdomen

VI.1

Contrast-Enhanced MR Angiography of the Abdominal Aorta

Philippe C. Douek

Introduction

X-ray angiography and more recently CT angiography have been considered the gold standard examinations for assessment of the abdominal aorta. However, the invasive nature of the investigation, the large amount of potentially nephrotoxic contrast media involved and the use for ionizing radiation have always been negative factors strengthening the call for a full non-invasive method for demonstration of the abdominal aorta and iliac arteries. Rapid advances in medical technology have made this possible in current clinical practice through magnetic resonance angiography (MRA). Major improvements in image acquisition times and reductions in the volumes of contrast agent utilized have made 3D CE MRA a fast, reproducible, and patient-friendly examination [1, 2]. A full MRA study of the abdominal aorta can require as few as 10 minutes of scanner time. The lack of ionizing radiation and use of non-nephrotoxic gadolinium-based contrast agents makes this exam considerably safer for patients.

A major factor that has driven the development and clinical use of CE MRA is the need to overcome the limitations of noncontrast gradient-echo time-of-flight (TOF) techniques. The drawbacks of TOF imaging include long imaging times, an inability to see in-plane and small vessels, and the loss of signal in aneurysmal vascular structures secondary to turbulent flow. The use of paramagnetic contrast agents and faster 3D gradient recalled echo techniques have provided a strong competitor to x-ray angiography and CT angiography as the first line of study for precise evaluation of the abdominal aorta. The aims of this chapter are to describe the technical approaches to CE MRA of the abdominal aorta and to provide an overview of the pertinent clinical applications in this vascular territory.

Normal Anatomy

The abdominal aorta begins at the aortic hiatus of the diaphragm, in front of the lower border of the body of the last thoracic vertebra, and, descending in front of the vertebral column, ends on the body of the fourth lumbar vertebra, typically a little to the left of the middle line, by dividing into the two common iliac arteries (Fig. 1). The shape of the abdominal aorta is slightly convex forward with the summit of the convexity corresponding to the third lumbar vertebra. Numerous branches give off from the abdominal aorta before it divides into the common iliac arteries. The common iliac arteries are about 5 cm in length and diverge from the termination of the aorta. They pass downward and laterally before dividing into the external iliac and hypogastric arteries opposite the intervertebral fibrocartilage between the last lumbar vertebra and the sacrum. The external iliac artery supplies the lower extremity while the hypogastric artery supplies the walls and viscera of the pelvis, the buttock, the generative organs, and the medial side of the thigh. The hypogastric artery is about 4 cm in length and smaller than the external iliac artery. After arising at the bifurcation of the common iliac opposite the lumbosacral articulation, it passes downward to the upper margin of the greater sciatic foramen where it divides into two large trunks, an anterior and a posterior trunk.

Imaging Technique

The sequences used for 3D CE MRA are spoiled gradient-recalled-echo (SGE) sequences with zero interpolation in the partition or the slice-selected direction. The abdominal aorta is generally well displayed with a contrast dose of 0.1 mmol/kg of gadobenate dimeglumine (Gd-BOPTA) or 0.2 mmol/kg of a non-protein interacting gadolinium

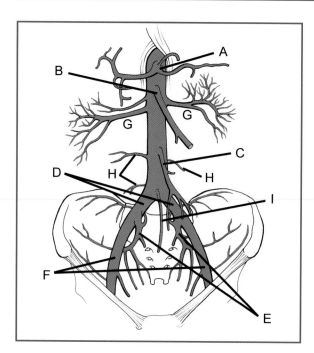

Fig. 1. Schematic drawing of the normal anatomy of the abdominal aorta
A Celiac artery
B Superior mesenteric artery
C Inferior mesenteric artery
D Common iliac arteries
E Internal iliac artery
F External iliac artery
G Renal arteries
H Lumbar arteries
I Medial sacral artery

contrast agent [3, 4]. One of the goals in optimizing the sequence parameters is to keep the overall image acquisition time to a minimum, so that acquisition can be achieved in a single breath-hold. This goal is further aided by short TR and TE values. The short TR permits an overall reduction of the imaging time while a short TE helps in minimizing T2* effects. Whenever feasible, the highest possible spatial resolution should be utilized. The speed of acquisition and the spatial resolution of 3D CE MRA are determined and ultimately limited by the performance characteristics of the gradient and other hardware of the scanner. Until comparatively recently, most improvements in performance were achieved by increasing the gradient strength of the scanner. However, the need to avoid neuromuscular stimulation from rapid gradient switching limits this approach. This limitation has inspired the development of techniques that acquire data much differently and/or more rapidly. These techniques improve the temporal resolution without compromising the spatial resolution and without requiring high gradient strengths. Among these newer approaches are time-resolved techniques which allow repeated acquisition of a volume of interest during the passage of the contrast agent bolus.

Parallel imaging

Parallel techniques [5, 6] use combinations of component coil signals in a radio-frequency (RF) coil array to substitute for omitted gradient steps. This reduces the burden on the gradients and allows multiple components of the spatial encoding required to generate an MR image to be performed in parallel. This technique has been shown to achieve a four- to eightfold reduction in image acquisition time, with no compromise in spatial resolution.

TRICKS

Time Resolved Imaging of Contrast Kinetics (TRICKS) [7] uses an increased sampling rate for lower frequencies, temporal interpolation of k-space views, and zero-filling in the slice-encoding direction. When appropriately combined, these elements permit reconstruction of a series of 3D image sets, having an effective temporal frame rate of one volume every two to six seconds, with no serious compromise in spatial resolution. Conversely, given the limited duration of the bolus of contrast agent in the arteries, and the potential for motion during MR angiography, there is a practical lower limit on the appropriate sampled voxel size. This lower limit on spatial resolution improves with field-of-view (FOV) minimization because less time is required to reach the desired sampling resolution. Furthermore, interference from venous signal intensity and respiratory motion can be minimized by using the elliptic centric view order, which makes longer acquisition times feasible. Consistent with this approach, a high-spatial-resolution MR angiographic technique with reduced FOV and slightly extended acquisition time can be used: 26.0 cm (x axis [superior to inferior]) x 19.0 cm (y axis [right to left]) x 6.4 cm (z axis [anterior to posterior]) and covered the region of interest in a total acquisition time of 40 seconds [8].

Additional sequences may be added to the standard protocol in specific cases [9]. When the abdominal aorta is being evaluated for aneurysm, additional images should be acquired to depict the outer wall of the aorta and give an estimate of the true size of the aneurysm. The size of the aneurysm may be underestimated on CE MRA, as it is primarily a luminogram similar to the conventional angiogram. Since the background is sup-

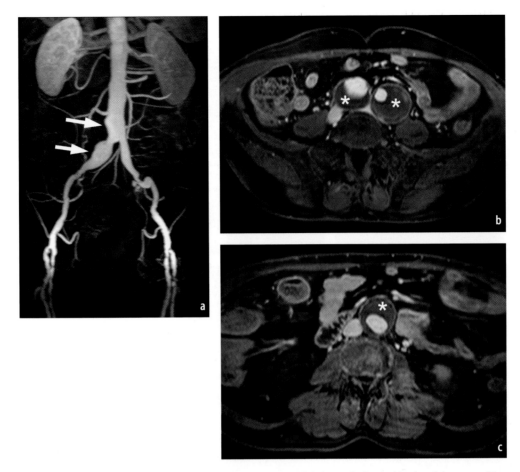

Fig. 2a-c. The MIP image (**a**) of a 3D CE MRA dataset (Gd-BOPTA, 0.1 mmol/kg) shows the luminal image of the aorta with extensive atherosclerotic disease of the iliac and femoral vessels and dilatation as well as wall irregularities of the distal abdominal aorta and right common iliac artery (*arrows*). Two post contrast T1w fat suppressed images at the level of the common iliac arteries just below the bifurcation (**b**) and at the level of the distal aorta (**c**), performed after the CE MRA study, demonstrate large aneurysm formation with thrombus formation (*asterisk*) of both common iliac arteries as well as of the distal abdominal aorta. Whereas the perfused lumen of the left iliac artery appears almost normal on the MIP image, the aneurysm is even larger compared with that of the right iliac artery [Images courtesy of Dr. G. Schneider]

pressed on CE MRA in order to depict the vessels accurately, it may become difficult to visualize the outer wall of the aneurysm even on native slices or MPR. This is often a major problem, especially when patients are being considered for endovascular stent graft placement, which requires outer-to-outer wall measurements for placement of a stent graft. The solution is to use either an additional black-blood imaging sequence (Fig. 2) for evaluation of the vessel wall [10] or a true fast imaging with steady-state precession technique (true FISP) that uses a fully balanced gradient waveform to recycle transverse magnetization [11] (Fig. 3). Contrast is determined on the basis of the ratio of T2 to T1 rather than on the basis of inflow effects, as in spoiled gradient-echo methods. This difference eliminates sensitivity to saturation effects from absent or slow flow. Postcontrast T1-weighted images with fat suppression may also be helpful in some conditions of the aorta such as arteritis, mycotic aneurysm, or graft infection [12].

Patient Preparation

As with all CE MRA techniques, an intravenous line should be placed in the arm before the patient enters the magnet. Breath holding is especially important for aortic imaging and significantly improves image quality; however, it may not be possible in every case. Supplemental oxygen and hyperventilation can also help improve breath-holding. Breath-holding needs to be incorporated between the start of contrast agent injection and the start of contrast-enhanced imaging. It is acceptable to use a body coil because it provides a large field of view with homogenous signal, however, a torso or body phased-array coil is recommended for use with parallel imaging sequences. Typically, an anteroposterior phased-array surface coil (torso array coil) is used for signal reception. The coil is placed around the patient to cover the vasculature from the proximal abdominal aorta to the level of the inguinal ligaments, including the renal and pelvic

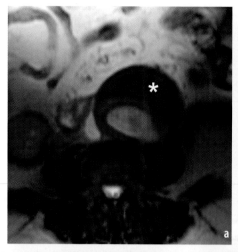
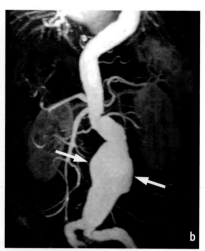
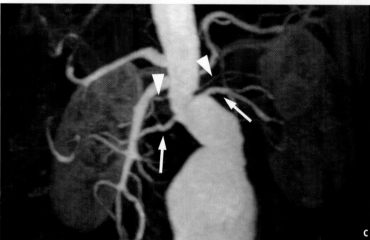

Fig. 3a-c. The true FISP image (**a**) acquired before contrast agent injection already demonstrates aneurysm formation and thrombosis (*asterisk*) in the infrarenal abdominal aorta. On the corresponding whole volume MIP image (**b**) of a 3D CE MRA dataset (Gd-BOPTA, 0.1 mmol/kg) extensive dilatation of the infrarenal aorta (*arrows*) and accessory renal arteries on both sides can be observed. The accessory renal arteries are even better displayed on a targeted MIP reformation (**c**) on which the accessory renal arteries are clearly identified (*arrows* = renal arteries, arrowheads = accessory renal arteries)

arteries. The arms of the patient should be placed either above the head or folded across the chest to avoid folding artefacts.

Clinical Applications

Aneurysms, aortic dissection and atherosclerosis including occlusive disease of the aorta are the most common indications for MR angiography of the abdominal aorta.

Abdominal Aortic Aneurysms

Abdominal aortic aneurysms (AAA) occur in 5-7% of the population older than 60 years of age. Although most patients with AAA are asymptomatic, they can present with symptoms of mass effect, compression of abdominal organs, or visceral or peripheral emboli originating from the wall of the aneurysm. Rarely, patients present with back pain, which can represent rupture of the aneurysm, a

surgical emergency. Patients older than 60 years of age who smoke and who are known to have atherosclerosis, hypertension, and/or chronic obstructive pulmonary disease are at increased risk for AAA. Routine screening of these patients by ultrasound is warranted. In the United States 15,000 deaths per year are attributed to abdominal aortic aneurysms. Classically, AAAs have been attributed to a weakening of the arterial wall as a result of atherosclerotic vascular disease caused by the atheromatous lesions seen on pathologic examination. Atherosclerotic aneurysms are typically fusiform (Fig. 4), although focal eccentric aneurysms due to atherosclerosis are occasionally encountered (Fig. 5). Recent evidence supports a multifactorial process in which atherosclerosis is involved. Other etiologic co-factors under investigation include changes in the matrix of the aortic wall with age, proteolysis, metalloproteinase changes, inflammation, infectious agents (Fig. 6) (e.g., syphilis, mycotic infections), and a genetic predisposition (e.g., Marfan syndrome, Ehlers-Danlos syndrome). Inflammatory aneurysms, once believed to be distinct entities, are currently

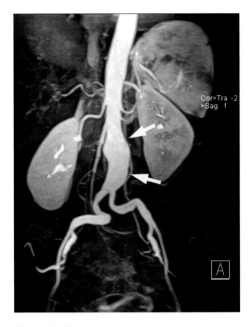

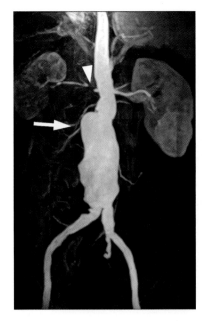

Fig. 4. Fusiform infrarenal aneurysm of the abdominal aorta (*arrows*) as displayed on a MIP reformation of a 3D CE MRA dataset (Gd-BOPTA, 0.1 mmol/kg) [Image courtesy of Dr. G. Schneider]

Fig. 5. Focal eccentric aneurysm (*arrow*) of the infrarenal abdominal aorta due to atherosclerosis, revealed on a MIP reformation of a 3D CE MRA dataset (Gd-BOPTA 0.1 mmol/kg). Note in addition the high grade stenosis of the right renal artery (*arrowhead*) [Image courtesy of Dr. G. Schneider]

considered one extreme in the spectrum of atherosclerotic aneurysms; these account for 3-10% of all AAAs. Clinical and imaging characteristics differentiate inflammatory from noninflammatory aneurysms. Mycotic aneurysms result from weakening of the vessel wall by a bacterial infection, causing saccular outpouching, most commonly involving the suprarenal portion of the aorta (Fig. 6). Contrast-enhanced MR angiography can demonstrate the aneurysm itself, whereas postcontrast T1-weighted imaging may demonstrate enhancement in and around the vessel wall [13].

Once an aneurysm is identified, it should be repaired or followed up with imaging, depending on the clinical scenario and the size of the aneurysm at the time of diagnosis. Most aneurysms (80%) demonstrate progressive enlargement. The natural history of AAAs is closely related to size. Rupture is uncommon if aneurysms are < 5 cm wide but dramatically more common if > 6 cm. Thus, elective surgical repair is usually recommended for all aneurysms > 6 cm in size unless surgery is contraindicated [14]. In patients who are good surgical risks, elective repair is generally recommended for

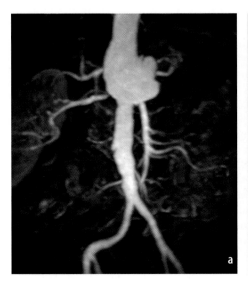

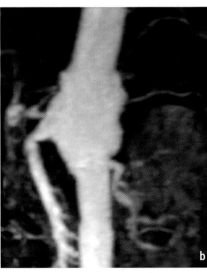

Fig. 6a, b. Mycotic aneurysm of the suprarenal portion of the aorta with involvement of the renal arteries, the superior mesenteric artery and the celiac artery. The whole volume MIP image (**a**) of a 3D CE MRA dataset (Gd-BOPTA 0.1 mmol/kg) shows an eccentric aneurysm with occlusion of the left renal artery. A subvolume MIP reformation in sagittal projection (**b**) additionally reveals occlusion of the celiac artery [Images courtesy of Dr. G. Schneider]

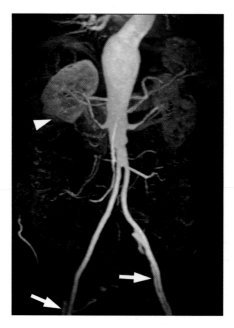

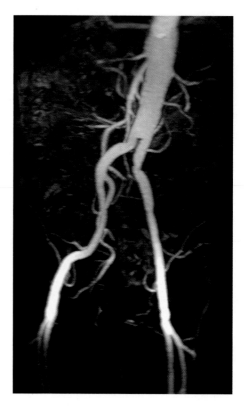

Fig. 7. Patient post surgery of an infrarenal AAA and graft anastomosis to both femoral arteries. The MIP reformation shows normal postsurgical proximal and distal anastomosis as well as a retrograde filling of the iliac arteries (*arrows*) which were bypassed during surgery. The graft was connected to the femoral arteries since an anastomosis at the level of the iliac arteries was not possible due to advanced atherosclerotic disease. Note the non-contrasted inferior pole of the right kidney (*arrowhead*) which is caused by occlusion of a lower pole artery of the right kidney during surgery and the additional development of a suprarenal aneurysm [Images courtesy of Dr. G. Schneider]

Fig. 8. Normal post surgical findings in a patient post AAA surgery without stenosis or aneurysm formation at the proximal or distal anastomosis (*arrows*) [Image courtesy of Dr. G. Schneider]

aneurysms between 5 and 6 cm in size for whom mortality is about 2 to 5%. Surgical repair consists of excision of the aneurysm and replacement with a synthetic conduit (Fig. 7); the graft may have to be carried into either or both iliac arteries if the aneurysm also involves these vessels (Fig. 8). Extension of the aneurysm above the renal arteries necessitates their reimplantation onto the synthetic graft or the creation of bypass grafts to them. Treatment of a mycotic aneurysm consists of vigorous antibiotic therapy directed at the specific organism, followed by excision of the aneurysm. Early diagnosis and treatment favourably influence outcome.

The Society for Vascular Surgery (SVS) and the International Society for Cardiovascular Surgery (ISCS) have suggested the classification of aneurysms by their site, origin, histologic features, and clinicopathologic manifestations. The morphologic features, including the maximum diameter in both the anteroposterior and lateral dimensions and the length of the aneurysm, and any involvement of major branch vessels should be reported (Fig. 9). All of these features can be identified and characterized with MR imaging [15, 16]. The shape of the aneurysm (fusiform or saccular)

and its relationship to branch vessels should be described (Fig. 10). Arterial wall complications such as expansion over time, compression or erosion into adjacent structures, rupture, dissection, and thrombotic occlusion should also be documented [17].

Many refinements in treatment technique have occurred, but none as significant as the stent-graft [18]. With the advent of the endoluminal repair of aneurysms [19], several additional morphologic characteristics should be recorded. These determine if endovascular repair is possible, and if so, what type of device can be used. These features include the following: greatest mural diameter, extent of aneurysm (e.g., length of proximal and distal neck, extension into iliac arteries), tortuosity of the aorta, anatomy of the iliac arteries (e.g., iliac artery occlusive disease, tortuosity, caliber, patency of internal iliac arteries and relation of aneurysm to the iliac arteries, presence of concomitant iliac artery aneurysms), presence and degree of intraluminal thrombus, presence and degree of calcification in the neck and iliac arteries, and anatomy of the femoral arteries (e.g., caliber, degree of calcification or occlusive disease) [20] (Fig. 11). Accurate

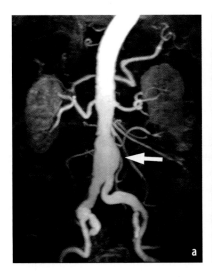
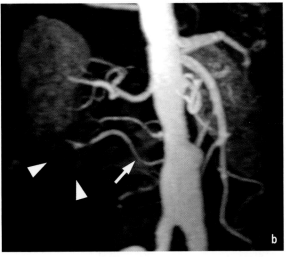

Fig. 9a, b. The MIP image (**a**) of a 3D CE MRA dataset (Gd-BOPTA, 0.1 mmol/kg) shows an infrarenal AAA (*arrow*) and possibly a reduced enhancement of the lower pole of the left kidney. On a subvolume MIP reformation (**b**) a lower pole artery of the left kidney (*arrow*) branching at the level of the AAA can be demonstrated, which is the reason for the delayed enhancement of the lower pole of the left renal artery (*arrowheads*) [Images courtesy of Dr. G. Schneider]

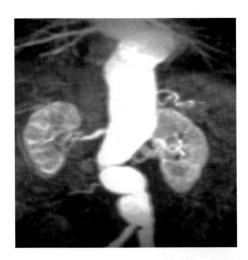

Fig. 10. A coronal arterial-phase MIP image from a 3D gadolinium-enhanced MR angiographic examination reveals a suprarenal extension of an abdominal aortic aneurysm

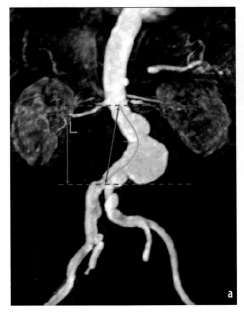

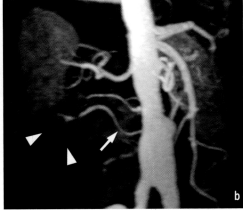

Fig. 11a, b. Pretreatment assessment of abdominal aortic aneurysm: Coronal (**a**) and sagittal (**b**) arterial-phase MIP images from a 3D gadolinium-enhanced MR angiographic examination reveal an infrarenal aneurysm. Evaluation of the extent of the aneurysm, the length and diameter of the proximal and distal neck, the extension into the iliac arteries as well as the tortuosity of the aorta in both planes is demonstrated

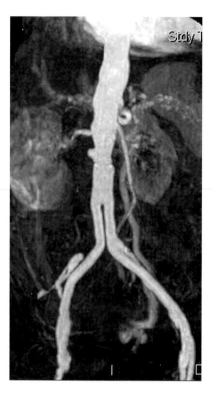

visualization of the visceral vessels is important in determining stenosis of these vessels. Evaluation of calcification may be difficult with MR and a CT without iodine injection is usually necessary for a complete preoperative evaluation of AAA.

It is preferable to perform follow-up imaging with a noninvasive test such as MRA. Standard follow-up is recommended at one month and 6 months after stent placement or after surgery (Fig. 12). The majority of endoleaks are of Type 2, which may be caused by backfilling of the aneurysm sac by either the lumbar arteries or the inferior mesenteric artery (Fig. 13). Aortic stent-grafts (AneuRx, Talent) produce minimal artifact from the nitinol within the stent-graft [21]. While this causes local distortion of the post-contrast images, vessel patency and endoleak can be visualized. Embolization coils cause major distortion artifacts, obscuring all adjacent organs, as well as vessel lumen patency.

Fig. 12. Post operative control of abdominal aortic aneurysm. Coronal arterial-phase MIP image from a 3D gadolinium-enhanced MR angiographic examination demonstrates the patency of the bypass with no anastomotic stenoses or aneurysm

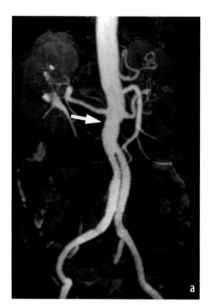
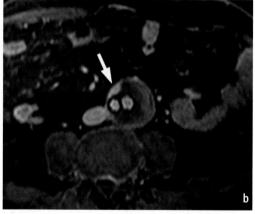

Fig. 13a, b. Type 2 endoleak in a patient post aortic stent-graft. Whereas the arterial phase MIP image (**a**) of a 3D CE MRA dataset (Gd-BOPTA, 0.1 mmol/kg) shows a normal appearance of the proximal anastomosis of the stent graft (*arrow*), the axial VIBE image (**b**) performed immediately after the CE MRA study shows backfilling of the aneurysm sac by lumbar arteries (*arrow*) [Images courtesy of Dr. G. Schneider]

Abdominal Aortic Dissection

Aortic dissection occurs when blood dissects into the media of the aortic wall through an intimal tear. It is generally secondary to hypertension. In young patients with aortic dissection, an underlying process such as Marfan syndrome should be investigated. Dissection originating in the infrarenal abdominal aorta is very rare and, given the vagueness of presenting symptoms of uncomplicated dissection, diagnosis is very difficult in the early stages. In the absence of a pulsatile abdominal mass, acute uncomplicated aortic dissection should be considered in the differential diagnosis of a sudden onset of abdominal and back pain [22].

Stanford type A dissections are treated in emergency by surgery while dissections arising distal to the left subclavian artery (Stanford type B) are usually treated medically [23]. However, delayed mortality caused by organ malperfusion is a major determinant of prognosis for both types of dissection. When an ischemic complication is clinically diagnosed, the mortality rate is of 50% in patients with type A dissection and 28 to 67% in patients with type B dissection. To manage such complications, minimum invasive endovascular approaches have been developed with promising results in selected patients. However, the success of such procedures is still dependent on early diagnosis.

An MR angiography study must evaluate the extent of the dissection, the sizes of the true and false lumina, the patency of the false lumen, and abdominal branch vessel involvement [24] (Fig. 14). The presence of a compressed true lumen, defined as dissection flap oriented concave to the false lumen, should be assessed. Branch lumen, including right and left renal arteries, celiac artery, mesenteric artery, and right and left common iliac arteries, is considered to be dissected when the branch arose from the false aortic lumen or when an intimal flap is shown to extend into the branch lumen (Fig. 15). The number of dissected aortic branches (i.e. renal, celiac, mesenteric and common iliac arteries) per patient should be noted. Association of significant visual lower enhancement of a segment or the entire parenchyma of a viscera in comparison with the contralateral paired viscera (for the kidney) is a sign of poorer prognosis (Fig. 16). Imaging should extend from the arch to the aortic bifurcation (Fig. 17). MIP images may not show the intimal flap; however, axial reformatted images from CE MRA are helpful for visualization of the intimal tear and re-entry sites. CE MRA is also helpful in postoperative follow-up [25]. It can accurately depict associated complications, including thrombosis, hemorrhage, aortoenteric fistula, and pseudoaneurysms. Potential drawbacks of MRI include false positives. On CE MRA these may include a central line artifact. This occurs when the acquisition is performed too early as the

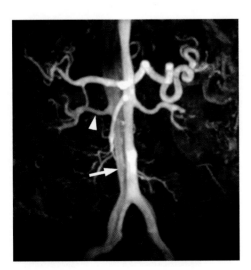

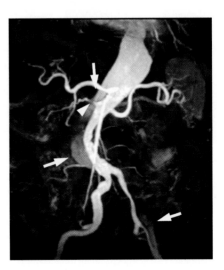

Fig. 14. The MIP image of a 3D CE MRA dataset (Gd-BOPTA, 0.1 mmol/kg) of a patient with chronic Stanford Type B dissection shows retrograde filling of the false lumen (*arrow*) from a re-entry in the iliac artery as well as branching of the right renal artery (*arrowhead*) from the false lumen [Image courtesy of Dr. G. Schneider]

Fig. 15. MIP reformation of a 3D CE MRA dataset (Gd-BOPTA, 0.1 mmol/kg) of a patient with chronic Stanford Type B dissection with multiple re-entries (*arrows*) and extension of the dissection membrane into the right renal artery (*arrowhead*) [Image courtesy of Dr. G. Schneider]

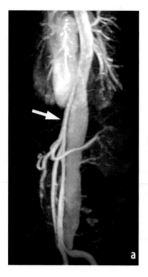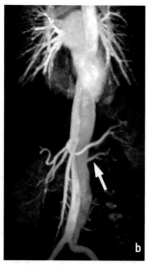

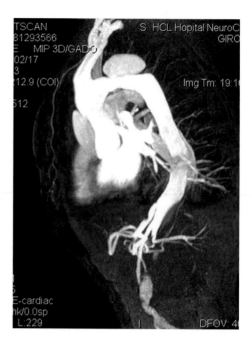

Fig. 16. Chronic Stanford Type B dissection. The sagittal MIP projection (a) shows the flattened true lumen anteriorly (*arrow* in **a**) from which the celiac artery and the superior mesenteric artery branch. In a slightly tilted projection (**b**) the origin of the left renal artery from the false lumen can be identified (*arrow* in **b**) [Image courtesy of Dr. G. Schneider]

Fig. 17. Parasagittal arterial-phase MIP image from a 3D gadolinium-enhanced MR angiographic examination demonstrates near occlusion of both the true and false lumens of a Stanford Type B dissection

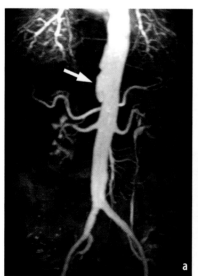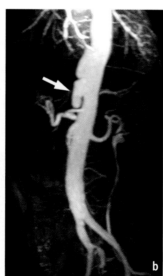

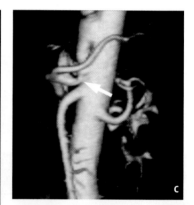

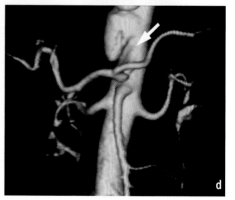

Fig. 18a-d. Penetrating atherosclerotic ulcer of the aorta at the level of the diaphragm. The coronal MIP projection (**a**) of a 3D CE MRA dataset (Gd-BOPTA, 0.1 mmol/kg) already demonstrates the outpouching (*arrow*) of the perfused lumen extending beyond the contour of the aorta. This is even better appreciated on a sagittal MIP reformation (*arrow* in **b**). Additional volume rendered images (**c, d**) are helpful to further evaluate the relationship between the penetrating atherosclerotic ulcer and the celiac artery, in this case demonstrating a short distance between the ulcer and the origin of the celiac artery (*arrow* in **d**) as well as a stenosis of the celiac artery approximately 1.5 cm from its origin [Image courtesy of Dr. G. Schneider]

concentration of intraortic gadolinium is rising. This artifact can be readily differentiated from an aortic dissection as it does not take a spiral course as with a true intimal flap.

Penetrating atherosclerotic ulcer is characterized by ulceration of an atherosclerotic plaque that penetrates through the intima into the media of the aortic wall. It typically affects elderly individuals with hypertension and extensive aortic atherosclerosis. It is seen as an outpouching extending beyond the contour of the aortic lumen and can become quite large (Fig. 18). A penetrating atherosclerotic ulcer is typically located in the descending aorta but can be seen in the abdominal aorta. It can be associated with a variable degree of hematoma within the aortic wall. Placement of an endovascular stent-graft is becoming a popular method of treating this entity, given that the disease tends to occur in elderly patients with comorbid conditions that put them at high surgical risk.

Occlusive Disease of the Aorta and Branches

The vast majority of stenotic (Fig. 19) and occlusive diseases of the aorta in the western world result from atherosclerosis. Occlusion of the abdominal aorta can be acute or chronic. Abrupt occlusion of the aortic bifurcation is rare. It is characterized by the sudden onset of pain, pallor, paralysis, and coldness in the legs. Usually a filling defect-meniscus on MIP projections indicates embolus. Urgent embolectomy is indicated and can usually be performed transfemorally. Chronic occlusion of the aortic bifurcation (Leriche's syndrome) is usually due to arteriosclerosis, is most frequently seen in the elderly, especially males with a history of smoking and manifests as intermittent claudication in the legs and buttocks and erectile impotence (Fig. 20). Leriche syndrome typically re-

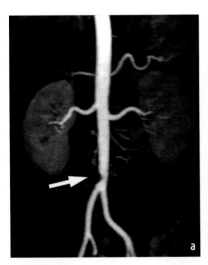
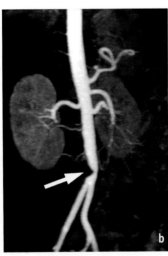

Fig. 19a, b. Stenosis of the abdominal aorta just above the level of the bifurcation in a young male with a history of smoking. The coronal (**a**) and parasagittal (**b**) MIP reformations of a 3D CE MRA dataset (Gd-BOPTA, 0.1 mmol/kg) show high grade stenosis of the aorta (*arrows*) in otherwise normal looking vessels of the abdomen [Image courtesy of Dr. G. Schneider]

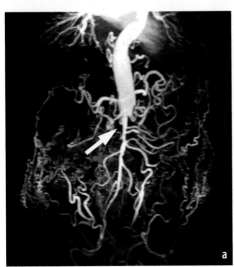
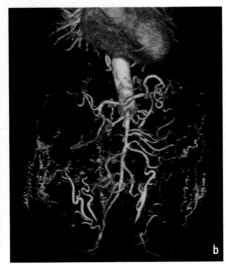

Fig. 20a, b. MIP reformation (**a**) and volume rendered image (**b**) of a 3D CE MRA dataset (Gd-BOPTA, 0.1 mmol/kg) show occlusion of the abdominal aorta (Leriche syndrome) just below the renal arteries (*arrow* in **a**). Note the extensive collaterals that developed due to the slow progression of the disease [Image courtesy of Dr. G. Schneider]

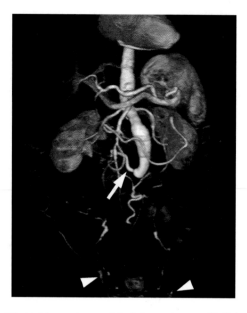

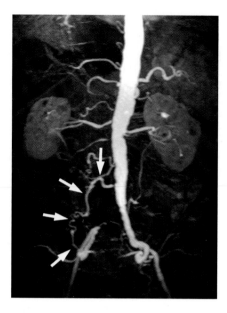

Fig. 21. Leriche syndrome of the infrarenal aorta with iliolumbar collaterals (*arrow*) and reconstitution of perfusion at the level of the femoral arteries (*arrowheads*). Volume rendered image from a 3D CE MRA dataset (Gd-BOPTA, 0.1 mmol/kg) [Image courtesy of Dr. G. Schneider]

Fig. 22. Occlusion of the right iliac artery at the level of the bifurcation with collateral pathways via the iliolumbar vessels (*arrows*). MIP reformation from a 3D CE MRA dataset (Gd-BOPTA, 0.1 mmol/kg) [Image courtesy of Dr. G. Schneider]

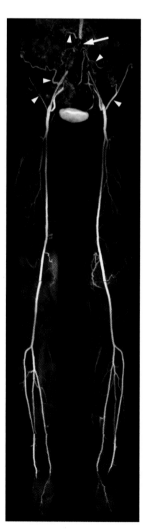

Fig. 23. Four station moving table MRA in a patient with Leriche syndrome. The assembly of the different MIP images of the four CE MRA stations (Gd-BOPTA, 0.15 mmol/kg) shows occlusion of the aorta (*arrow*) with extensive collateralization (*arrowheads*) from lumbar and gluteal as well as inferior epigastric arteries. Note that the complete run-off vessels are displayed revealing no further high-grade stenosis [Image courtesy of Dr. G. Schneider]

sults in extensive collateral development and filling of the distal vessels with reconstitution at the iliac or common femoral arteries (Fig. 21). Collateral pathways include the Arc of Riolan, the marginal artery of Drummond, iliolumbar collaterals (Fig. 22), superior and inferior epigastric arteries, and gluteal collaterals. CE MRA represents an ideal imaging technique for evaluation of patients with suspected abdominal aortic occlusion [26, 27]. Conventional angiography is difficult in these patients, since access from the femoral arteries is limited. It is therefore necessary to perform arterial puncture of the brachial artery, a technique that is associated with a higher incidence of complications than catheterization procedures from the femoral artery. CE MRA is also preferable for these patients because the gadolinium chelates utilized are not associated with a significant risk of nephrotoxicity, as opposed to the iodinated contrast agents used in conventional angiography and CTA. Furthermore, MRA provides an excellent imaging technique for imaging the vessels distal to the aortic occlusion [28]. In this case, moving table MRA is also performed to evaluate the superficial femoral arteries and the infrapopliteal vessels (Fig. 23). This information is important, since the surgeon needs to know of the status of the distal runoff vessels. Understanding this anatomy is especially important for the femoral vessels, which serve as the distal terminus of the aortal-to-femoral bypass grafts.

The differential diagnosis for aortic occlusion

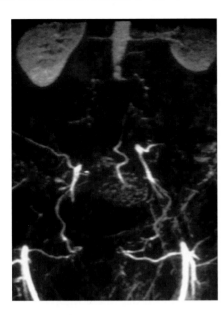

Fig. 24. A coronal oblique MIP image from an arterial-phase gadolinium-enhanced MR angiographic examination reveals occlusion of the abdominal aorta below the origin of the renal arteries in a patient with Takayasu arteritis

includes aortic dissection with occlusion of true lumen by enlarging false lumen, and various coarctation syndromes (e.g., neurofibromatosis, Williams' syndrome, Takayasu's arteritis) (Fig. 24). Radiation-induced and giant cell arteritis are other relatively frequent causes of aortic diseases. In Takayasu's disease, also called *pulseless syndrome*, the aortic arch vessels are primarily affected, although the thoracic and abdominal aorta and pulmonary arteries may also be involved. The aorta may become inflamed by various processes. Inflammatory aortic diseases usually involve all three layers of the aorta (i.e., intima, media, adventitia), and the inflammatory infiltrate may vary from predominantly round cells in Takayasu's arteritis to giant cells in giant cell arteritis. Inflammation may occlude affected arteries or weaken vessel walls with subsequent aneurysm formation. Postcontrast T1-weighted images are important for the evaluation of arteritis, which may exhibit enhancing wall thickening in its early stages. The soft-tissue differentiation possible with MR imaging is valuable for the differentiation of active versus quiescent forms of Takayasu disease.

Pitfalls

Due to the sometimes tremendous tortuosity of the abdominal aorta in patients with atherosclerotic disease, the 3D dataset of the CE MRA study may exclude some relevant arterial territories due to incomplete coverage. As in imaging of the thoracic aorta, it is usually advisable to perform extensive localizer imaging before positioning the slab of the CE MRA study in order to avoid incomplete coverage of the arterial vessels.

Another advantage of extensive localizer imaging is the detection and localization of aortic aneurysms which is important for the timing of the CE MRA study. Either the test bolus or the interactive observation of the arrival of the contrast agent in the region of interest should be done at the level of the aneurysm to achieve complete enhancement of both the aneurysm itself and of the distal vessel territories. If the bolus is timed for the enhancement of the aorta proximal to the aneurysm both the aneurysm and the distal vessels may only fill partially with contrast agent which may result either in missing the full display of the vessel or in ringing artifacts. Frequently, it may take 5 sec or more for an aneurysm to fill completely.

Apart from ringing artifacts in the aortic lumen due to incorrect timing, other artifacts which may occur include blurring of branching vessels due to respiratory motion. Although this can often be avoided by performing the CE MRA study in apnea, in some patients that are unable to follow a breath-hold command these kinds of artifacts cannot be avoided.

References

1. Prince MR, Narasimham DL, Stanley JC et al (1995) Breath-hold gadolinium-enhanced MR angiography of the abdominal aorta and its major branches. Radiology 197:785-792
2. Douek P, Revel D, Chazel S et al (1995) Fast MR angiography of the aorto-iliac arteries and arteries of the lower extremitiy: value of bolus-enhanced, whole volume subtraction technique. Am J Roengenol 165:431-437
3. Knopp MV, Schoenberg SO, Rehm C et al (2002) Assessment of Gadobenate Dimeglumine (Gd-BOPTA) for MR Angiography: Phase I Studies. Invest Radiol 37:706-715
4. Prokop M, Schneider G, Vanzulli A et al. Contrast-enhanced MR angiography of the renal arteries: blinded multicenter crossover comparison of gadobenate dimeglumine and gadopentetate dimeglumine. Radiology (in press)
5. Weiger M, Pruessmann KP, Kassner A et al (2000) Contrast-enhanced 3D MRA using SENSE. J Magn Reson Imaging 12:671-677
6. Sodickson DK, McKenzie CA, Li W et al (2000) Contrast-enhanced 3D MR angiography with simultaneous acquisition of spatial harmonics: A pilot study. Radiology 217:284-289
7. Korosec FR, Frayne R, Grist TM et al (1996) Time resolved contrast-enhanced 3D MR angiography. Magn reson Med 36:345-351
8. Wilman AH, Riederer SJ, King BF et al (1997) Fluo-

roscopically triggered contrast-enhanced three-dimensional MR angiography with elliptical centric view order: application to the renal arteries. Radiology 205:137-146

9. Matsunaga N, Hayashi K, Okada M et al (2003) Magnetic resonance imaging features of aortic diseases. Top Magn Reson Imaging 14:253-266

10. Tatli S, Lipton MJ, Davison BD et al (2003) From the RSNA refresher courses: MR imaging of aortic and peripheral vascular disease. Radiographics 23 Spec No:S59-78

11. Carr JC, Finn JP (2003) MR imaging of the thoracic aorta. Magn Reson Imaging Clin N Am 11:135-148

12. Venkataraman S, Semelka RC, Weeks S et al (2003) Assessment of aorto-iliac disease with magnetic resonance angiography using arterial phase 3-D gradient-echo and interstitial phase 2-D fat-suppressed spoiled gradient-echo sequences. J Magn Reson Imaging 17:43-53

13. Gilfeather M, Holland GA, Siegelman ES et al (1997) Gadolinium-enhanced ultrafast three-dimensional spoiled gradient-echo MR imaging of the abdominal aorta and visceral and iliac vessels. Radiographics. 17:423-432

14. Farner MC, Carpenter JP, Baum RA et al (2003) Early changes in abdominal aortic aneurysm diameter after endovascular repair. J Vasc Interv Radiol 14:205-210

15. Haulon S, Lions C, McFadden EP et al (2001) Prospective evaluation of magnetic resonance imaging after endovascular treatment of infrarenal aortic aneurysms. Eur J Vasc Endovasc Surg 22:62-69

16. Ludman CN, Yusuf SW, Whitaker SC et al (2000) Feasibility of using dynamic contrast-enhanced magnetic resonance angiography as the sole imaging modality prior to endovascular repair of abdominal aortic aneurysms. Eur J Vasc Endovasc Surg 19:524-530

17. Bendib K, Berthezene Y, Croisille P et al (1997) Assessment of complicated arterial bypass graft: Value of contrast-enhanced subtraction magnetic resonance angiography. J Vasc Surg 26:1036-42

18. Faries PL, Dayal R, Rhee J et al (2004) Stent graft treatment for abdominal aortic aneurysm repair: recent developments in therapy. Curr Opin Cardiol 19:551-557

19. Parodi JC (1995) Endovascular repair of abdominal aortic aneurysms and other arterial lesions. J Vasc Surg 21:549-555

20. Eugster T, Bolli M, Pfeiffer T et al (2004) The incidence of iliac aneurysms in patients with abdominal aortic aneurysms: comparison of four centers in Europe and the USA. Vasa 33:68-71

21. Maintz D, Kugel H, Schellhammer F et al (2001) In vitro evaluation of intravascular stent artifacts in three-dimensional MR angiography. Invest Radiol 36:218-224

22. Kasher JA, El-Bialy A, Balingit P (2004) Aortic dissection: a dreaded disease with many faces. J Cardiovasc Pharmacol Ther 9:211-218

23. Duebener LF, Lorenzen P, Richardt G et al (2004) Emergency endovascular stent-grafting for life-threatening acute type B aortic dissections. Ann Thorac Surg 78:1261-1266

24. Kunz RP, Oberholzer K, Kuroczynski W et al (2004) Assessment of chronic aortic dissection: contribution of different ECG-gated breath-hold MRI techniques. AJR Am J Roentgenol 182:1319-1326

25. Cesare ED, Giordano AV, Cerone G et al (2000) Comparative evaluation of TEE, conventional MRI and contrast-enhanced 3D breath-hold MRA in the post-operative follow-up of dissecting aneurysms. Int J Card Imaging 16:135-147

26. Ruehm SG, Weishaupt D, Debatin JF (2000) Contrast-enhanced MR angiography in patients with aortic occlusion (Leriche syndrome). J Magn Reson Imaging 11:401-410

27. Naganawa S, Koshikawa T, Kato K et al (2001) Aortoiliac stenooculusive disease and aneurysms: screening with non-contrast enhanced two-dimensional cardiac gated cine phase contrast MR angiography with multiple velocity encoded values and cardiac gated two-dimensional time-of-flight MR angiography. Radiat Med 19:99-105

28. Ho KY, Leiner T, de Haan MW et al (1998) Peripheral vascular tree stenoses: evaluation with moving-bed infusion-tracking MR angiography. Radiology 206:683-692

VI.2

MR Angiography of the Renal Arteries

Honglei Zhang, Stefan Schoenberg and Martin R. Prince

Introduction

Renal artery stenosis causes renal ischemia, hypertension and when bilateral, progressive ischemic nephropathy [1]. Although patients with renal artery stenosis can be managed conservatively, renal revascularization is indicated in patients with refractory hypertension on a multidrug regimen and in patients with declining renal function. Angioplasty, stent implantation or surgery may relieve the hypertension and improve renal function as long as the kidney is revascularized before ischemic nephropathy becomes irreversible.

Given the devastating consequences of uncontrolled renovascular hypertension and renal failure, it is helpful to diagnose renal artery stenosis as early as possible. Conventional angiography with measurements of pressure proximal and distal to stenosis is the gold standard for diagnosing renovascular disease. Unfortunately, this procedure is of limited value as a screening examination because of its invasiveness and the need for radiation exposure and nephrotoxic iodinated contrast media.

Within the past decade, several less-invasive techniques have been developed to detect and assess renal arterial disease [2-4]. Doppler ultrasonography and captopril renography have focused on detecting the hemodynamic effects of a functionally significant renal artery stenosis, whereas computed tomography (CT) and magnetic resonance (MR) angiography are more effective at detecting renal artery morphological changes, using a subjective impression of stenosis severity to predict functional significance. Because it is essential to identify the location and features (i.e. length, severity, relationship to aortic plaque and branch vessels) of a stenosis when planning revascularization, there has been a tendency to favor contrast-enhanced MRA and CTA over functional techniques such as ultrasound and nuclear medi-

cine. However, for optimum management of renovascular hypertension, clinicians need both functional and anatomic data. Functional information is important because there may not be any benefit from dilating a severe stenosis when ischemic nephropathy or other concomitant nephropathy is already end-stage. Indeed, an unnecessary renal revascularization procedure may further compromise a patient with borderline renal function and accelerate their need for renal dialysis secondary to interventional complications such as iodinated contrast nephrotoxicity, cholesterol emboli or renal artery dissection.

Arterial narrowing does not reduce blood flow until it reaches a hemodynamically significant degree, which creates a pressure gradient. The widely accepted criterion for diagnosing significant stenosis is a caliber decrease of greater than 75%. Unfortunately, a major shortcoming of this reference standard is that it neglects the influence of renal blood flow. A morphologically severe stenosis might not induce a pressure gradient if the artery has slow flow due to renal parenchymal impairment [5].

Fortunately, MR angiography can be combined with a variety of pulse sequences for assessing organ function that can help determine which patients/kidneys can benefit from renal revascularization. The combination of gadolinium enhanced MR angiography with functional pulse sequences offers more complete and accurate information for a highly effective renovascular disease screening exam.

Normal Anatomy

Normally, each kidney is supplied by a single renal artery originating from the side of the aorta, immediately below the superior mesenteric artery typically at the level of L2 (Fig. 1). Each renal ar-

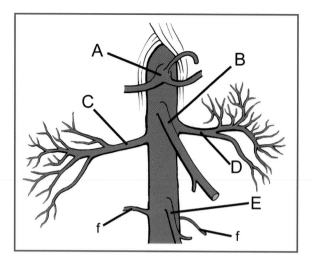

Fig. 1. Normal Anatomy
A Coeliac trunc
B Superior mesenteric artery
C Right renal artery
D Left renal artery
E Inferior mesenteric artery
f Lumbar arteries

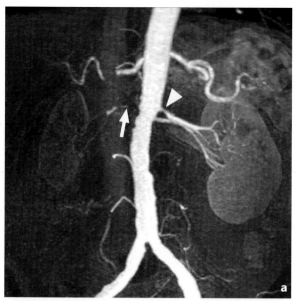

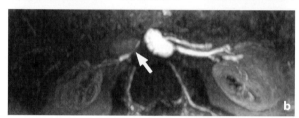

Fig. 2a, b. Renal MRA with single dose Gd-BOPTA during a 30-second breath-hold shows an occluded right renal artery (*arrows* in **a**, **b**) and two left renal arteries. The superior left renal artery (*arrowhead* in **a**) has a moderate stenosis

tery courses posteriorly to reach the kidneys, with the right longer and lower than the left, given the relatively inferior position of the right kidney. The right renal artery courses behind the inferior vena cava, the right renal vein, the head of the pancreas, and the descending part of the duodenum. The left renal artery lies posterior to the left renal vein, the body of the pancreas and the splenic vein, and is crossed by the inferior mesenteric vein.

The renal artery divides into four or five branches before reaching the renal hilum. The first branch is into the anterior and posterior division, usually occurring just prior to the renal hilum. The posterior division may be smaller and supplies a large portion of blood flow to the posterior portion of the kidney. The anterior division continues before dividing into the apical, upper, middle, and lower anterior segmental arteries at the renal hilum. These segmental arteries course through the renal sinus and branch into the lobar arteries.

Normal Variants

Aberrant or accessory renal arteries may arise off the aorta or iliac arteries. They are present in up to 25% of patients, originating above or below the main renal artery (Fig. 2a, b). Accessory renal arteries will be seen coursing into the renal hilum usually perfusing the upper or lower polar regions. If an aberrant artery enters the upper or lower pole directly, without passing through the renal hilum, it is called a polar artery (Fig. 3). These aberrant

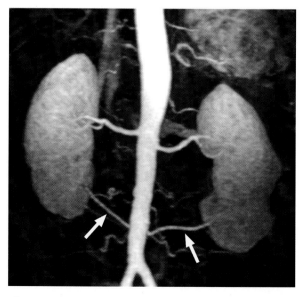

Fig. 3. Two lower polar arteries (*arrows*) in a 42-year-old male with hypertension. No renal artery stenosis is present (Gd-BOPTA, 0.1 mmol/kg) [Image courtesy of Dr. G. Schneider]

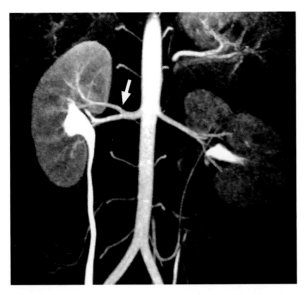

Fig. 4. Renal MRA shows early branching of the right renal artery (*arrow*). This is a relative contraindication to donation

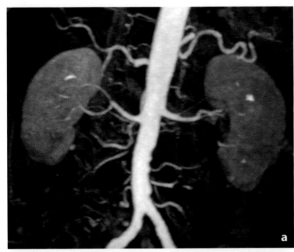

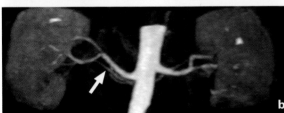

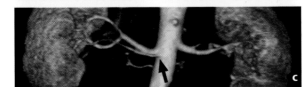

Fig. 5a-c. CE-MRA study of a potential living kidney donor with an accessory renal artery on the right and early branching of the left renal artery (**a-c**). On the whole volume MIP the additional renal artery is hard to detect (**a**) whereas on the subvolume reconstructions (**b**, **c**) it is clearly depicted (*arrows*). Note that the origin of the accessory renal artery on the left is much better appreciated on the surface rendered image (*black arrow* in **c**). (Gd-BOPTA, 0.1 mmol/kg) [Image courtesy of Dr. G. Schneider]

renal arteries may arise more anteriorly from the aorta and have a more anterior course for example coursing anterior to the IVC on the right. Early arterial branching is another common variant for which detection is necessary in patients undergoing evaluation for donor nephrectomy (Fig. 4). Branching within 2 cm of the main renal artery origin is considered "early" and may complicate harvesting as a donor kidney (Fig. 5a-c). Contrast-enhanced 3D MRA permits detailed assessment of the normal and variant vascular anatomy in most cases (Fig. 6).

Renal MR Angiography Techniques

Non-Contrast-Enhanced Renal MRA

Many renal MR angiography techniques have been described. Standard non-contrast, flow sensitive sequences include time-of-flight (TOF) and phase contrast (PC) MRA. The image quality of these flow-based techniques is limited by diminished flow in patients with vascular stenosis or parenchymal disease and by motion artifacts due to respiration during acquisition times that are too long for breath-holding. Proximal stenoses (where there is less respiratory motion) are better depicted than distal disease [6]. It is possible to excite blood proximal to the renal arteries and then image the blood after it flows into the renal arteries but this is also limited in patients with slow flow. Black blood MRA [7] and navigator-gated, balanced fast field echo projection MRA with aortic

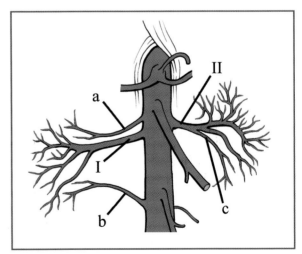

Fig. 6. Normal variants of renal vasculature
I Right renal artery
II Left renal artery
a Accessory right renal artery
b Right lower polar artery
c Early left renal artery branching

spin labeling [8] offer better visualization of the renal arteries without requiring contrast agents, but again these techniques are limited in patients with disease that disturbs normal renal blood flow.

Contrast-Enhanced Renal MRA

Gadolinium-based contrast material shortens the T1 relaxation time of blood, thereby increasing intravascular signal for high signal-to-noise ratio (SNR), high resolution arteriograms during breath-holding. Most of the published studies of 3D Gd renal MRA have been performed on high field 1.5 Tesla MR scanners. This reflects the importance of high SNR, which scales roughly linearly with field strength. Low field MR scanners at 0.5 Tesla or less have about 1/3 of the SNR and thus are less likely to provide as much vascular detail. It is expected that 3 Tesla MR scanners will offer further improvements in image quality, however, at present this is traded off against the lack of suitable coils and design deficiencies in the currently available 3T MR systems. MR scanners with high gradient performance enable breath-hold acquisitions with smaller voxel sizes for higher spatial resolution data and improved visualization of vascular detail.

Coils

Phased array coils increase the SNR for imaging renal arteries in small or average-sized patients. Coil arrays also allow for implementation of parallel imaging techniques that can shorten data acquisition time, increase resolution or both [9]. Large patients, > 100 kg, may have to be imaged with a body coil built into the wall of the magnet since phased array coils have a limited depth of penetration.

Patient Preparation

It is important to first evaluate the patient's ability to hold his or her breath. The patient's breath-hold capacity dictates MRA scan duration, which should be prescribed to be short enough to enable patient compliance and successful breath-holding. Scan parameters should then be adjusted for the highest possible spatial resolution for sufficient anatomic coverage of the aorta, iliac and renal arteries back to at least mid-kidney. Patients who have a respiratory rate of less than 20 breaths per minute (bpm) can easily suspend breathing for 30-40 seconds which makes high resolution renal MRA easy. But in patients who can only hold their breath for 15 or 20 seconds, it may become neces-

sary to compromise on the desired spatial resolution and coverage. Oxygen may help patients who are dyspneic to double their breath-holding capacity. Even when patients are holding their breath there may still be motion of the kidneys [10]. Thus, it is important to ensure that patients hold their abdomen still in addition to holding their breath. Patients with a respiratory rate greater than 25 breaths per minute are not likely to be able to hold their breath for more than a few seconds. In these patients where breath-holding is difficult or unrealistic, it is preferable to perform a one-minute long scan with higher SNR and free breathing. These very dyspneic patients tend to have scarred lungs that do not allow much respiratory motion anyway. In the future, intravascular contrast agents in combination with navigator-gated MRA techniques may allow even higher-resolution MRA with free-breathing.

It is better to start the intravenous line (IV) in the right arm because this provides a more direct path to the central circulation when compared to the left arm. In older patients, the left brachiocephalic vein may get pinched in between the sternum and an ectatic and tortuous aorta thereby interfering with the bolus injection of contrast. IV tubing should be used that allows the simultaneous attachment of two syringes for the contrast agent and saline flush. Suitable tubing is provided with MR power injectors. For manual injection there is an optimized tubing system (SmartSet, TopSpins, Ann Arbor, MI) designed for MRA which has one-way valves that automatically switch between Gd injection and saline flush. Manual injection is recommended in pediatric patients, patients with tenuous IV lines and in patients in whom power injection via central lines may not be safe.

Renal MRA Protocols

At our institution, the renal MRA protocol comprises the following sequences:
- Sagittal black blood sequence (~ 4 minutes) or a 3-plane gradient echo localizer (30 seconds).
- Axial and coronal T2-weighted single shot fast spin echo (1 minute).
- Coronal 3D dynamic Gd-enhanced acquisitions (20 to 30 seconds per phase) repeated during arterial and venous phases with 2 separate breath-holdings. State-of-the-art is a matrix of 512 x 192, ~30° flip angle (60-75° when there is a non-magnetic stent) with 2-3 mm thick slices zero-filled down to 1-1.5 mm. Higher resolution is possible using parallel imaging techniques such as SENSE or auto-SMASH based techniques like GRAPPA. Coronal acquisition with a field of view of 32-40 cm is gener-

ally sufficient to cover a region from the diaphragm down to the common femoral arteries. With parallel imaging, however, it may be necessary to use a slightly larger field-of-view to make sure there is no wrap around artifact in the left-right (phase) direction since this interferes with the parallel data deconvolution. Auto-SMASH-based techniques are less susceptible to these artifacts than SENSE-based techniques. Zero filling of the MR Fourier data is important for reducing partial volume effects and eliminating stair-step artifact on reformations and other reconstructions.

- Axial 3D phase contrast (~7 minutes with velocity encoding @ 30-50 cm/second).
- Post Gd coronal 3D of the renal collecting system (~30 seconds).

The total imaging time is about 15 minutes, giving a total examination time of about 30 minutes with patient set up, breath-holding instruction, etc.

An optional sequence for measuring blood flow in the renal artery is 2D cine phase contrast MRA. Although this requires EKG gating, peripheral gating works nearly as well and is easier to set-up. Advanced scanners nowadays offer easy-to-use EKG-gating. Cine phase contrast images are acquired perpendicular to each renal artery in the sagittal oblique orientation with a 5-6 mm slice thickness positioned proximal to stenoses to avoid turbulent dephasing jets. The temporal and spatial resolution must be adapted to make the scan short enough to acquire in two breath-holds: one breath-hold for each renal artery. For measurement of renal blood flow, it is better to sacrifice spatial resolution in order to preserve temporal resolution. SNR can be maximized by acquiring the phase contrast data after gadolinium administration. Velocity is measured in the slice direction. It is necessary to select a velocity encoding (venc) value which is equal to or higher than the peak renal artery velocity, typically 75 to 100 cm/second. The optimal venc will be lower in older patients or in patients with renal failure. Some additional pulse sequencing is described below under functional information.

Gadolinium Dose

The standard dose of gadolinium contrast agent for renal MRA is 0.2 mmol/kg (~30 mL) with 40 mL saline flush both injected at a rate of 2 mL/second. Favorable results with 0.1 mmol/kg have been reported with Gd-BOPTA (Fig. 7a, b), which has a two-fold higher relaxivity compared with other gadolinium compounds [11-13].

Bolus Timing

In order to get maximum arterial Gd concentration during the center of k-space, perfect bolus timing is essential. There are several reliable and precise techniques available for determining contrast travel time from IV site to renal arteries in order to correctly coordinate the initiation of bolus injection with initiation of scanning. The most widely used techniques involve a test bolus to measure the contrast travel time, using an automatic pulse sequence that monitors signal in the aorta and then initiates imaging after contrast is detected arriving in the aorta (Fluoroscopic triggering, Bolustrak, Carebolus or MR SmartPrep). An alternative procedure that reduces the need for accurate bolus timing is time-resolved imaging. It is useful to ask the manufacturer of your equipment which technique works best. Time-resolved MRA with a temporal resolution of about 7 seconds per 3D acquisition and a single dose of contrast material has been reported to detect unilateral renal artery stenosis with sensitivity of 75% and specificity of 96% [14]. Time-resolved MRA may have less spatial resolution but it is particularly useful in high flow lesions such as arteriovenous fistulae or renal vascular malformations. More sophisticated time-resolved techniques under development with oversampling of the center of k-space and sliding window reconstruction such as TRICKS (time-resolved imaging of contrast kinetics) potentially offer high temporal resolution without compromising spatial resolution.

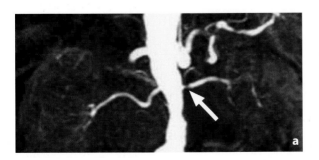
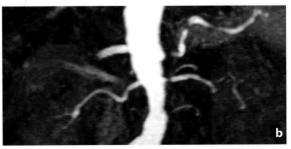

Fig. 7a, b. CE renal MRA with single dose (0.1 mmol/kg) Gd-BOPTA (**a**) versus double dose (0.2 mmol/kg) of Gd-DTPA (**b**). Equivalent diagnostic information of renal artery stenosis (*arrow* in **a**) is obtained at half the dose [Images courtesy of Dr. G. Schneider]

Image Post-processing and Interpretation

Compared to conventional angiography, which has a limited number of projections, MR angiography produces a 3D data set that can be reconstructed into an unlimited number of projections using different slab thicknesses, orientations and rendering methods. These optimized projections are created by post-processing the 3D MRA data on a specialized computer workstation. Post-processing substantially improves image quality and visualization of the vessel lumenal details. Maximum intensity projection (MIP), multiplanar reformatting (MPR) and 3D surface or volume rendering (VR) are the most commonly used post-processing techniques. Reformations and MIPs are essential for optimal assessment of vascular anatomy and grading the severity of stenoses. Subvolume MIPs may be oriented to display bifurcations and branch vessels in profile. This is important because atherosclerotic disease tends to be most severe at branch points. In evaluating renal artery stenosis, oblique coronal and oblique axial MIPs are the most valuable views. Source images must still be reviewed to detect mural thrombus, renal masses, retroperitoneal fibrosis, vasculitis and other mural or parenchymal abnormalities [15].

Examples for Various Clinical Indications and Pathologies

Atherosclerotic Renal Artery Stenosis

Atherosclerosis is the most common cause of renal artery stenosis. Clinical features that are suspicious for renal artery stenosis include abrupt-onset or accelerated hypertension at any age, hypertension at a young age, unexplained acute or chronic azotemia, azotemia induced by an angiotensin-converting enzyme (ACE) inhibitors, asymmetric renal dimensions, and congestive heart failure with normal ventricular function. Elderly patients with generalized atherosclerosis and hypertension often have atherosclerotic renal artery stenosis. Typically the aorta is atherosclerotic (Fig. 2) and disease in the aorta extends into the renal artery origins, thereby compromising renal blood flow. These atherosclerotic stenoses are often progressive, tend to involve the ostium or proximal third of the renal artery, and are frequently eccentric. It is important to mention that atherosclerotic stenoses my as well be found in accessory renal arteries (Fig. 8a-c) which are typically hard to diagnose on ultrasound. Hypertension in these patients may not be entirely renin-dependent (i.e., essential hypertension). Renal artery revascularization with stenting may be considered for refractory severe hypertension, and would be expected

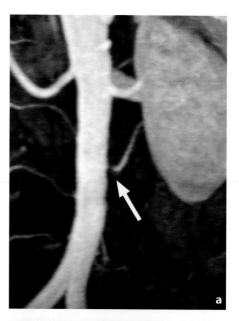

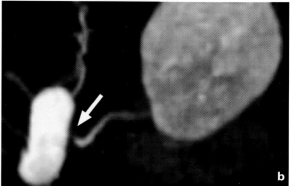

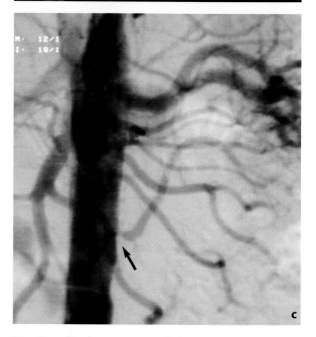

Fig. 8a-c. Renal artery stenosis of a lower polar artery (Gd-BOP-TA, 0.1 mmol/kg). On the whole volume MIP a stenosis of a lower polar artery is evident (*arrow* in **a**). This is even better displayed in a targeted subvolume MIP (*arrow* in **b**) with good correlation with conventional angiography (**c**) [Images courtesy of Dr. G. Schneider]

to improve blood pressure control and modestly reduce medication requirements. Curing hypertension with renal revascularization in these patients is less likely.

Fibromuscular Dysplasia (FMD)

The second most common cause of renal artery stenosis is fibromuscular dysplasia (FMD). FMD affects younger patients and women more frequently than men. One study reports FMD in as many as 10% of cases of renal artery stenosis [16] but our observation is that it is rare, which may reflect our older patient population. Patients with pure renin-dependent (renovascular) hypertension are common with renal FMD and may be cured with angioplasty in over 80% of cases. In contrast to atherosclerotic stenoses, FMD tends to affect the mid- and distal renal artery (Fig. 9). Initial medical therapy for renovascular hypertension associated with FMD is an ACE inhibitor. Early detection and intervention are recommended for FMD because it responds well to balloon angioplasty and procedural morbidity is low in these typically younger patients. Three-dimensional CE MRA permits visualization of renal artery pathology affecting both the proximal as well as the distal renal arteries if spatial resolution is sufficient. In our experience, FMD is always well seen on 3D phase contrast MRA as a signal void from turbulent dephasing caused by the multiple webs (Fig. 10a-c). However, intrarenal segmental renal arteries may be missed on renal 3D CE MRA due to motion of the kidneys, parenchymal enhancement and limited spatial resolution.

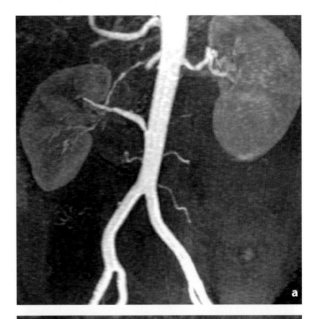

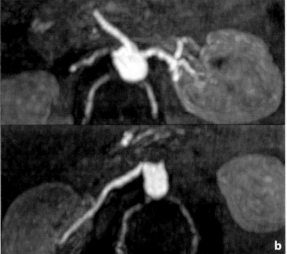

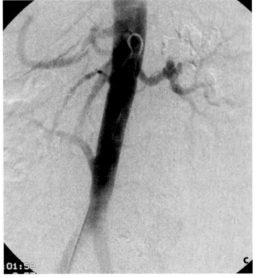

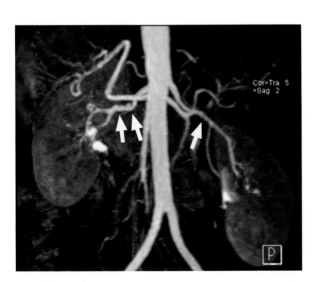

Fig. 9. High resolution CE MRA (Gd-BOPTA, 0.1 mmol/kg) in a patient with fibromuscular dysplasia (FMD). Note the multiple irregular dilatations and stenoses of the renal arteries (*arrows*) [Images courtesy of Dr. G. Schneider]

Fig. 10a-c. Renal MRA with single dose Gd-BOPTA (0.1 mmol/kg) shows fibromuscular dysplasia (FMD) of both renal arteries

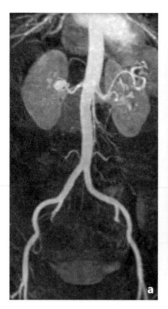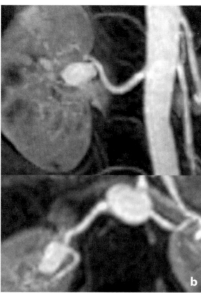

Fig. 11a, b. CE MRA in a patient with Kawasa-ki's disease in childhood. CE MRA shows a persistent distal right renal artery aneurysm

Renal Artery Aneurysm

Aneurysm of the renal artery is rare. It can occur as a manifestation of atherosclerotic disease, FMD, neurofibromatosis, and polyarteritis nodosa. Renal artery aneurysms can be classified as extraparenchymal (saccular, fusiform, false/dissecting) or intraparenchymal. The incidence of hypertension in patients with renal artery aneurysms may reach 90%; however, this may reflect the importance of hypertension for ordering diagnostic angiography. On 3D CE MRA, aneurysms involving the main and proximal segmental renal arteries are seen well (Fig. 11a, b). However, the smaller, intraparenchymal aneurysms of polyarteritis nodosa may not be reliably detected. Viewing reformations and source images is crucial for determining whether the aneurysm is saccular or fusiform. This may help to determine appropriate treatments for the patients, including surgery, transcatheter embolization, stent-graft or frequent follow-up imaging to assess for growth.

Renal Artery Dissection

Renal artery dissection is typically found in patients with dissection of the aorta and involvement of the renal artery. 3D CE MRA can noninvasively evaluate for involvement of the renal arteries in aortic dissection (Fig. 12a, b) and help planning interventional therapy. Due to the 3D dataset optimal projections for depiction of the dissection membrane can be chosen, however it is always advisable to review the raw data as well.

Renal Vascular Malformation

Renal arteriovenous malformations (AVMs) and fistulae are abnormal communications between the intrarenal arterial and venous systems. Renal AVMs are usually identified during the evaluation of gross hematuria. Two types of congenital renal AVMs are described, including cirsoid AVM and cavernous congenital AVM which is the less common type. Acquired AVM or fistula can occur following trauma, especially from renal biopsy. Angiographic embolization is the preferred treatment for symptomatic AVMs. MRA is especially useful in those patients who cannot tolerate iodine-based contrast. In one study, the values for sensitivity, specificity, and accuracy using 3D PC MRA to diagnose renal vascular malformation were 78%, 100%, and 91%, respectively [17].

AVM's may as well be found in patients with re-

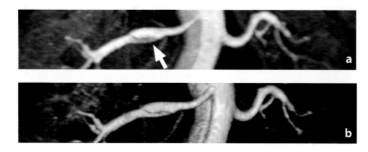

Fig. 12a, b. Dissection of the aorta with involvement of the renal artery. Both the MIP image (**a**) and the surface rendered image (**b**) display the involvement of the renal artery (*arrow* in **a**). [Images courtesy of Dr. G. Schneider]

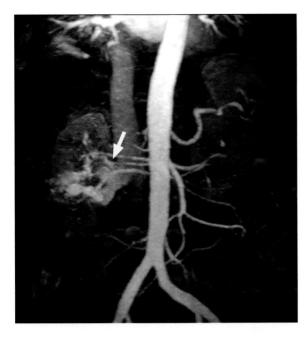

Fig. 13. AVM in a patient with renal cell carcinoma (RCC) (Gd-BOPTA, 0.1 mmol/kg). The right kidney shows 3 renal arteries of which the middle artery shows an AV-shunt (*arrow*) [Images courtesy of Dr. G. Schneider]

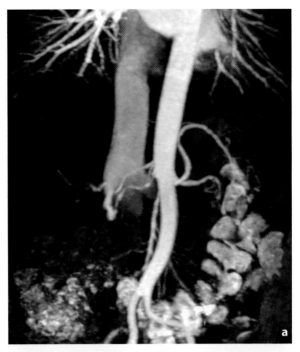

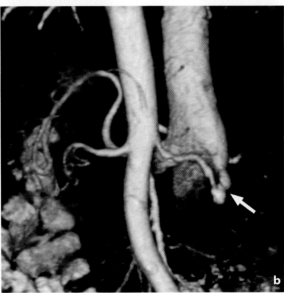

Fig. 14a, b. AVM of the renal artery post nephrectomy and ligation of combined artery and vein (Gd-BOPTA, 0.1 mmol/kg). Note that the relationship between the renal artery and the vein on the MIP image (**a**) is not clear but is easily understood on the surface rendered image (*arrow* in **b**) [Images courtesy of Dr. G. Schneider]

nal tumors, in which due to tumor necrosis direct connections between larger intrarenal arteries and veins may occur (Fig. 13). In the same way AV malformations may be found rarely post nephrectomy (Fig. 14a, b) if during surgery separate ligation of the artery and the vein is not performed.

Renal Transplant

The most common cause for deteriorating renal function in renal transplant patients is rejection. However, the possibility of transplant renal artery stenosis must also be considered, especially if there is associated new onset or severe hypertension. Early diagnosis of arterial stenosis is essential to salvage a failing renal allograft (Fig. 15a, b). Digital subtraction angiography is the gold standard for evaluation of these vascular complications, but the invasiveness and particularly the risk of potential nephrotoxicity to the already compromised kidney due to the iodinated contrast medium make DSA less suitable for renal transplant follow-up. MRA has been shown to be a reliable method of diagnosing transplant renal artery stenosis (Table 4).

The transplant renal artery examination is performed in a manner similar to native renal artery imaging but shifted lower into the pelvis to cover the transplant kidney and in-flow from the iliac arteries. Three-dimensional contrast MRA is performed in the coronal plane encompassing the lower abdominal aorta and extending down to below the femoral heads. The transplanted artery is usually anastomosed to the ipsilateral external iliac artery using an end-to-side anastomosis or to the

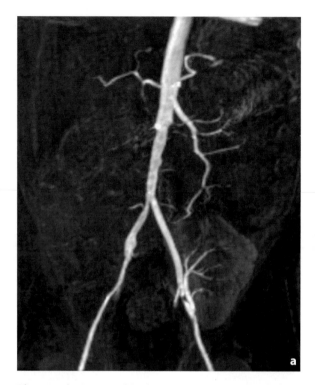
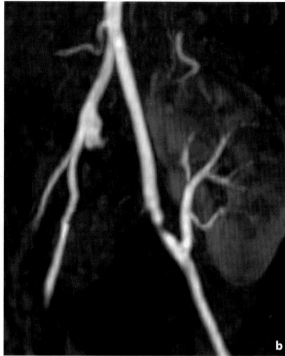

Fig. 15a, b. Stenosis of the iliac artery in a patient with ipsilateral transplant kidney

internal iliac artery using an end-to-end anastomosis. Generally, about 40 sections (interpolated
to 80 sections with zero padding), each 2-3 mm or
less, are sufficient to include the aorta, iliac arteries
and the entire transplant kidney. The posterior
coverage must be sufficient to include tortuous iliac arteries. Post contrast T1-weighted images within 5-10 minutes of intravenous Gd injection should
be acquired to assess renal excretory function and
to demonstrate perfusion defects, masses, infarction, peri-transplant fluid collections, and hydronephrosis. T2-weighted imaging with fat saturation is also helpful. Vascular clips in the surgical
bed may produce metallic artifact on MRA (Fig.
16). This potential pitfall can be avoided by recog-
nizing its characteristic MR imaging appearance
and correlating the imaging findings with CT or
conventional radiography.

Nevertheless an origin of an accessory renal artery or a renal artery in congenital malformations
(Fig. 17a, b) from the iliac arteries may as well be
found, thus it is always important to include the iliac arteries in the field-of-view.

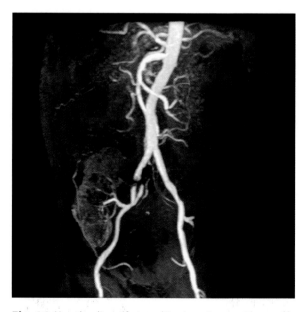

Fig. 16. Vascular clip artifact resulting in an image with an artificial occlusion of the right iliac artery. However due to the normal
enhancement of the distal vessel it is obvious that the occlusion is
artificial

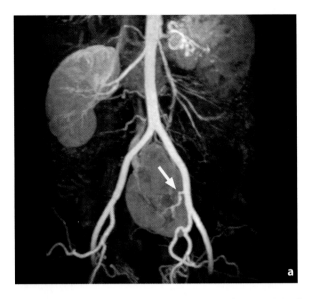
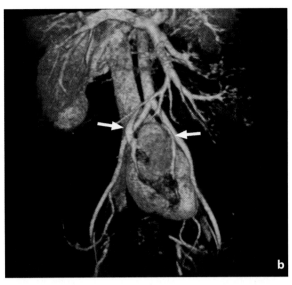

Fig. 17a, b. Congenital pelvic kidney with a renal artery arising from the left common iliac artery (Gd-BOPTA, 0.1 mmol/kg). Whereas a first arterial acquisition (**a**) clearly displays the origin of the renal artery (*arrow*) the venous phase image (**b**) nicely displays two renal veins and their complex relationship to the iliac arteries and aortic bifurcation [Images courtesy of Dr. G. Schneider]

Renal Donors

Defining renal vascular anatomy is essential for the evaluation of potential living-related kidney donors because anatomic variants occur in an estimated 12% to 44% of cases. Accessory arteries perfusing more than 5% of the renal parenchyma must not be sacrificed. But multiple arterial anastomoses may result in an increased risk of thrombosis, malperfusion, and finally rejection. Early branching renal arteries may also complicate harvesting and implantation of the renal allograft. Thus, failure to identify accessory renal arteries before surgery can complicate the transplantation procedure and may compromise the outcome. Accurate determination of the number, length, and location of renal arteries is essential for proper surgical planning, especially with the minimally invasive techniques. It is also important to identify anatomic variations in the renal venous and parenchymal anatomy (Fig. 18).

CE MRA is ideal for assessing renal vessels and renal parenchyma in potential living kidney donors [18-22]. CE MRA shows the arterial system, venous system, and collecting system as well as the kidney parenchyma using multi-phase coronal 3D CE MRA. It may be helpful to follow Gd injection with 10 mg lasix to more completely fill out the colleting systems on a 10-minute delayed image for MR urographic evaluation. In interpreting MRA images, it is necessary to analyze source images and data in the reformation mode. The data must be viewed in both the coronal and axial planes. Axial reformation allows easy differentia-

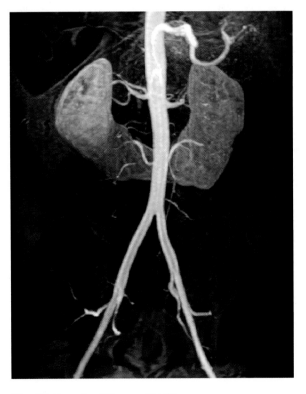

Fig. 18. Horseshoe kidney on CE MRA

tion between lumbar arteries, accessory renal arteries, and overlying mesenteric arterial branches. MRA provides sufficient information about the renal arterial anatomy and is superior in diagnosing the anatomy of the renal veins in the evaluation of living kidney donors [23, 24]. One potential limita-

Table 1. Sensitivity and specificity of renal MR angiography without contrast agents

Technique	Author	Year	# Patients	Sensitivity (%)	Specificity (%)
2D TOF	Kent [49]	1991	23	100	94
2D TOF	Debatin [50]	1991	33	53	97
2D TOF	Servois [51]	1994	21	70	78
2D TOF	Hertz [52]	1994	16	91	94
3D TOF	Loubeyre [53]	1994	53	100	76
3D TOF	Nelson [54]	1999	5	71	95
2D PC	Debatin (50)	1991	33	80	91
3D PC	De Cobelli [55]	1996	50	94	94
Cine PC	Silverman [56]	1996	37	100	93
3D PC	de Haan [57]	1996	38	93	95
3D PC	Miller [58]	1999	32	93	81
3D PC – PSL*	Westenberg [59]	1999	17	Correlation coefficient = 0.90	
Cine-PC	Lee [40]	2000	35	50	78
Cine-PC +ACE**				67	84
T2 dark blood	Tello [7]	2003	16	96	92

* post-stenotic signal loss
** angiotensin-converting enzyme

tion is the inability of MR to detect renal calculi, however these are rare in the asymptomatic renal donor population.

Pitfalls and Limitations

Pacemakers, aneurysm clips and orbit metal fragments are contraindications of MR examination. Patients with severe claustrophobia may require sedation (Valium 5-10 mg or Xanax 1-2 mg po to be taken 30 minutes prior to MRI). Ferromagnetic stents (eg. Palmaz stent) are impossible to be imaged because of the artifact they produce. However, non-magnetic stents made of nitinol or platinum may be imaged successfully although there is some radiofrequency shielding by the stent mesh, which acts like a Faraday Cage. This can be overcome by using more radiofrequency (RF) power, which is achieved by raising the flip angle of the RF pulse. A flip angle of 60-75° has worked for platinum-iridium, nitinol and tantalum stents. Respiratory motion blur obscures renal arterial detail so breath-holding is essential.

Accuracy of Renal MRA Techniques in Literature

Table 1 shows sensitivity and specificity data reported for diagnosing renal artery stenosis using non-contrast MR angiography. Many of the limitations due to flow and saturation artifacts on flow-based techniques are eliminated by using gadolinium contrast to enhance the renal MRA examina-

tion. Gadolinium contrast agents enormously increase the SNR allowing for higher resolution in short scan times. Using conventional angiography as a reference standard, the reported sensitivity and specificity of renal MRA with gadolinium enhancement for diagnosing renal artery stenosis are 88-100% and 70-100% respectively (Table 2) with similar interobserver variability [25], especially for severe stenoses greater than 70%. Accuracy can be improved by evaluation of the vessel area on multiplanar reformats. This requires high-resolution renal 3D CE MRA with parallel imaging. MRA thus avoids invasive diagnostic procedures [26]. In addition, renal MRA eliminates the need for aortography at the time of subsequent angioplasty [27] and thereby dramatically reduces iodinated contrast load and radiation exposure during renal revascularization. By showing the precise location of each renal artery and the angle arising from the aorta, catheter manipulation during renal revascularization may be minimized, thereby potentially reducing the procedural risk of cholesterol emboli.

A recent meta-analysis compared MRA, CTA, ultrasound, captopril renography and captopril test for diagnosing renal artery stenosis [28]. Gadolinium-enhanced MRA and CTA with iodinated contrast were found to be highly and comparably accurate with a 0.99 area under the receiver-operator curve (ROC). Ultrasound, time-of-flight MRA, and captopril renography were significantly less accurate. Compared to CE MRA, ultrasound is more operator-dependent with inferior sensitivity; renal scintigraphy is also significantly less accurate, especially in patients with impaired renal function; CTA is as accurate as MRA, but us-

Table 2. Sensitivity and specificity of contrast- enhanced renal MRA

Technique	Author	# Patients	Sensitivity (%)	Specificity (%)
3D Gd	Prince [60]	19	100	93
3D Gd	Grist [61]	35	89	95
3D Gd	Snidow [62]	47	100	89
3D Gd	Holland [63]	63	100	100
3D Gd	Steffens [64]	50	96	95
3D Gd	Rieumont [65]	30	100	71
3D Gd	De Cobelli [66]	55	100	97
3D Gd	Bakker [67]	50	97	92
3D Gd	Hany [68]	103	93	90
3D Gd	Thornton [69]	62	88	98
3D Gd	Schoenberg [70]	26	94-100	96-100
3D Gd	Thornton [71]	42	100	98
3D Gd + PC	Cambria [72]	25	97	100
3D Gd	Ghantous [73]	12	–	100
3D Gd	Gilfeather [25]	54	Overestimate 21%, underestimate 14% SD: MRA = 6.9%, Angio = 7.5%	
3D Gd	Marchand [74]		88-100	71-100
3D Gd	Shetty [39]	51	96	92
3D Gd	Winterer[75]	23	100	98
3D blood pool	Weishaupt [76]	20	82	98
3D Gd	Bongers [77]	43	100	94
Time-resolved	Volk [78]	40	93	83
3D Gd at 1T	Oberholzer [79]	23	96	97
3D Gd	Korst [80]	38	100	85
3D Gd	De Corbelli [81]	45	94	93
3D Gd	Mittal [15]	26	96	93
3D Gd	Voiculescu [82]	36	96	86
3D Gd	Qanadli [3]	41	97	64
3D Gd	Hood [83]	21	100	74
3D Gd + cine PC	Schoenberg [38]	23	97% agreement with DSA	
Time-resolved	Krause [14]	71	75	95.7
3D Gd	Willmann [84]	46	92-93	99-100
3D Gd	Coenegrachts [85]	25	100	98

es ionizing radiation as well as nephrotoxic contrast material, which are considered less favorable, particularly in patients at risk for renal insufficiency. However, CTA may be preferred when there are contraindications to MR such as a pacemaker, orbital metal fragment, severe claustrophobia or brain aneurysm clip.

In addition to diagnosing renal artery stenosis, 3D CE MRA identifies concomitant vascular conditions including aorto-iliac occlusive disease, ulcerated atherosclerotic plaques, the angle of the renal artery with respect to the aorta, early renal artery branching and accessory renal arteries which may influence planning for interventional procedures. Furthermore, MRA can be combined with additional pulse sequences that enable assessment of kidney function and hemodynamic significance of borderline renal artery stenosis.

Functional Assessment of renal Artery Stenosis

In addition to depicting lumenal anatomy, MRA data is analyzed for evidence of diminished or asymmetrical renal function, which occur in the setting of hemodynamically significant renal artery stenosis.

Symmetry of Renal Length and Parenchymal Thickness

Normal kidneys measure 11-13 cm in length with a tendency for the right kidney to be slightly smaller (up to 1 cm) compared to the left. Typical parenchymal thickness is 1.7 ± 0.3 cm [29]. Parenchymal volume is a more accurate parame-

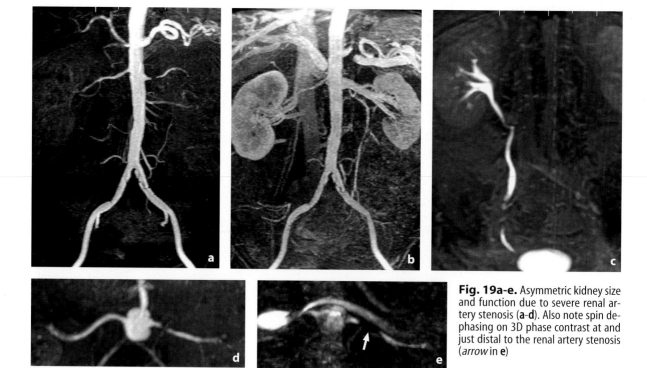

Fig. 19a-e. Asymmetric kidney size and function due to severe renal artery stenosis (**a-d**). Also note spin dephasing on 3D phase contrast at and just distal to the renal artery stenosis (*arrow* in **e**)

ter. Hemodynamically significant renal artery stenosis reduces perfusion pressure within the kidney, causing it to decrease in length and volume (Fig. 19). Chronic ischemia destroys nephrons resulting in gradual renal atrophy, further reducing length, parenchymal thickness and volume. Whenever a kidney with a stenotic renal artery is more than 1 cm smaller than the contralateral kidney, the possibility of hemodynamic significance should be considered with greater suspicion. In one study, renal volume measurements showed high sensitivity (91%) and negative predictive value (80%) in predicting the outcome of percutaneous transluminal renal angioplasty (PTRA) [30].

Post-stenotic Dilatation

Post-stenotic dilatation of greater than 20% is commonly seen with severely stenotic renal arteries [31]. The association between significant renal artery stenosis causing post-stenotic fusiform aneurysm and hypertension can be attributed to activation of the renin-angiotensin system, with increased angiotensin II levels resulting in fluid retention and vasoconstriction. Also when the renal artery lumen narrows, blood flow accelerates to maintain the same volume flow across a narrower cross sectional area. This accelerated jet flow tends to impact a spot on the artery wall distal to the stenosis, eventually producing post-stenotic dilatation. It may not be present in stenoses that are so

severe that only a weak jet can make it through the stenosis.

Symmetry of Gd Excretion

A delayed scan (about 10 minutes after administration of contrast material) can be used to assess the excretory function of kidneys (Fig. 19). On older scanners with longer echo times, the highly concentrated Gd in collecting systems may shorten the T2 so much that the MR signal dephases faster than the TE, thereby reducing the utility of the delayed scan. However, on state-of-the-art MR scanners with TE < 1 msec, it is possible to capture the signal from highly concentrated Gd in the urine. Asymmetrical signal intensity in collecting systems is a reliable indicator of unilateral renal dysfunction that may result from ischemia [32]. In the ischemic kidney, glomerular filtration of Gd is maintained by activating the renin-angiotensin system. But there is greater reabsorption of water for maintenance of high blood pressure. This results in hyperconcentration of Gd contrast within urine on the ischemic side (Fig. 20a, b) [32].

Spin Dephasing on 3D Phase Contrast

On 3D phase contrast (3D PC) MRA with flow encoding in all three axes, image intensity corresponds to how fast the blood is flowing. Flowing

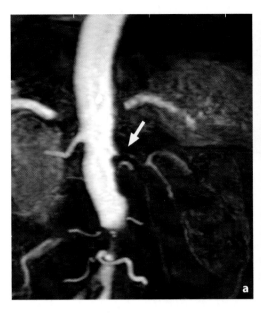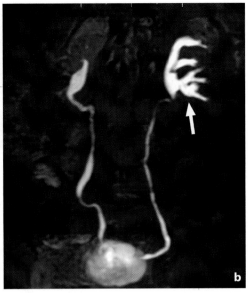

Fig. 20a, b. Hyper-concentration of urine (*arrow* in **b**) due to ipsilateral severe renal artery stenosis (*arrow* in **a**)

blood is bright while stationary tissues are dark. With mild stenoses, flow accelerates and creates a blooming effect, making the stenosis appear less severe (Fig. 19); when a stenosis reaches critical severity (> 70% narrowing), flow accelerated through the tight stenosis becomes disorganized, separated, swirling and turbulent. This chaotic, accelerated flow occurs when there is a pressure gradient [33]. Flow jets created by pressure gradients also dephase and destroy MR phase coherence causing loss of MR signal (Fig. 19). This dephasing is especially prominent on 3D PC MRA due to the relatively long echo times and the motion of protons during the application of flow-encoding gradients. On 3D PC images, the underestimation of mild stenoses and overestimation of severe stenoses (with pressure gradients) was formerly considered a disadvantage of flow sensitive MRA. However, by facilitating differentiation of unimportant mild stenoses from hemodynamically significant stenoses it can also be considered an advantage. An in-vitro study [33] shows that the degree of this spin dephasing is directly correlated with the trans-stenotic pressure gradient. This raises the exciting possibility of using the information on spin dephasing to estimate pressure gradients. More dephasing indicates a more significant stenosis. Combining 3D CE MRA information with 3D PC MRA offers more accurate grading of renal artery stenosis and facilitates clinical decision-making (Table 3).

Renal Artery Flow Measurement on 2D Cine Phase Contrast Sequence

Cine PC can non-invasively measure renal artery blood flow. A 2D cine PC sequence can also be performed after gadolinium-enhanced MRA to take advantage of the increased SNR provided by paramagnetic contrast agents [34]. Using cardiac gating and breath-holding, cine phase contrast offers both high spatial and temporal resolution [35]. Flow volume data per unit time as well as a velocity-time curve for a region of interest can be derived from phase contrast images (Fig. 21). The re-

Table 3. General guide for grading renal artery stenoses

Grade	3D Gd MRA	3D PC MRA	Recommendation
Normal	Normal	Normal	Leave alone, medication
Mild stenosis	Stenosis	Normal	Leave alone, medication
Moderate stenosis	Stenosis	+/- dephasing	DSA + pressure measurement
Severe stenosis	Stenosis	+ dephasing	Angioplasty
Occluded	occlusion	Occlusion	Surgery or Medicine

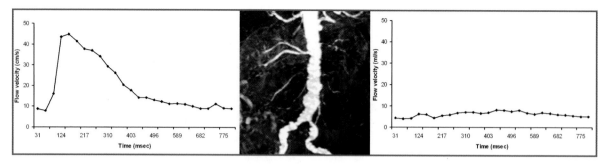

Fig. 21. Flow measurement with 2D cine phase contrast obtained post gadolinium. Note the difference between the flow profile of the normal right and high grade stenotic left renal artery

sults from this technique show high accuracy and excellent correlation with flow measurements in animal models and indirect techniques such as clearance of p-aminohippurate [36] and ^{133}Xenon washout measurements [37]. On PC-flow curves, the characteristic changes of significant renal artery stenosis include delay and sometimes complete loss of the early systolic peak with reduction in renal capillary resistance [38]. A renal flow index less than 1.5 ml/min/cm^3 predicts successful outcome of revasculization [30].

Combining cine PC data with MR angiography reduces interobserver variability on stenosis grading [38]. Cine PC may be useful for follow-up of patients with metallic stents. Although susceptibility artifacts from the stent may impair assessment of vessel patency on traditional CE MRA, cine PC detection of decreased flow beyond the stent may help to detect stenosis within the stent [39]. Cine PC renal blood flow measurements obtained before and after pharmacologic intervention provides even more physiological data. For example, an ACE inhibitor will dramatically reduce flow to the ischemic kidney but has only a minor and symmetrical effect when stenoses are not hemodynamically significant [4]. However, different studies have reported controversial results in evaluating the significance of ACE inhibitors [40]. Fur-

ther experiments are needed to clarify their usefulness and accuracy.

Corticomedullary Differentiation

On T1-weighted images, the renal cortex is brighter than the medulla. Loss of corticomedullary differentiation (CMD) on unenhanced T1-weighted images is a nonspecific marker of renal dysfunction. Although this can occur with any renal disease, it is expected in ischemic nephropathy. Following gadolinium injection, reduction of CMD (Fig. 19) also results from the decreased blood flow that is more pronounced in cortex than medulla [41].

Time-resolved Cortical and Medullary Enhancement

Whereas contrast arrival time at the cortex is similar for normal and ischemic kidneys, the transit time from cortex to medulla is much longer (40 seconds vs 15 seconds) for kidneys with renal vascular disease and decreased function [42]. Thus, medullary enhancement in ischemic kidneys is characteristically delayed and decreased compared to normal kidneys. Recently Lee et al. reported us-

Table 4. Sensitivity and specificity of contrast-enhanced renal MRA for assessing transplant renal arteries

Technique	Author	Year	# Patients	Sensitivity (%)	Specificity (%)
TOF	Gedroyc [86]	1992	50	83	97
3D TOF	Smith [6]	1993	34	100	95
3D Gd	Johnson [87]	1997	11	67	88
3D PC				60	76
2D TOF				47	81
3D Gd + PC				100	100
3D Gd	Luk [88]	1999	9		100
3D Gd	Ferrieros [89]	1999	24	100	98
3D Gd	Chan [90]	2001	17	100	75
3D Gd	Huber [91]	2001	41	100	100

ing MR renography with low dose Gd contrast (2 mL) to assess contrast enhancement of renal cortex and medulla [43]. After an initial vascular phase (20 seconds), dysfunctional kidneys demonstrate markedly less medullary enhancement during the tubular phase (1 to 4 minutes), reflecting diminished glomerular filtration.

Gadolinium Clearance Rate

Animal experiments have shown a statistically significant decrease of Gd extraction fraction in kidneys with renal artery stenosis [44]. Combining renal artery flow measurements with an additional pulse sequence to measure Gd concentration in the renal artery (input) and renal vein (output) permits exact calculation of the gadolinium clearance rate for each kidney [45]. Since gadolinium is filtered but not excreted or reabsorbed, this corresponds directly with creatinine clearance.

Diffusion-weighted MR Imaging

Diffusion-weighted imaging is feasible for assessment of vascular related renal dysfunction. Larger B factors are necessary to eliminate the confounding influences of glomerular filtration, tubular reabsorption, tubular secretion and urine flow on the apparent diffusion coefficient (ADC) [46]. The cortex of ischemic kidneys shows lower ADC values than that of the contralateral ones because significantly reduced blood flow may have more physiological impact on cortex than medulla. In acute or chronic renal failure caused by other factors, both cortex and medulla show reduced ADC values [47].

Renovascular vs Parenchymal Renal Disease: Quantitative Perfusion Imaging

Renal artery stenosis comprises only one entity in a large complex of overlapping diseases that ranges from essential hypertension to primary parenchymal disease. A high incidence of coexisting renoparenchymal disease explains why many patients do not improve after revascularization. Parenchymal disease is a result of both primary causes such as diabetes or glomerulonephritis as well as secondary causes resulting from long standing renal artery stenosis. Recently, the possibility to perform quantitative perfusion measurements of the kidney in patients with renal artery stenosis has provided a means to acquire an independent measure of parenchymal blood flow in the renal cortex as well as the medulla [48]. Absolute quantification of parenchymal blood

flow is possible with intravascular contrast agents using T2* based MR techniques. Faster MR techniques such as dynamic saturation recovery perfusion imaging allow semiquantitative assessment of renoparenchymal perfusion, which can be integrated into a comprehensive MR exam to differentiate renovascular from renoparenchymal disease.

Future Trends

MRA resolution continues to improve with the use of faster gradients and parallel imaging techniques (Fig. 22). However, a really exciting area of development involves the contribution of functional information to enable more comprehensive assessments of renal physiology in individual patients and individual kidneys. MR spectroscopy, quantitative perfusion imaging and oxygen saturation may add information to help answer the question of which patients with renal artery stenosis will benefit from renal revascularization. MR spectroscopy takes advantage of the unique spin resonance of common organic molecules to determine their relative concentration in tissue. It can be applied to hydrogen protons as well as to isotopes of sodium, phosphorus, carbon and a host of other atoms. Blood oxygen saturation determinations based upon T2 shifts in whole blood which corre-

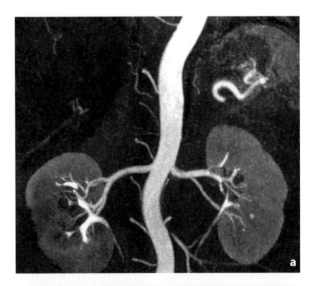
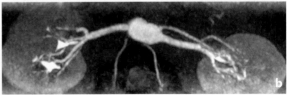

Fig. 22a, b. High resolution MRA using GRAPPA (Gd-BOPTA, 0.1 mmol/kg)

spond to the hemoglobin oxidation status may also be useful. Ischemic organs tend to extract more oxygen which results in decreased oxygen saturation in the venous blood coming from the organ. However, these and all of the other functional methods require further study to determine their relative importance for predicting hemodynamically significant stenosis and the potential benefit of revasculization.

References

1. Coen G, Calabria S, Lai S et al (2003) Atherosclerotic ischemic renal disease. Diagnosis and prevalence in a hypertensive and/or uremic elderly population. BMC Nephrol 4:2
2. Nelemans PJ, Kessels AG, De Leeuw P et al (1998) The cost-effectiveness of the diagnosis of renal artery stenosis. Eur J Radiol 27:95-107
3. Qanadli SD, Soulez G, Therasse E et al (2001)Detection of renal artery stenosis: prospective comparison of captopril-enhanced Doppler sonography, captopril-enhanced scintigraphy, and MR angiography. AJR Am J Roentgenol 177:1123-1129
4. Soulez G, Oliva VL, Turpin S et al (2000) Imaging of renovascular hypertension: respective values of renal scintigraphy, renal Doppler US, and MR angiography. Radiographics 20:1355-1368
5. Wikstrom J, Holmberg A, Johansson L et al (2000) Gadolinium-enhanced magnetic resonance angiography, digital subtraction angiography and duplex of the iliac arteries compared with intra-arterial pressure gradient measurements. Eur J Endovasc Surg 19:516-523
6. Smith HJ, Bakke SJ (1993) MR angiography of in situ and transplanted renal arteries. Early experience using a three-dimensional time-of-flight technique. Acta Radiol 34:150-155
7. Tello R, Mitchell PJ, Witte DJ et al (2003) T2 dark blood MRA for renal artery stenosis detection: preliminary observations. Comput Med Imaging Graph 27:11-16
8. Spuentrup E, Manning WJ, Bornert P et al (2002) Renal arteries: navigator-gated balanced fast field-echo projection MR angiography with aortic spin labeling: initial experience. Radiology 225:589-596
9. van den Brink JS, Watanabe Y, Kuhl CK et al (2003) Implications of SENSE MR in routine clinical practice. Eur J Radiol 46:3-27
10. Vasbinder GB, Maki JH, Nijenhuis RJ et al (2002) Motion of the distal renal artery during three-dimensional contrast-enhanced breath-hold MRA. J Magn Reson Imaging 16:685-696
11. Kroencke TJ, Wasser MN, Pattynama PM et al (2002) Gadobenate dimeglumine-enhanced MR angiography of the abdominal aorta and renal arteries. AJR Am J Roentgenol 179:1573-1582
12. Knopp MV, Schoenberg SO, Rehm C et al (2002)Assessment of gadobenate dimeglumine for magnetic resonance angiography: phase I studies. Invest Radiol 37:706-715
13. Prokop M, Schneider G, Vanzulli A et al. Contrast-enhanced MR angiography of the renal arteries: blinded multicenter crossover comparison of 0.1 mmol/kg gadobenate dimeglumine (Gd-BOPTA) and 0.2 mmol/kg gadopentetate dimeglumine (Gd-DTPA). Radiology In press
14. Krause UJ, Pabst T, Kostler H et al (2002) Time-resolved MR angiography of the renal artery: morphology and perfusion. Rofo Fortschr Geb Rontgenstr Neuen Bildgeb Verfahr 174:1170-1174
15. Mittal TK, Evans C, Perkins T et al (2001) Renal arteriography using gadolinium enhanced 3D MR angiography-clinical experience with the technique, its limitations and pitfalls. Br J Radiol 74:495-502
16. Surowiec SM, Sivamurthy N, Rhodes JM et al (2003) Percutaneous Therapy for Renal Artery Fibromuscular Dysplasia. Ann Vasc Surg in press
17. Takebayashi S, Ohno T, Tanaka K et al (1994) MR angiography of renal vascular malformations. J Comput Assist Tomogr 18:596-600
18. Bakker J, Ligtenberg G, Beek FJ et al (1999) Preoperative evaluation of living renal donors with gadolinium-enhanced magnetic resonance angiography. Transplantation 67:1167-1172
19. Fink C, Hallscheidt PJ, Hosch WP et al (2003) Preoperative evaluation of living renal donors: value of contrast-enhanced 3D magnetic resonance angiography and comparison of three rendering algorithms. Eur Radiol; 13:794-801
20. Halpern EJ, Mitchell DG, Wechsler RJ et al (2000) Preoperative evaluation of living renal donors: comparison of CT angiography and MR angiography. Radiology 216:434-439
21. Liem YS, Kock MC, Ijzermans JN et al (2003) Living renal donors: optimizing the imaging strategy–decision- and cost-effectiveness analysis. Radiology 226:53-62
22. Rankin SC, Jan W, Koffman CG (2001) Noninvasive imaging of living related kidney donors: evaluation with CT angiography and gadolinium-enhanced MR angiography. AJR Am J Roentgenol 177:349-355
23. Hussain SM, Kock MC, IJzermans JN et al (2003) MR imaging: a "one-stop shop" modality for preoperative evaluation of potential living kidney donors. Radiographics 23:505-520
24. Giessing M, Kroencke TJ, Taupitz M et al (2003) Gadolinium-enhanced three-dimensional magnetic resonance angiography versus conventional digital subtraction angiography: which modality is superior in evaluating living kidney donors. Transplantation 76:1000-1002
25. Glifeather M, Yoon HC, Siegelman ES et al (1999) Renal artery stenosis: evaluation with conventional angiography versus Gadolinium-enhanced MR angiography. Radiology 210:367-372
26. Omary RA, Baden JG, Becker BN et al (2000) Impact of MR angiography on the diagnosis and management of renal transplant dysfunction. J Vasc Interv Radiol 11:991-996
27. Sharafuddin MJ, Stolpen AH, Dixon BS (2002)Value of MR angiography before percutaneous transluminal renal artery angioplasty and stent placement. J Vasc Interv Radiol 13:901-908
28. Vasbinder GB, Nelemans PJ, Kessels AG et al (2001) Diagnostic tests for renal artery stenosis in patients suspected of having renovascular hypertension: a meta-analysis. Ann Intern Med 135:401-411
29. Dong Q, Schoenberg SO, Carlos RC et al (1999) Diagnosis of renal vascular disease with MR angiography. RadioGraphics 19:1535-1554

30. Binkert CA, Debatin JF, Schneider E et al (2001) Can MR measurement of renal artery flow and renal volume predict the outcome of percutaneous transluminal renal angioplasty. Cardiovasc Intervent Radiol 24:233-239

31. Prince MR, Schoenberg SO, Ward JS et al (1997) Hemodynamically significant atherosclerotic renal artery stenosis: MR angiographic features. Radiology 205:128-136

32. Walsh P, Rofsky NM, Krinsky GA et al (1996) Asymmetric signal intensity of the renal collecting systems as a sign of unilateral renal artery stenosis following administration of gadopentetate dimeglumine. J Comput Assist Tomogr 20:812-814

33. Mustert BR, Williams DM, Prince MR (1998) In vitro model of arterial stenosis: correlation of MR signal dephasing and trans-stenotic pressure gradients. Magn Reson Imaging 16:301-310

34. Prince MR, Grist TM, Debatin JF (2003) 3D contrast MR angiography: Springer

35. Schoenberg SO, Essig M, Bock M et al (1999) Comprehensive MR evaluation of renovascular disease in five breath holds. J Magn Reson Imaging 10:347-356

36. Schoenberg SO, Knopp MV, Bock M et al (1997) Renal artery stenosis: grading of hemodynamic changes with cine phase-contrast MR blood flow measurements. Radiology 203:45-53

37. de Haan MW, van Engelshoven JM, Houben AJ et al (2003) Phase-contrast magnetic resonance flow quantification in renal arteries: comparison with 133Xenon washout measurements. Hypertension 41:114-118

38. Schoenberg SO, Knopp MV, Londy F et al (2002) Morphologic and functional magnetic resonance imaging of renal artery stenosis: a multireader tricenter study. J Am Soc Nephrol 13:158-169

39. Shetty AN, Bis KG, Kirsch M et al (2000) Contrast-enhanced breath-hold three-dimensional magnetic resonance angiography in the evaluation of renal arteries: optimization of technique and pitfalls. J Magn Reson Imaging 12:912-923

40. Lee VS, Rofsky NM, Ton AT et al (2000) Angiotensin-converting enzyme inhibitor-enhanced phase-contrast MR imaging to measure renal artery velocity waveforms in patients with suspected renovascular hypertension. AJR Am J Roentgenol 174:499-508

41. Chung JJ, Semelka RC, Martin DR (2001) Acute renal failure: common occurrence of preservation of corticomedullary differentiation on MR images. Magn Reson Imaging 19:789-793

42. Ros PR, Gauger J, Stoupis C et al (1995) Diagnosis of renal artery stenosis: feasibility of combining MR angiography, MR renography, and Gadopentetate-based measurement of glomerular filtration rate. AJR Am J Roentgenol 165:1447-1451

43. Lee VS, Rusnek H, Johnson G et l (2001) MR renography with low-dose Gadopentetate Dimeglumine: feasibility. Radiology 221:371-379

44. Coulam CH, Lee JH, Wedding KL et al (2002) Noninvasive measurement of extraction fraction and single-kidney glomerular filtration rate with MR imaging in swine with surgically created renal arterial stenoses. Radiology 223:76-82

45. Niendorf ER, Grist TM, Lee FT et al (1998) Rapid in vivo measurement of single-kidney extraction fraction and glomerular filtration rate with MR imaging. Radiology 206:791-798

46. Namimoto T, Yamashita Y, Mitsuzaki K et al (1999) Measurement of the apparent diffusion coefficient in diffuse renal disease by diffusion-weighted echo-planar MR imaging. J Magn Reson Imaging 9:832-837

47. Toyoshima S, Noguchi K, Seto H et al (2000) Functional evaluation of hydronephrosis by diffusion-weighted MR imaging: relationship between apparent diffusion coefficient and split glomerular filtration rate. Acta Radiol 41:642-646

48. Schoenberg SO, Aumann S, Just A et al (2003) Quantification of renal perfusion abnormalities using an intravascular contrast agent (Part 2): results in animals and patients with renal artery stenosis. Magn Reson Med

49. Kent KC, Edelman RR, Kim D et al (1991) Magnetic resonance imaging: a reliable test for the evaluation of proximal atherosclerotic renal arterial stenosis. J Vasc Surg 13:311-318

50. Debatin JF, Spritzer CE, Grist TM et al (1991) Imaging of the renal arteries: value of MR angiography. AJR Am J Roentgenol 157:981-990

51. Servois V, Laissy JP, Feger C et al (1994) Two-dimensional time-of-flight magnetic resonance angiography of renal arteries without maximum intensity projection: a prospective comparison with angiography in 21 patients screened for renovascular hypertension. Cardiovasc Intervent Radiol 17:138-142

52. Hertz SM, Holland GA, Baum RA et al (1994) Evaluation of renal artery stenosis by magnetic resonance angiography. Am J Surg 168:140-143

53. Loubeyre P, Revel D, Garcia P et al (1994) Screening patients for renal artery stenosis: value of three-dimensional time-of-flight MR angiography. AJR Am J Roentgenol 162:847-852

54. Nelson HA, Gilfeather M, Holman JM et al (1999) Gadolinium-enhanced breathhold three-dimensional time-of-flight renal MR angiography in the evaluation of potential renal donors. J Vasc Interv Radiol 10:175-181

55. De Cobelli F, Mellone R, Salvioni M et al (1996) Renal artery stenosis: value of screening with three-dimensional phase-contrast MR angiography with a phased-array multicoil. Radiology 201:697-703

56. Silverman JM, Friedman ML, Van Allan RJ (1996) Detection of main renal artery stenosis using phase-contrast cine MR angiography. AJR Am J Roentgenol 166:1131-1137

57. de Haan MW, Kouwenhoven M, Thelissen RP et al (1996) Renovascular disease in patients with hypertension: detection with systolic and diastolic gating in three-dimensional, phase-contrast MR angiography. Radiology 198:449-456

58. Miller S, Hahn U, Schick F et al (1999) [Diagnosis of renal artery stenosis in 1.0 T using 3D phase contrast magnetic resonance angiography and dynamic contrast medium perfusion]. Rofo Fortschr Geb Rontgenstr Neuen Bildgeb Verfahr 170:163-167

59. Westenberg JJ, van der Geest RJ, Wasser MN et al (1999) Stenosis quantification from post-stenotic signal loss in phase-contrast MRA datasets of flow phantoms and renal arteries. Int J Card Imaging 15:483-493

60. Prince MR, Narasimham DL, Stanley JC et al (1995)

Breath-hold gadolinium-enhanced MR angiography of the abdominal aorta and its major branches. Radiology 197:785-792

61. Grist TM, Swan JS, Korosec FR (1996) Investigators refine MR angio methods. Diagn Imaging (San Franc) 18:45-50

62. Snidow JJ, Johnson MS, Harris VJ et al (1996) Three-dimensional gadolinium-enhanced MR angiography for aortoiliac inflow assessment plus renal artery screening in a single breath hold. Radiology 198:725-732

63. Holland GA, Dougherty L, Carpenter JP et al (1996) Breath-hold ultrafast three-dimensional gadolinium-enhanced MR angiography of the aorta and the renal and other visceral abdominal arteries. AJR Am J Roentgenol 166:971-981

64. Steffens JC, Link J, Grassner J et al (1997) Contrast-enhanced, K-space-centered, breath-hold MR angiography of the renal arteries and the abdominal aorta. J Magn Reson Imaging 7:617-622

65. Rieumont MJ, Kaufman JA, Geller SC et al (1997) Evaluation of renal artery stenosis with dynamic gadolinium-enhanced MR angiography. AJR Am J Roentgenol 169:39-44

66. De Cobelli F, Vanzulli A, Sironi S et al (1997) Renal artery stenosis: evaluation with breath-hold, three-dimensional, dynamic, gadolinium-enhanced versus three-dimensional, phase-contrast MR angiography. Radiology 205:689-695

67. Bakker J, Beek FJ, Beutler JJ et al (1998) Renal artery stenosis and accessory renal arteries: accuracy of detection and visualization with gadolinium-enhanced breath-hold MR angiography. Radiology 207:497-504

68. Hany TF, Leung DA, Pfammatter T et al (1998) Contrast-enhanced magnetic resonance angiography of the renal arteries. Original investigation. Invest Radiol 33:653-659

69. Thornton J, O'Callaghan J, Walshe J et al (1999) Comparison of digital subtraction angiography with gadolinium-enhanced magnetic resonance angiography in the diagnosis of renal artery stenosis. Eur Radiol 9:930-934

70. Schoenberg SO, Bock M, Knopp MV et al (1999) Renal arteries: optimization of three-dimensional gadolinium-enhanced MR angiography with bolus-timing-independent fast multiphase acquisition in a single breath hold. Radiology 211:667-679

71. Thornton MJ, Thornton F, O'Callaghan J et al (1999) Evaluation of dynamic gadolinium-enhanced breath-hold MR angiography in the diagnosis of renal artery stenosis. AJR Am J Roentgenol 173:1279-1283

72. Cambria RP, Kaufman JL, Brewster DC et al (1999) Surgical renal artery reconstruction without contrast arteriography: the role of clinical profiling and magnetic resonance angiography. J Vasc Surg 29:1012-1021

73. Ghantous VE, Eisen TD, Sherman AH et al (1999) Evaluating patients with renal failure for renal artery stenosis with gadolinium-enhanced magnetic resonance angiography. Am J Kidney Dis 33:36-42

74. Marchand B, Hernandez-Hoyos M, Orkisz M et al (2000) [Diagnosis of renal artery stenosis with magnetic resonance angiography and stenosis quantification]. J Mal Vasc 25:312-320

75. Winterer JT, Strey C, Wolffram C et al (2000) [Preoperative examination of potential kidney transplantation donors: value of gadolinium-enhanced 3D MR angiography in comparison with DSA and urography]. Rofo Fortschr Geb Rontgenstr Neuen Bildgeb Verfahr 172:449-457

76. Weishaupt D, Ruhm SG, Binkert CA et al (2000) Equilibrium-phase MR angiography of the aortoiliac and renal arteries using a blood pool contrast agent. AJR Am J Roentgenol 175:189-195

77. Bongers V, Bakker J, Beutler JJ et al (2000) Assessment of renal artery stenosis: comparison of captopril renography and gadolinium-enhanced breath-hold MR angiography. Clin Radiol 55:346-353

78. Volk M, Strotzer M, Lenhart M et al (2000) Time-resolved contrast-enhanced MR angiography of renal artery stenosis: diagnostic accuracy and interobserver variability. AJR Am J Roentgenol 174:1583-1588

79. Oberholzer K, Kreitner KF, Kalden P et al (2000) [Contrast-enhanced MR angiography of abdominal vessels using a 1.0 T system]. Rofo Fortschr Geb Rontgenstr Neuen Bildgeb Verfahr 172:134-138

80. Korst MB, Joosten FB, Postma CT et al (2000) Accuracy of normal-dose contrast-enhanced MR angiography in assessing renal artery stenosis and accessory renal arteries. AJR Am J Roentgenol 174:629-634

81. De Cobelli F, Venturini M, Vanzulli A et al (2000) Renal arterial stenosis: prospective comparison of color Doppler US and breath-hold, three-dimensional, dynamic, gadolinium-enhanced MR angiography. Radiology 214:373-380

82. Voiculescu A, Hofer M, Hetzel GR et al (2001) Noninvasive investigation for renal artery stenosis: contrast-enhanced magnetic resonance angiography and color Doppler sonography as compared to digital subtraction angiography. Clin Exp Hypertens 23:521-531

83. Hood MN, Ho VB, Corse WR (2002) Three-dimensional phase-contrast magnetic resonance angiography: a useful clinical adjunct to gadolinium-enhanced three-dimensional renal magnetic resonance angiography. Mil Med 167:343-349

84. Willmann JK, Wildermuth S, Pfammatter T et al (2003) Aortoiliac and renal arteries: prospective intraindividual comparison of contrast-enhanced three-dimensional MR angiography and multi-detector row CT angiography. Radiology 226:798-811

85. Coenegrachts KL, Hoogeveen RM, Vaninbroukx JA et al (2004) High-spatial-resolution 3D balanced turbo field-echo technique for MR angiography of the renal arteries: initial experience. Radiology 231:237-242

86. Gedroyc WM, Negus R, al-Kutoubi A et al (1992) Magnetic resonance angiography of renal transplants. Lancet 339:789-791

87. Johnson DB, Lerner CA, Prince MR et al (1997) Gadolinium-enhanced magnetic resonance angiography of renal transplants. Magn Reson Imaging 15:13-20

88. Luk SH, Chan JH, Kwan TH et al (1999) Breath-hold 3D gadolinium-enhanced subtraction MRA in the detection of transplant renal artery stenosis. Clin Radiol 54:651-654

89. Ferreiros J, Mendez R, Jorquera M et al (1999) Using gadolinium-enhanced three-dimensional MR an-

giography to assess arterial inflow stenosis after kidney transplantation. AJR Am J Roentgenol 172:751-757

90. Chan YL, Leung CB, Yu SC et al (2001) Comparison of non-breath-hold high resolution gadolinium-enhanced MRA with digital subtraction angiography in the evaluation on allograft renal artery stenosis. Clin Radiol 56:127-132

91. Huber A, Heuck A, Scheidler J et al (2001) Contrast-enhanced MR angiography in patients after kidney transplantation. Eur Radiol 11:2488-2405

VI.3

MR Angiography of the Mesenteric Arteries

Mathias Goyen

Introduction

MR-based imaging has been used for the assessment of the mesenteric vasculature since the early 1990s; the resolution of 3D contrast MR angiography in its most recent implementation is sufficient to accurately evaluate the origins of the splanchnic arteries, including the celiac artery (CA) and superior mesenteric artery (SMA).

Normal Anatomy

The blood supply to the intestinal tract is derived from the three major anterior branches of the abdominal aorta: the celiac artery (celiac trunk), the superior mesenteric artery (SMA), and the inferior mesenteric artery (IMA) (Figs. 1, 2). However, a multitude of variants exist (see Fig. 10). Contrast-enhanced 3D MRA (CE-MRA) allows the detailed assessment of the normal and abnormal vascular anatomy in the majority of cases [1-4].

Celiac Artery

The CA arises from the ventral surface of the aorta at the T12-L11 interspace (Fig. 1a). It supplies the upper abdominal viscera. In 65% of patients, the celiac artery classically branches into three major vessels: the splenic artery, common hepatic artery, and left gastric artery. In 35% of patients, the branching pattern of the celiac artery is variable. The splenic, common hepatic, or left gastric artery may arise directly from the aorta or from the superior mesenteric artery. The proper hepatic artery typically divides into the left and right hepatic artery. This branching pattern is present in 50% of all individuals. The remaining 50% have replaced or accessory hepatic arterial branches. The gastroduodenal artery arises from the common hepatic artery in approximately 75% of patients and usually has two main branches: the superior pancreaticoduodenal artery and the right gastroepiploic artery. The superior pancreaticoduodenal artery forms an anastomotic arcade with the inferior pancreaticoduodenal artery.

Superior Mesenteric Artery

The SMA arises from the ventral aspect of the aorta approximately 1 cm below the origin of the CA (Fig. 1b). Rarely, a single celio-mesenteric trunk arises directly from the aorta. The inferior pancreaticoduodenal artery typically is the first branch of the SMA. The jejunal and ileal artery branches usually originate from the left side of the superior mesenteric artery. A distinguishing feature of the jejunal and ileal branches is the presence of arcades, which anastomose with adjacent branches. The most distal arcades run along the mesenteric border of the bowel and give off the straight vasa rectae, which reach the antimesenteric border [5-7]. The middle colic artery, the right colic artery, and the ileocolic artery are not visualized routinely with MRA.

Inferior Mesenteric Artery

The inferior mesenteric artery (IMA) (Fig. 1c) arises from the ventral aspect of the aorta approximately at the level of the L3 vertebral body and measures between 1.2 and 5.5 mm in diameter at its origin. This makes it difficult to image consistently with MRA [6]. The first branch of the IMA is typically an ascending branch, which represents the left colic artery. The inferior mesenteric artery then gives off the sigmoid branches. More distally, the IMA becomes the superior rectal artery.

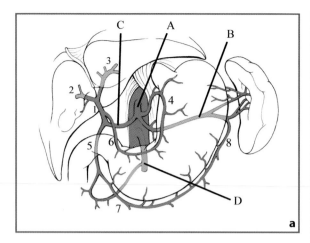

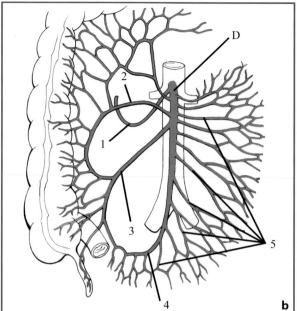

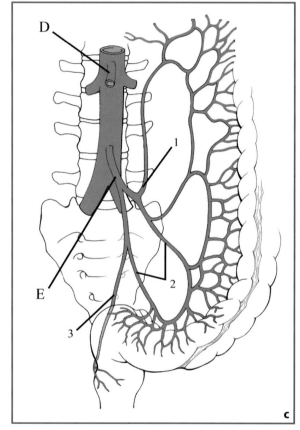

Fig. 1a-c. Normal anatomy of the mesenteric arteries

a Celiac trunk
A Celiac artery (CA)
B Splenic artery
C Common hepatic artery
D Superior mesenteric artery (SMA)

1 Proper hepatic artery
2 Right hepatic artery
3 Left hepatic artery
4 Left gastric artery
5 Gastroduodenal artery
6 Right gastric artery
7 Right gastroepiploic artery
8 Left gastroepiploic artery

b Superior mesenteric artery
D Superior mesenteric artery (SMA)

1 Gastroduodenal artery
2 Medial colic artery
3 Right colic artery
4 Iliocolic artery
5 Jejunal- and ilieal arteries

c Inferior mesenteric artery
D Superior mesenteric artery (SMA)
E Inferior mesenteric artery (IMA)

1 Left colic artery
2 Sigmoid arteries
3 Superior rectal artery

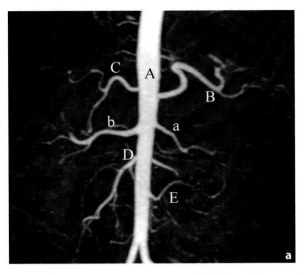 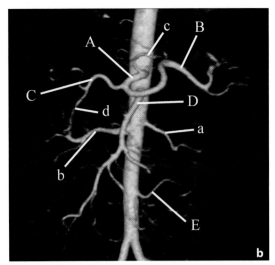

Fig. 2a, b. MIP (**a**) and volume rendered (**b**) displays of a 3D CE MRA data set acquired in the early arterial phase demonstrate the arterial vascular anatomy in the abdomen. Beyond the aorta and both renal arteries, branches of the celiac trunk and the superior mesenteric artery are well depicted [Images courtesy of Dr. G. Schneider]

A Celiac artery (CA)
B Splenic artery
C Common hepatic artery
D Superior mesenteric artery (SMA)
E Inferior mesenteric artery (IMA)
a Right renal artery
b Left renal artery
c Left gastric artery
d Gastroduodenal artery

MRA Techniques

Patient preparation for MRA is not as important as it is for catheter-based arteriography, computed tomography, and ultrasound in patients suspected of having chronic mesenteric ischemia. Patients do not need to fast prior to the MR examination. Glucagon (0.5 to 1 mg IV or IM) has been proposed as a means for reducing bowel motion and augmenting celiac flow. However, with a fast scanner capable of high resolution imaging during a breath-hold, arresting bowel motion is not necessary. A high caloric meal prior to the examination can transiently increase splanchnic flow, thereby enhancing visibility of the smaller branch vessels. Patients with chronic abdominal symptoms, suspected of acute mesenteric ischemia, should be considered surgical emergencies. MRA should only be performed in patients presenting with an acute abdomen under unusual circumstances and only if adequate monitoring is available. A surgeon should be nearby in the event that the patient rapidly decompensates and requires immediate surgical exploration.

Patients suspected of chronic mesenteric ischemia are often very thin, and thus well-suited to imaging with surface array coils, such as a body array or torso phased array coil. Large patients may be easier to image using the body coil. The pa-

tient is placed in the supine position. The arms may be in a comfortable position by the patient's side during the initial localizer sequence but will need to be elevated above the head for the 3D contrast-enhanced MRA acquisition in the coronal plane. Elevating the arms helps to minimize aliasing and ensures a downhill path for the gadolinium thereby maintaining a tight bolus [8].

Time-of-Flight MRA

Time-of-flight (TOF) MR techniques are not employed for evaluation of the mesenteric arteries for a number of reasons. Images have to be acquired orthogonal to flow, meaning that depiction of the ostia of both the celiac artery and SMA is prone to error because the flow within the aorta is at right angles to that in the proximal part of both vessels. This creates artifacts at the vessel origins where most of the pathology in patients with chronic mesenteric ischemia occurs. Due to the anatomic predisposition of the celiac artery and the SMA it is not possible to optimize a single TOF sequence for depiction of the two arteries. In addition, misregistration artifacts may arise in patients with limited breath-holding capabilities because of the need to acquire images during suspended respiration.

Phase-Contrast MRA

Phase-contrast (PC) MRA techniques can be used to assess the mesenteric vasculature using either 3D [9] or 2D approaches [10-13]. An advantage of the 3D-technique is that images can be acquired in any plane [9]. However, as scan times are long, this technique is prone to respiratory motion artifacts. In addition, ghost artifacts caused by diminished and reversed flow during systole, can hamper image quality. Although this latter limitation can be addressed by means of cardiac triggering, a further increase in scan time results and respiratory motion artifacts remain a problem.

Two-dimensional cardiac-gated PC MRA techniques have been implemented with the mesenteric vasculature to provide functional information [10-13]. This approach segments the phase data acquired at different points throughout the cardiac cycle to provide quantitative flow measurements including flow velocities and flow volume.

Contrast-Enhanced MRA

With the introduction of CE-MRA, it became feasible to generate high-quality images of the mesenteric vasculature [14-16]. Imaging in the coronal plane permits evaluation of the aorta, splanchnic arteries and portal vein in one examination. A partition thickness of 3 or 4 mm or even 5 mm is acceptable if zero padding is available for interpolation. In the absence of an interpolation algorithm, the slice thickness should be kept to less than 3 mm. To determine stenotic disease of the proximal mesenteric arteries, imaging in the sagittal plane is preferred. Aliasing is not as severe for scans in the sagittal plane, so it is possible to prescribe a rectangular field-of-view with a high spatial resolution acquisition matrix (e.g. 512 x 256). If using a slower MR system, it is advantageous to acquire in the sagittal plane so that fewer sections or partitions are required to cover the aorta, celiac SMA, and IMA. Generally, a short duration breath-hold scan performed in the sagittal plane is superior to a longer duration coronal acquisition which is hampered by respiratory motion. Imaging parameters should be adjusted to allow for a breath-held data acquisition. Axial imaging may be useful if the primary goal is evaluation of the hepatic arteries, hepatic parenchyma and portal vein (see chapter VI.4). One difficulty with the axial orientation is aliasing in the slice direction which tends to be severe with the extremely short RF pulses used in 3D CE-MRA. To minimize aliasing a coil whose S-I dimension is only slightly larger than the S-I dimension of the imaging volume should be used. Also fat saturation or chemically selective fat inversion pulses should be considered. These will help minimize unwanted signal from pericardial and abdominal fat wrapping onto the bottom and top of the image volume. A 3D CE-MRA image data set should be collected before, during, and after completion of the IV contrast administration. Precontrast images should be checked to ensure the imaging volume is positioned correctly. These images can also be used subsequently for digital subtraction to improve image contrast.

Proper gadolinium bolus timing is essential for arterial phase acquisitions. This is accomplished with automatic triggering (SmartPrep or Care Bolus) or fluoroscopic triggering (BolusTrack) or with a test bolus to the mid-abdominal aorta. After arterial phase imaging, a delayed image data set is useful for showing the portal venous and hepatic venous anatomy (see Chapter VI 4: Portal Venous System).

Arterial phase 3D CE-MRA is best evaluated by first acquiring multiple overlapping MIP reconstructions in the coronal plane. Subsequently, reformations and subvolume MIPs can be reconstructed in perpendicular planes through each major abdominal aortic branch vessel, including the celiac trunk, SMA and IMA. It is also useful to assess the iliac arteries, especially the internal iliac arteries, as they may represent an important collateral pathway in patients with chronic mesenteric ischemia.

Complementary Sequences

T1- and T2-weighted images covering the liver and upper abdomen may be acquired prior to contrast injection to search for other pathologies that might account for the patient's abdominal symptoms. The amount of abdominal intraperitoneal and subcutaneous fat can be assessed on these images. Most patients with mesenteric ischemia will have a scaphoid abdomen and less than 15 mm of subcutaneous fat over the rectus abdominis muscles.

3D CE-MRA permits a morphologic analysis of the mesenteric arteries. The high incidence of visceral artery stenosis in an asymptomatic population makes it difficult to determine the clinical significance of a morphologic finding. For patients with mesenteric artery stenosis or an equivocal history of mesenteric ischemia it may be difficult to predict whether correcting the mesenteric artery stenosis will alleviate symptoms. Functional MR imaging may complement 3D CE-MRA in this regard. A cine phase contrast sequence can be employed to assess blood flow in the superior mesenteric vein (SMV) following caloric stimulation. In patients with mesenteric ischemia the increased post-prandial blood-flow within the SMV is out of proportion to that in the SMA. This effect is due to recruitment of collateral flow. By exploiting the known paramagnetic effect of deoxyhemoglobin, Li et al showed close correlation between T2 measurements of blood in the SMV and oxygen saturation in an *in vivo* animal model [12]. Identifying low oxygen saturation in the SMV compared to the IVC suggests ischemia.

When the CA and SMA are patent, the possibility of branch vessel stenosis and regional ischemia can be assessed by looking at bowel wall enhancement (see below). Bowel mucosa normally enhances greatly immediately following gadolinium administration. Regional areas of diminished or delayed bowel enhancement are suggestive of regional ischemia. The combination of morphologic 3D CE MRA of the splanchnic vasculature with functional assessment of mesenteric flow holds considerable promise as the emerging modality of choice for evaluation of patients with suspected mesenteric ischemia.

Clinical Examples for Various Clinical Indications and Pathologies

3D CE MRA is capable of displaying the main visceral vessels with excellent diagnostic accuracy. However, the spatial resolution achievable with selective catheter angiography remains superior for

smaller branch vessels. Accordingly, current clinical applications of 3D CE MRA in the splanchnic circulation focus on clinical situations that require assessment of the proximal celiac axis and SMA. Typical pathologies are mesenteric ischemia, visceral artery aneurysms, tumor encasement, anatomic variations (see sub-chapter), and pre/post liver transplantation.

Mesenteric Ischemia

Selective angiography has been considered the gold standard for the diagnosis of chronic mesenteric ischemia [17]. The demonstration of significant stenoses in two of the three main mesenteric vessels in conjunction with appropriate clinical symptoms verifies the diagnosis of mesenteric ischemia [3] (Fig. 3). MRA has the potential to become a definitive noninvasive tool for the diagnosis of chronic mesenteric ischemia. It can provide information about patency and stenosis in mesenteric vessels and is becoming a modality of choice for the selection of patients suspected of having mesenteric ischemia who may benefit from surgery.

Chronic mesenteric ischemia generally occurs when there is insufficient blood supply to the intestine during periods of high metabolic demand, such as following a meal. It is most commonly caused by severe stenosis or occlusion of at least two of the three main splanchnic arteries. The clinical syndrome of mesenteric ischemia is rare. Symptoms may include abdominal pain, weight loss and food aversion [3,18-19]. Atherosclerosis of the splanchnic arteries is considered to be the main pathophysiologic mechanism for chronic mesenteric ischemia [1, 5]. However, the diagnosis of mesenteric ischemia is frequently perplexing in clinical practice. Reflecting the risks associated with arterial catheterization, the clinical diagnosis of mesenteric ischemia has been mostly one of exclusion. The median time-delay between clinical presentation and diagnosis is 18 months for patients with new symptoms and one month for patients with recurrent symptoms. Symptoms of mesenteric ischemia may overlap with those of more common intestinal disorders such as peptic ulcer or chronic cholecystitis. Recent advances in MR technology permit adequate assessment of the splanchnic arterial system [2,9,16, 20-21]. Hence, MRA in combination with flow quantification [10,12-13,22] or oximetry [23] has been proposed for the diagnosis of mesenteric ischemia. However, despite the availability of non-invasive MRA, a reliable diagnosis remains difficult in a high percentage of cases: atherosclerotic changes are often based on the level of arterioles and therefore cannot be captured by luminographic procedures

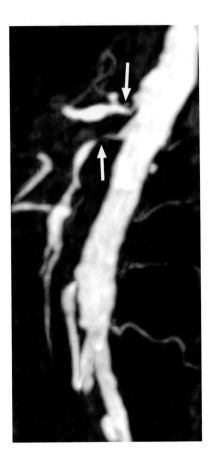

Fig. 3. MIP display of a 3D CE MRA data set acquired in the early arterial phase; the sagittal, reformatted view reveals stenoses (*arrows*) of the celiac trunk and SMA

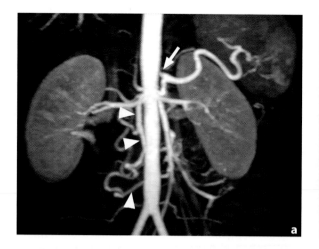
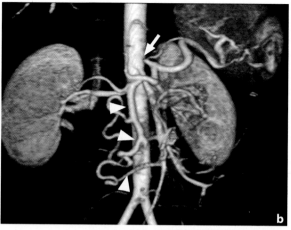

Fig. 4a, b. MIP (**a**) and volume rendered (**b**) displays of a 3D CE MRA data set (0.1 mmol/kg Gd-BOPTA) in the early arterial phase showing a high-grade stenosis of the celiac trunk (*arrow*). Collateral flow from the SMA via the gastroduodenal artery (*arrowheads*) is noted, indicated by the enlarged diameter of the gastroduodenal artery. In general, an enlarged, pronounced gastroduodenal artery on CE MRA images is almost pathognomonic for a stenosis of either the celiac trunk or the SMA [Images courtesy of Dr. G. Schneider]

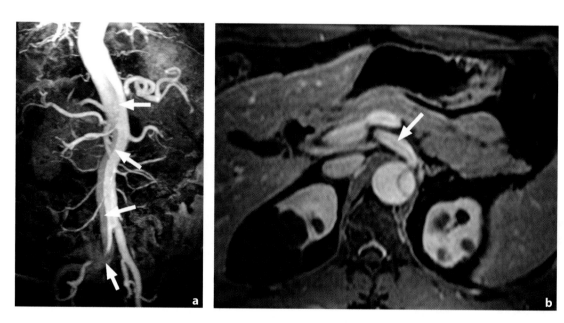

Fig. 5a, b. Patient with aortic dissection extending into the SMA. On the whole volume MIP (**a**) of the 3D CE MRA data set (0.1 mmol/kg Gd-BOPTA) the dissection membrane extending into the right iliac artery can be appreciated (*arrows*), however the involvement of the SMA is difficult to evaluate. Nevertheless extension of the dissection membrane into the SMA (*arrow*) can be appreciated with an additional VIBE sequence (**b**), performed immediately after the CE MRA study [Image courtesy of Dr. G. Schneider]

[24]. In addition, the mesenteric circulation is frequently supported by arterial collaterals. Therefore, completely asymptomatic patients can be seen even though severe stenotic changes are present in the main mesenteric vessels [25-26] (Fig. 4). A solution to this problem might be the evaluation of mesenteric ischemia using perfusion values of the small bowel wall before and after caloric stimulation (see below). Mesenteric ischemia may occur in conjunction with aortic dissection due to extension of the dissection membrane into a mesenteric artery. Typically, clinically relevant involvement is due to an extension of the dissection into the SMA (Fig. 5). Acute onset of symptoms due to mesenteric ischemia is found in conjunction with thromboembolic events, in which the lack of collaterals indicates an acute (Fig. 6) stage. In contrast, those cases in which a collateral supply is already visible are examples of a subacute stage (Fig. 7).

Finally, mesenteric ischemia may also be present in the context of inflammatory diseases, which can occur as part of a vascular inflammation syndrome such as Takayasu arteritis (Fig. 8).

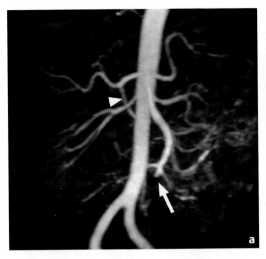
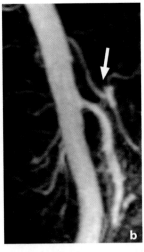

Fig. 6. A contrast enhanced MRA study (0.1 mmol/kg Gd-BOPTA) in a patient with left atrial thrombus formation and sudden onset of abdominal pain shows peripheral embolization of the SMA (*arrow* in **a**) and acute thromboembolic occlusion of the celiac artery (*arrow* in **b**). Note the absence of collateral vessels but a dilated gastroduodenal artery (*arrowhead* in **a**) [Image courtesy of Dr. G. Schneider]

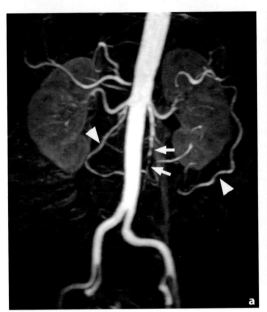
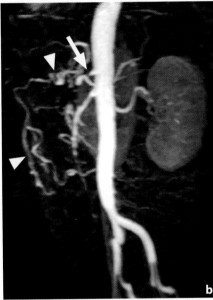

Fig. 7. MIP display of a 3D CE MRA data set (0.1 mmol/kg Gd-BOPTA) of the mesenteric arteries shows multiple wall irregularities of the SMA indicating recurrent thromboembolic events (*arrows* in **a**). Furthermore, occlusion of the celiac artery can be noted (*arrow* in **b**). In contrast to the case in Fig. 6 collateral vessels (*arrowheads*) have developed in this patient due to recurrent, subacute emboli [Image courtesy of Dr. G. Schneider]

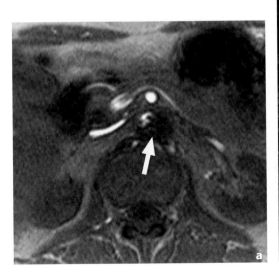
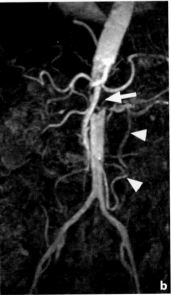

Fig. 8. Involvement of the mesenteric arteries in a patient with Takayasu arteritis. The True-FISP axial image (**a**) reveals an almost complete occlusion of the abdominal aorta (*arrow*). The high grade stenosis (*arrow*) is confirmed on a whole volume MIP reconstruction (**b**) of the 3D CE MRA data set (0.1 mmol/kg Gd-BOPTA). Additionally, the Arc of Riolan (*arrowheads*) is visible which on CE MRA images typically indicates stenosis either of the SMA or the IMA since it serves as a collateral between these vessels [Image courtesy of Dr. G. Schneider]

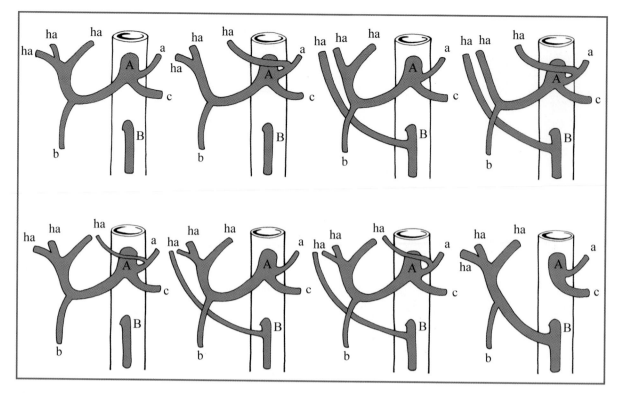

Fig. 9. Schematic representation of variants of the hepatic vasculature.

A   Celiac artery
B   Superior mesenteric artery
a   Left gastric artery
b   Gastroduodenal artery
c   Splenic artery
ha   Hepatic arteries

Aneurysms

Aneurysmal dilatation of the proximal celiac or SMA can occur in patients with aortic aneurysms. Abdominal aortic aneurysms (AAA) are more commonly associated with iliac, common femoral, and popliteal artery aneurysms. Isolated aneurysms can also involve the splenic, hepatic, gastro-duodenal, gastric, gastro-epiploic, and inferior mesenteric arteries. Splenic artery aneurysms are the most common, particularly in post-partum women or secondary to weakening of the splenic artery from pancreatitis. SMA aneurysms are often mycotic as a result of proximity to the small intestine. Aneurysmal dilatation of the celiac axis may occur secondary to post-stenotic dilatation related to either atherosclerotic narrowing of the origin or narrowing from extrinsic compression by the median arcuate ligament.

Tumor Encasement

Tumors may enhance rapidly during the arterial phase, or, if hypovascular, the tumor may blend in with surrounding tissues making it difficult to identify. Retroperitoneal masses, and particularly pancreatic adenocarcinoma, may surround, encase, and narrow or even occlude the splanchnic arteries and portal venous system. Masses arising in the head of the pancreas tend to encase the SMA, SMV, and portal vein. Lesions in the body and tail of the pancreas tend to narrow the splenic vein. The characteristic serrated lumen of arterial encasement seen with conventional angiography is generally not appreciated on MRA due to its lower resolution. Large masses may also displace the mesenteric arteries without encasement. For example, this displacement may occur with pancreatic pseudocyst, hematoma, or abscess.

Anatomic Variations / Pre and Post Liver Transplantation

Variations in the splanchnic arterial anatomy occur in more than 40% of patients (Fig. 9). For this reason, pre-operative vascular planning for hepatic resections, liver transplantations, resection of retroperitoneal masses, chemoinfusion pump

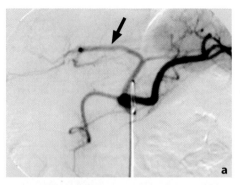
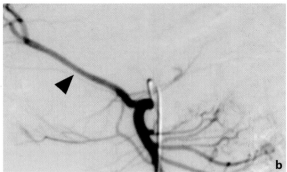
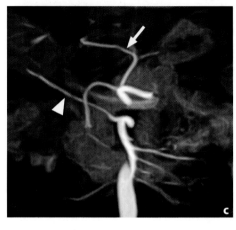

Fig. 10a-c. DSA (**a**, **b**) as well as the coronal MIP image (**c**) obtained from an arterial phase breath-hold FLASH 3D acquisition reveal a Michels class VIII hepatic arterial variant – the left hepatic artery arises from the left gastric artery (*arrows*) and the right hepatic artery arises from the superior mesenteric artery (*arrowheads*)

placement, surgical shunting, or other abdominal operations may require mapping of the visceral arterial anatomy. Generally, this is done by conventional angiography for the fine detail necessary to identify variations involving tiny arteries. To evaluate the splanchnic artery origins and major branches, 3D CE MRA is frequently sufficient. When patients are undergoing renal revascularization, it is important to know the splanchnic arterial anatomy in case a spleno-renal or hepato-renal bypass is needed to avoid clamping the aorta. The most common variation is a replaced (17%) or accessory (8%) right hepatic artery, most commonly from the SMA (Fig. 10). Less common variations include the left hepatic artery arising from the left gastric artery (Fig. 11), the common hepatic artery arising from the SMA (2.5%) or directly from the aorta (2%), the left gastric artery arising from the aorta (1%-2%), or a celiaco-mesenteric trunk (<1%). Other even more complex variations may also occur.

Gastrointestinal Bleeding

The development of blood pool MR contrast agents may make it possible to replicate the concept of labeled red cell nuclear medicine examinations using 3D CE MRA. Although MR blood pool agents are experimental, the higher SNR and resolution of MR compared to nuclear medicine makes this a promising future technique for use in patients suspected of gastrointestinal (GI) bleeding. Arterial and venous mesenteric anatomy can be evaluated during the arterial and venous phases of blood pool contrast agent injection. By periodically re-imaging the patient over time, the accumulation of blood in the GI tract can be imaged to identify the site of GI bleeding. Just as with labeled red cells, when bleeding is intermittent, the patient can be scanned periodically, every hour or two until a bleeding episode is detected. The 3D-nature of MR imaging makes it easier to identify the specific loop of bowel that is bleeding [27-28].

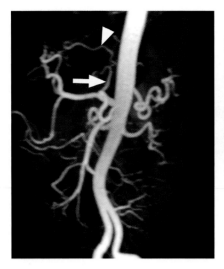 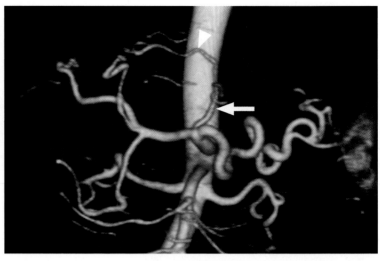

Fig. 11. Left hepatic artery (*arrowhead*) arising from the left gastric artery (*arrow*) on a CE MRA MIP reconstruction (**a**) and on a volume rendered image (**b**) (0.1 mmol/kg Gd-BOPTA). Note that the vessels are better appreciated on the volume rendered image [Image courtesy of Dr. G. Schneider]

Pitfalls and Limitations

Celiac Pseudostenosis

Extrinsic compression of the celiac axis by the median arcuate ligament can simulate a celiac axis stenosis. Often this has a characteristic appearance in which the celiac axis is pulled inferiorly. This extrinsic compression varies with respiration, and thus may appear more or less severe, depending on the patient's degree of inspiration or expiration. Although usually asymptomatic, there have been reports of relief of abdominal symptoms following surgical release of a severe extrinsic compression.

Motion Artifacts

Respiratory motion during the acquisition may obscure the SMA, particularly along its more distal intraperitoneal course. Respiratory motion may also compromise visualization of the hepatic and splenic arteries. When the 3D MRA data set is corrupted by respiratory motion it may be repeated during the equilibrium phase. Alternatively, a postcontrast 3D phase contrast MRA technique (VENC = 40-50 cm/s) can provide diagnostic evaluation of the celiac and SMA origins.

Surgical Clip Artifacts

Surgical clips in the region of interest (such as those used for cholecystectomy) can cause signal voids resulting in hampered or non-diagnostic im-

age quality of the neighboring vessels. To verify the presence of a clip, analysis of the source images for metallic susceptibility artifacts is most helpful. Clips can usually be recognized by their characteristic dark-bright appearance on MR images. If in doubt, it is helpful to perform a plain film of the abdomen to confirm the presence of surgical clips. Clip artifacts can be minimized by using the widest possible bandwidth to obtain the shortest possible echo time.

Limited Spatial Resolution

Small emboli in the distal splanchnic arterial branches cannot be excluded by 3D CE MRA due to insufficient spatial resolution, i.e. mesenteric ischemia cannot be absolutely excluded. An infarction of a limited part of the bowel can be caused by a small embolus which remains undetected on the 3D MRA examination. However, segmental ischemia of the bowel may be detected by identifying the absence of the normal mucosal enhancement on delayed images or perfusion images (see below). Also tiny aneurysms due to vasculitis are generally not resolved on 3D CE MRA images. In addition, intrinsic spatial resolution limitations of MRA may also make it difficult to assess the IMA.

Accuracy of Mesenteric MRA in the Literature

MR-based assessment of mesenteric artery stenosis is most reliably accomplished by 3D CE MRA

Table 1. Accuracy of MRA for mesenteric vessels

Investigator	Year	No. Patients	Technique	Sensitivity (%)	Specificity (%)
Carlos et al (38)	2002	26	3D Gd	96	95
Meaney et al (16)	1997	14	3D Gd	100	95
Wasser et al (9)	1996	10	3D PC	-	-
Miyazaki et al (39)	1995	100	2D TOF	80	33
Prince et al (15)	1995	43	3D Gd	94	98
Durham et al (40)	1993	28	2D TOF	60	96

but can also be demonstrated by TOF and PC-MRA. Table 1 provides a summary of published studies. Assessment of the functional significance is usually based on the presence of severe stenosis or occlusion of at least two of the splanchnic arteries. However, mesenteric blood flow can be measured with a 2D PC technique. Further functional information can be obtained from determination of *in vivo* oximetry.

Phase-Contrast MRA

Wasser et al [9] reported their experience with a systolically-gated phase contrast MRA technique in patients with suspected mesenteric ischemia. Only 66% of stenoses seen on catheter-based arteriography could be visualized by MRA, and false-positive results were encountered. The limitations included problems with phase ghosting, motion artifacts and uncertainty as to the choice of the appropriate velocity-encoding (VENC) gradient value.

Contrast-Enhanced MRA

Due to its non-invasive character, MRI has become an attractive alternative for the evaluation of the visceral vessel system. Meaney et al. examined 65 patients with suspected mesenteric ischemia using a 3D CE MRA technique [16]. Overall significant stenoses of the celiac artery and the superior mesenteric artery were identified in 14 patients and correlated with catheter-based angiography. A total of 28 of 30 arteries with correlation were correctly graded; therefore, despite disagreement between MRA and catheter-based arteriography in two patients, the sensitivity of CE MRA was 100% for the diagnosis of mesenteric ischemia while the specificity was 95%. The authors concluded that 3D CE MRA is accurate for the evaluation of the origins of the mesenteric and celiac arteries, but that the spatial resolution is too low for reliable assessment of the IMA. In addition, delineation of the small mesenteric branch vessels was shown to be hampered by the limited spatial resolution of MRA [29].

To be considered also is that development of a strong collateral circulation can prevent major abdominal symptoms in patients with severe alterations of the mesenteric arteries [25,26,29-30]. Thus, other parameters need to be defined for the assessment of chronic mesenteric ischemia (see below).

In a study aimed at optimizing an "all-in-one" imaging protocol for the assessment of potential living donors for liver transplants [31] 3D MRA was shown to be useful in depicting vascular anomalies with regard to the aortic branch vessels. In this study 3D FLASH data sets of the hepatic vasculature were collected before and after intravenous administration of Gd-BOPTA (Multi-Hance®, Bracco Imaging SpA, Milan/Italy) at a dose of 0.2 mmol/kg bodyweight in 38 potential liver donors. After exclusion of patients as potential donors because of insufficient liver mass of the left hepatic lobe (n=5), presence of hepatic pathologies (n=9) or dilated biliary ducts (n=4), 20 patients were available for assessment. 3D CE MRA depiction of the hepatic arterial morphology was shown to correlate with conventional DSA in each of these 20 patients. Specifically, 3D CE MRA correctly identified 3 left hepatic arteries originating from the left gastric artery, 3 aberrant right hepatic arteries originating from the SMA, 2 aberrant origins of both hepatic arteries and one common hepatic artery originating from the SMA.

Vascular complications of liver transplantation are another indication for visceral artery imaging. Stafford-Johnson et al [32] reported on the utility of a contrast-enhanced 3D MRA technique for the evaluation of vascular complications following liver transplantation. In 9 of 11 patients MR-based findings could be confirmed by surgery or catheter-based arteriography. In the remaining two patients, 3D CE MRA overestimated a hepatic artery stenosis in one patient while in the other patient a severe stenosis on 3D CE MRA was subsequently shown to represent three discrete tandem lesions.

In patients with intra-abdominal neoplasms CE MRA can be used for staging purposes prior to surgery. Gaa et al [33] reported promising results using a comprehensive "all-in-one" approach for assessing patients with pancreatic cancer.

Functional Assessment of Mesenteric Flow / Oxymetry

MR flow quantification has been proposed as an indirect parameter for the evaluation of mesenteric ischemia [10,11,13]. Using phase-contrast MRI, flow characteristics of the SMA, CA and IMA can be qualitatively and quantitatively assessed. Thus, a reciprocal correlation between the degree of stenoses in the SMA and the flow augmentation after a caloric stimulation could be determined [10]. Other authors prefer flow quantification of the SMV, which is an accurate predictor of flow in the visceral arteries and can therefore capture changes in each of the three main arterial branches [13, 30]. However, flow measurements are only an indirect parameter for the blood supply of the small bowel.

Perfusion MRI of the Small Bowel to Assess Mesenteric Ischemia

Perfusion imaging as a noninvasive method has been widely used for the determination of myocardial blood flow [34]. Cardiac perfusion examinations are usually performed during baseline conditions as well as during pharmacologically induced hyperemia [35, 36]. Thus, a "myocardial perfusion reserve" can be determined, which accurately depicts individual graded coronary lesions [35]. This pathophysiological background can be transferred from myocardial perfusion to visceral perfusion, since processes in coronary artery disease are fairly comparable to those in mesenteric ischemia. Instead of increasing the blood flow and heart activity by the intravenous application of pharmaceutical drugs, the blood flow and "bowel activity" can be enlarged by the oral administration of a high caloric foodstuff. In fact, the reserve capacity of bowel wall perfusion, which is comparable to the myocardial perfusion reserve, has proven to be a reliable parameter for the differentiation between healthy volunteers and patients with mesenteric ischemia. The baseline examination alone without caloric stimulation should not be considered for the assessment of mesenteric ischemia as in our experience there have hardly been any differences between our reference and patient groups. Interestingly, both for the examination with caloric stimulation as well as for the examination concerning the reserve capacity, differences turned out to be most significant during the first pass of the intravenous contrast material. Hence evaluation of dynamic perfusion MRI should be based mainly on this first pass period.

Perfusion MRI of the bowel wall is a feasible method for the assessment of mesenteric ischemia [37]. Among its advantages is its non-invasiveness.

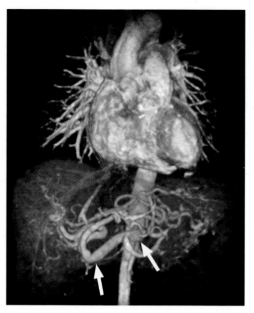

Fig. 12. Volume rendered 3D CE MRA data set (0.1 mmol/kg Gd-BOPTA) in a patient with Osler's disease. Multiple diffusely distributed hepatic arterio-venous malformations lead to hepatic shunting resulting in an enlarged celiac trunk and hepatic artery (*arrows*) [Image courtesy of Dr. G. Schneider]

In addition, direct information of the bowel wall can be obtained. Although only patients with proven artherosclerosis of the SMA were examined, the concept should be suitable for the evaluation of changes to each of the mesenteric arteries. To this end, the perfusion values of the colonic wall should be analyzed to exclude or confirm pathologies of the IMA.

Conclusion

Contrast-enhanced MRA is useful for evaluating a wide spectrum of abdominal pathologies (Fig. 12). In many centers worldwide, it is the technique of choice for evaluating patients with suspected chronic mesenteric ischemia, assessing the operability of patients with pancreatic cancer, and for investigating the portal system. Evolving indications include the assessment of liver transplant patients before and after transplant and of living related liver transplant donors.

References

1. Hagspiel KD, Leung DA, Angle JF et al (2002) MR angiography of the mesenteric vasculature. Radiol Clin North Am 40:867-886
2. Baden JG, Racy DJ, Grist TM (1999) Contrast-enhanced three-dimensional magnetic resonance angiography of the mesenteric vasculature. J Magn Reson Imaging 10:369-375

3. Meaney JF (1999) Non-invasive evaluation of the visceral arteries with magnetic resonance angiography. Eur Radiol 9:1267-1276

4. Vosshenrich R, Fischer U (2002) Contrast-enhanced MR angiography of abdominal vessels: is there still a role for angiography? Eur Radiol 12:218-230

5. Hagspiel KD, Angle JF, Spinosa DJ et al (1999) Mesenteric ischemia: angiography and endovascular interventions. In: Longo W, Peterson GJ, Jacobs DL, editors. Intestinal ischemia disorders: pathophysiology and management. St. Louis: Quality Medical Publishing: 105-154

6. Kadir S (1986) Esophago-gastrointestinal angiography. In: Kadir S, Editor. Diagnostic angiography. Philadelphia: WB Saunders Co.: 338-376

7. Michels NA (1955) Blood supply and anatomy of the upper abdominal organs. Philadelphia: JB Lipincott Co.

8. Prince MR, Grist TM, Debatin JF (2003) Mesenteric Arteries. In: Prince MR, Grist TM, Debatin JF. 3D Contrast MR Angiography. Springer Berlin Heidelberg New York

9. Wasser MN, Geelkerken RH, Kouwenhoven M et al (1996) Systolically gated phase-contrast MRA of mesenteric arteries in suspected mesenteric ischemia. J Comput Assist Tomogr 20:262-268

10. Li KCP, Whitney WS, Mc Donnell C et al (1994) Chronic mesenteric ischemia: evaluation with phase-contrast cine MR imaging. Radiology 190:175-179

11. Naganawa S, Cooper TG, Jenner G et al (1994) Flow velocity and flow measurement of superior and inferior mesenteric artery with cine phase contrast magnetic resonance angiography. Radiat Med 12:213-220

12. Li KCP, Hopkins KL, Dalman RL et al (1995) Simultaneous flow measurements within the superior mesenteric vein and artery with cine phase-contrast MR imaging: value in diagnosis of chronic mesenteric ischemia. Radiology 194:327-330

13. Burkart DJ, Johnson CD, Reading CC et al (1995) MR measurements of mesenteric venous flow: prospective evaluation in healthy volunteers and patients with chronic mesenteric ischemia. Radiology 194:801-806

14. Prince MR, Yucel EK, Kaufman JA et al (1993) Dynamic gadolinium-enhanced 3D abdominal MR arteriography. J Magn Reson Imaging 3:877-881

15. Prince MR, Narasimham DL, Stanley JC et al (1995) Breath-hold gadolinium-enhanced MR arteriography of the abdominal aorta and its major branches. Radiology 197:785-792

16. Meaney JFM, Prince MR, Nostrand TT et al (1997) Gadolinium-enhanced magnetic resonance angiography in patients with suspected chronic mesenteric ischemia. J Magn Reson Imaging 7:171-176

17. Char D, Hines G (2001) Chronic mesenteric ischemia: diagnosis and treatment. Heart Dis 4:231-235

18. Williams LF Jr (1988) Mesenteric ischemia. Surg Clin North Am 68:331-353

19. Moawad J, Gewertz BL (1997) Chronic mesenteric ischemia. Clinical presentation and diagnosis. Surg Clin North Am 77:357-369

20. Ernst O, Asnar V, Sergent G et al (2000) Comparing contrast-enhanced breath-hold MR angiography and conventional angiography in the evaluation of mesenteric circulation. AJR Am J Roentgenol 174(2):433-439

21. Hany TF, Schmidt M, Schoenenberger AW (1998) Debatin JF. Contrast-enhanced three-dimensional magnetic resonance angiography of the splanchnic vasculature before and after caloric stimulation. Invest Radiol 33:682-668

22. Debatin JF (1998) MR quantification of flow in abdominal vessels. Abdom Imaging 23:485-495

23. Li KC, Dalman RL, Chen IY et al (1997) Chronic mesenteric ischemia: use of in vivo MR imaging measurements of blood oxygen saturation in the superior mesenteric vein for diagnosis. Radiology 204:71-77

24. Tassi G, Maggi G, de Nicola P (1985) Microcirculation in the elderly. Int Angiol 4:275-283

25. Cunningham CG, Reilly LM, Stoney R (1992) Chronic visceral ischemia. Surg Clin North Am 72:231-44

26. Kurland B, Brandt LJ, Delany HM (1992) Diagnostic tests for intestinal ischemia. Surg Clin North Am 72:85-105

27. Hilfiker PR, Zimmermann-Paul GG, Schmidt M et al (1998) Detection of intestinal and peritoneal bleeding with a new MR blood pool agent in conjunction with fast 3D MRI: preliminary experience from an experimental study. Radiology 209:769-774

28. Weishaupt D, Hetzer FH, Ruehm SG et al (2000) Three-dimensional contrast-enhanced MRI using an intravascular contrast agent for detection of traumatic intra-abdominal hemorrhage and abdominal parenchymal injuries: an experimental study. Eur Radiol 10:1958-1964

29. Laissy JP, Trillaud H, Douek P (2002) MR angiography: noninvasive vascular imaging of the abdomen. Abdom Imaging 27:488-506

30. Chow LC, Chan FP, Li KC (2002) A comprehensive approach to MR imaging of mesenteric ischemia. Abdom Imaging 27(5):507-516

31. Goyen M, Barkhausen J, Debatin JF et al (2000) Right-lobe living related liver transplantation: evaluation of a comprehensive magnetic resonance imaging protocol for assessing potential donors. Liver Transpl 8:241-250

32. Stafford-Johnson DB, Hamilton BH, Dong Q et al (1998) Vascular complications of liver transplantation: evaluation with gadolinium-enhanced MR angiography. Radiology 207:153-160

33. Gaa J, Wendl M, Georgi M (1997) New concepts in MR imaging of pancreas carcinoma: the "all-in-one" approach. In: Oudkerk M, Edelman RR (eds) High power gradient MR imaging. Blackwell, London, 425-430

34. Wilke NM, Jerosch-Herold M, Zenovich A et al (1999) Magnetic resonance first-pass myocardial perfusion imaging: clinical validation and future applications. J Magn Reson Imaging 10:676-685

35. Nagel E, Underwood R, Pennell D et al (1998) New developments in non-invasive cardiac imaging: critical assessment of the clinical role of cardiac magnetic resonance imaging. Eur Heart J 19:1286-1293

36. Penzkofer H, Wintersperger BJ, Knez A et al (1999) Assessment of myocardial perfusion using multisection first-pass MRI and color-coded parameter maps: a comparison to 99mTc Sesta MIBI SPECT and systolic myocardial wall thickening analysis.

Magn Reson Imaging 17:161-170
37. Lauenstein TC, Herborn CU, Gohde SC et al (*in press*) Perfusion MRI of the small bowel wall for the diagnosis of mesenteric ischemia – a feasibility study J Magn Reson Imaging
38. Carlos RC, Stanley JC, Stafford-Johnson D et al (2001) Interobserver variability in the evaluation of chronic mesenteric ischemia with gadolinium-enhanced MR angiography. Acad Radiol 8:879-887
39. Miyazaki T, Yamashita Y, Shinzato J et al (1995) Two-dimensional time-of-flight magnetic resonance angiography in the coronal plane for abdominal disease: its usefulness and comparison with conventional angiography. Br J Radiol 68:351-357
40. Durham JR, Hackworth CA, Tober JC et al (1993) Magnetic resonance angiography in the preoperative evaluation of abdominal aortic aneurysm. Am J surg 166:173-177

VI.4

MR Angiography of the Portal Venous System

Mathias Goyen

Introduction

Three-dimensional (3D) contrast-enhanced (CE) magnetic resonance (MR) portography is a quick and robust means of evaluating the portal venous system offering some advantages over currently used imaging modalities including catheter-based digital subtraction angiography (DSA), computed tomography, ultrasonography and non-enhanced MR angiography with time-of-flight (TOF) and phase contrast (PC) techniques [1]. With 3D CE MR portography a first-pass study of the mesenteric vasculature is performed (see. VI 3.) after rapid bolus injection of gadolinium-based contrast agent. Repeated sequences allow depiction of the intra- and extrahepatic portal venous anatomy. The images can then be reconstructed by means of maximum-intensity-projection (MIP) postprocessing, and a subtraction technique can be employed to eliminate arterial enhancement and demonstrate portosystemic shunts. The coronal source images simultaneously demonstrate parenchymal lesions of the liver, pancreas, biliary tract and spleen. Precise and reliable assessment of the portal venous system in patients with hepatic cirrhosis and portal hypertension is essential before liver transplantation, non-surgical transjugular shunting or surgical portosystemic shunting. Especially in patients with portal hypertension and a history of gastro-esophageal bleeding it is mandatory to determine whether the portal venous system is patent or the portal vein or its main branches are thrombosed [2].

Normal Anatomy

The mesenteric venous anatomy (Fig. 1) parallels the arterial distribution (see VI.3) [3-4]. The portal vein is formed by the splenic and superior mesenteric veins. The pancreatic, left gastroepiploic, short gastric, and inferior mesenteric veins and splenic vein branches drain into the main splenic vein. The inferior mesenteric vein receives its supply from the left colic, sigmoid and superior hemorrhoidal veins. It usually joins the splenic vein prior to the junction of the splenic vein with the superior mesenteric vein. The superior mesenteric vein receives its contribution from jejunal, ileal

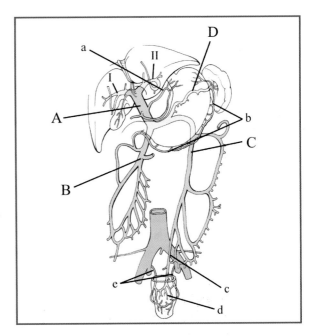

Fig. 1. Normal anatomy of the portal venous system
A Portal vein
B Superior mesenteric vein
C Inferior mesenteric vein
D Lienal vein

I   Right branch of the portal vein
II Left branch of the portal vein

a Coronary and pyloric veins
b Right and left gastroepiploic veins
c Superior hemorrhoidal vein
d Hemorrhoidal plexus
e Middle and inferior hemorrhoidal veins

Table 1. Overview of MR-contrast agents currently approved in Europe

Commercial Name	Laboratory Name	Generic Name	Manufacturer	T1 relaxivity* mmol^{-1} sec^{-1}
Magnevist®	Gd-DTPA	Gadopentetate dimeglumine	Schering	4.8
Gadovist®	Gd-BT-DO3A	gadolinium-DO3A-butriol	Schering	5.6
Dotarem®	Gd-DOTA	Gadoterate meglumine	Guerbet	–
Omniscan®	Gd-BMA	Gadodiamide	Amersham Health	4.4
ProHance®	Gd-HP-DO3A	Gadoteridol	Bracco	4.9
MultiHance®	**Gd-BOPTA**	**Gadobenate dimeglumine**	**Bracco**	**9.7**

* in plasma at 0.47 T and 20 mHz

right colic, and middle colic veins. The coronary veins (right and left gastric veins) usually drain directly into the portal vein. The portal vein then divides into the right and left portal branches at the porta hepatic. Approximately one half of patients have the portal vein bifurcation outside the liver capsule. A common normal variant of the portal venous system is trifurcation of the main portal vein, which is present in about 8% of patients. In these patients, the main portal vein divides into the right posterior segmental branch, the right anterior segmental branch, and the left portal vein.

MRA Techniques

When performing 3D CE MR portography some important technical issues have to be considered. By the time a conventional extracellular MR-contrast agents reaches the portal vein, it is considerably diluted. This dilution is caused by the contrast extraction at the capillary level for redistribution into the extracellular compartment and Gd extraction in the liver [5]. Table 1 lists the MR contrast agents currently available in Europe and elsewhere for CE-MRA. Current commercially available gadolinium-based agents are extracellular in nature and most have similar T1 relaxivity values of between approximately 4.4 and 5.6 mmol^{-1} sec^{-1}. The one agent with truly unique physicochemical properties among the contrast agents listed in Table 1 is gadobenate dimeglumine (MultiHance®, Gd-BOPTA, Bracco Imaging SpA, Milan, Italy) which is currently approved in Europe and elsewhere for MR imaging of the CNS and liver and under investigation for applications in CE-MRA. Gadobenate dimeglumine differs from the other agents in two major respects. Firstly, unlike the other available gadolinium–based contrast agents which are excreted exclusively by glomerular filtration through the kidneys [6-9], Gd-BOPTA is eliminated from the body through both the renal (96-98% of the injected dose) and hepatobiliary (2-4% of the injected dose) pathways [10, 11]. Secondly, due to a unique capacity among current agents for weak and transient interaction with serum albumin [12], Gd-BOPTA possesses a T1 relaxivity in plasma (9.7 mmol^{-1} sec^{-1}) which is approximately twice that of most of the conventional gadolinium chelates [13].

These facts have to be taken into account when determining the contrast dosage. Thus, when using conventional extracellular MR-contrast agents (i.e. agents with no albumin binding) a dosage of 0.2 mmol/kg body weight is recommended for dedicated portal vein imaging. This dosage can be lowered when employing Gd-BOPTA [14].

A rather lower flip angle of 20°–30° is advantageous as it improves visualization of the diluted gadolinium in the portal vein. The images can be acquired in a coronal or axial slice orientation. Coronal imaging has the advantage of including the mesenteric arteries including the inferior mesenteric artery on the arterial phase (see chapter VI.3) and also including the superior and inferior mesenteric veins and retroperitoneal collaterals. The axial plane has the advantage of imaging the main portal vein and its branches "in-plane", which usually results in higher resolution compared to reformations. Another advantage of the axial acquisition is the fact that the entire liver is depicted allowing the detection and characterization of hepatic tumors. Finally, axial imaging has a smaller field-of-view without wraparound artifacts if frequency encoding is right-to-left. However, one limitation of the axial plane is wrap-around in the slice direction (superior to inferior). Bright fat adjacent to the imaging volume hampers image quality. This problem can be eliminated by utilizing a fat suppression technique and by using an imaging volume that matches the entire volume of the coil sensitivity. In this way, tissue above and below the coil will have limited signal to wrap into the image volume [5].

3D axial imaging volumes can easily be prescribed from coronal localizers. The axial 3D volume should extend from just above where hepatic veins enter the inferior vena cava down to well below the spleno-portal confluence. On slower MR scanners it may be necessary to use a slice thickness of 5-6 mm to obtain adequate coverage.

When imaging in the coronal plane, it is crucial

to extend sufficiently anteriorly to include the entire portal and mesenteric venous system in the imaging volume. For planning of the 3D acquisition the portal vein should be readily identified on the localizer. Usually the main portal vein is depicted well on axial T1, T2 or gradient echo images.

High-performance gradient MR-scanners in combination with partial Fourier imaging can provide up to 50 imaging sections in a convenient 20 second breath-hold. MR scanners with inferior gradient performance may require thicker sections of up to 4 or 5 mm in order to extend far enough anteriorly (for coronal volumes) to include the portal vein and still be fast enough to be acquired during a breath-hold.

For portal venous phase imaging the breath-hold interval needs to be kept rather short. A patient who can suspend breathing for 40 seconds during the arterial phase may be too winded for another 40-second breath-hold during the portal venous phase. Therefore, it is best to keep the acquisition time under 30 seconds per phase to enable patients to suspend breathing twice in a row with only a few seconds rest in between [5].

Analysis of the portal venous and equilibrium phase images can be accomplished rapidly by performing a series of overlapping thick maximum-intensity-projections (MIP). Volume rendering may not work as well because of hepatic parenchymal enhancement.

Complementary Sequences

A PC-MR scan can be employed to determine the direction of portal venous blood flow. A single 5-10 mm thick 2D phase contrast image is acquired in an axial or oblique plan, perpendicular to the portal vein. Typical imaging parameters are: 28 ms/6 ms TR/TE/Flip = 28/6/45° and VENC = 40 cm/s. On 2D phase contrast velocity map images, background tissues are gray, while blood flow is shown as either bright vixels or black pixels, depending on their direction of flow. By convention, flow in the superior-to-inferior (S/I), right-to-left (R/L), and anterior-to-posterior (A/P) directions is bright, whereas flow in the opposite direction is displayed as dark on velocity-encoded 2D phase contrast images. Through plane flow can similarly be mapped on oblique acquisitions. In order to interpret flow data correctly, the orthogonal plane coming closest to the scan obliquity needs to be determined. Alternatively, if the portal vein is more vertical than horizontal, a straight axial 2D phase contrast image can be acquired and the flow direction compared to the aorta and inferior vena.

For patients with limited breath-holding capabilities who could not suspend breathing during the portal venous phase, axial 2D gradient echo images can be acquired post-gadolinium during either short periods of apnea (5s) or quiet respiration. Paramagnetic contrast within the vascular system enhances time-of-flight image quality allowing use of relatively thick, 5-8 mm slices. For non-breath-held scans a sufficient number of averages, in conjunction with respiratory ordered phase encoding, will usually result in diagnostic image quality [5].

Patients with suspected parenchymal pathology benefit from T1- and T2-weighted spin echo imaging prior to contrast injection. These images can be used as a guide to ensure inclusion of all pathology in 3D contrast MRA data sets. For patients with suspected biliary obstruction or pancreatitis, a HASTE or single shot fast spin echo MRCP-type sequence in coronal or coronal oblique planes is also useful and can generally be performed in a single breath-hold or during quiet respiration.

Clinical Examples for Various Clinical Indications and Pathologies

3D CE MR portography can demonstrate the intrahepatic and extrahepatic portal venous system as well as hepatic veins. Its advantages over DSA include its large field of view, its short imaging time, and its noninvasive nature and low risk of complications, which permit repeated studies. Clinical applications of 3D CE MR portography include portal hypertension (portosystemic shunt, portal vein obstruction, hepatic vein obstruction), hepatic encephalopathy, ascending portal thrombophlebitis, hepatocellular carcinoma and pancreatobiliary tumors, gastrointestinal hemorrhage, and differentiation of splanchnic arterial disease from portal venous disease [1, 15]. In patients with portal hypertension, 3D MR portography can be used to evaluate portosystemic shunt, hepatopetal collateral pathways, and obstruction of the portal or hepatic veins. In planning treatment for hepatic encephalopathy, it is important to identify the causative portosystemic shunt. In suspected cases of ascending portal thrombophlebitis, it is important to assess the severity of portal vein obstruction as well as portal collateral vessels. In patients with hepatocellular carcinoma or pancreatobiliary tumors, one must determine the presence or absence of portal vein invasion when planning treatment.

Portal Hypertension

DSA in patients with portal hypertension is often performed to measure portal venous pressures and the portal-systemic pressure gradient. These measurements can not be made directly using

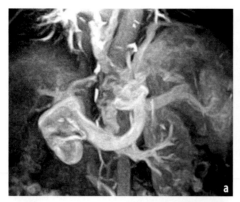
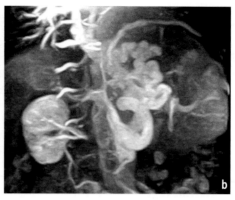
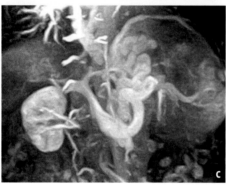

Fig. 2a-c. 44-year-old patient with hepatic cirrhosis and repeated gastrointestinal haemorrhage. Three rotated MIP displays of the portal venous phase 3D data set depict the portal venous morphology to good advantage. The splenic vein is dilated and is draining into a convolute of gastroesophageal collaterals which can be seen to extent to the distal oesophagus. Contrast-enhanced 3D MRA provides an excellent mean for non-invasively evaluating the portal venous system. Use of Gd-BOPTA (MultiHance®, Bracco) provides optimal image quality of the portal venous system owing to the transient albumin-binding of this particular contrast agent. Gastro-oesophageal collaterals are well visualized. Lack of enhancement of the intrahepatic portal venous system suggests retrograde flow in the portal vein with portal systemic shunting to the gastro-esophageal collaterals. Based on these imaging data this patient underwent TIPS (Transjugular-Intrahepatic-Portosystemic-Shunting) in combination with embolisation of the gastro-oesophageal-collaterals

MRI. However, for patients who require a portal-systemic shunt, 3D contrast MRA can be a useful guide for shunt planning (Fig. 2). MRA accurately assesses the patency of both spontaneous (Fig. 3) and surgical shunts (Figs. 4, 5) as long as metallic clips do not obscure portal venous anatomy. In conjunction with PC-MRA-techniques, shunt volumes can be determined non-invasively. TIPS shunts are more difficult to assess due to metallic stents. Most often, a stainless steel Wall stent is used to bridge the portal and systemic venous system. Even with echo times of less than 1 ms, the lumen of this metal stent cannot be evaluated by MRA.

Liver Transplantation

Imaging proof of a patent portal vein is required for a patient to be placed on the liver transplant waiting list. Ultrasound can image the portal vein but is not 100% reliable. When ultrasound fails to adequately visualize the portal vein, 3D CE MRA offers a safe, accurate, and comprehensive assessment of portal venous anatomy without requiring iodinated contrast [16, 17]. 3D CE MRA also evaluates the splenic vein, superior mesenteric vein (SMV), inferior mesenteric vein, IVC and potential varices (Fig. 6). Following liver transplantation, rising liver function tests may raise a suspicion of al-

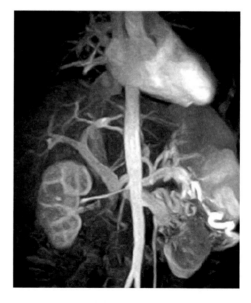

Fig. 3. Spontaneous spleno-renal shunt: 66-year-old woman with progressive toxic-induced hepatic cirrhosis. The patient was referred to MRA for evaluation of the liver. MIP display of a 3D MRA data set acquired the portal venous phase demonstrate a spontaneous splenorenal shunt. The left renal vein is dilated. No gastro-oesophageal varices are identified. Contrast enhanced 3D MRA is ideally suited for non-invasively assessing the portal venous system. Complex vascular morphology is comprehensively depicted owing to the inherent 3-dimensionality of the technique. In this patient the presence of gastro-oesophageal varices can be largely excluded. Most of the portal venous blood appears to be shunted through a spontaneous splenorenal shunt which is well demonstrated

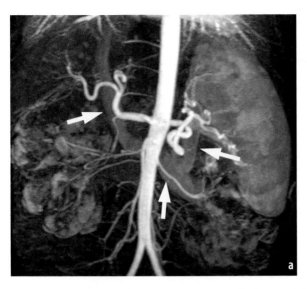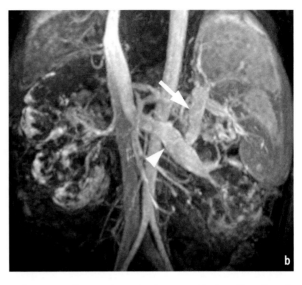

Fig. 4a, b. 13-year old female patient with surgical splenorenal shunt due to portalvenous hypertension caused by hereditary liver fibrosis in multicystic kidney disease. The arterial phase image (**a**) already shows an early enhancement of some venous structures (*arrows*) which in the portalvenous phase (**b**) can be identified as the splenic vein (*arrow*) connected to the left renal vein (*arrowhead*). The study confirms patency of the surgical splenorenal shunt without stenosis at the site of anastomosis. Note the enlarged kidneys on both sides due to polycystic kidney disease [Images courtesy of Dr. G. Schneider]

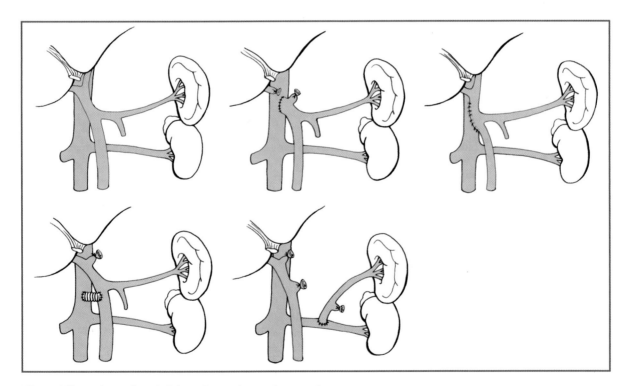

Fig. 5. Different forms of surgical shunts in portalvenous hypertension

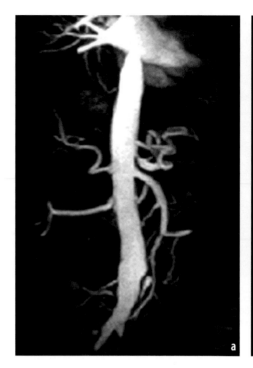
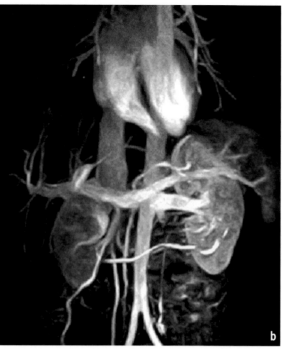

Fig. 6 a, b. 51-year-old woman with progressive hepatic failure referred to MRI of the liver to exclude hepatic disease. Oblique map display of the arterial phased 3D data set (**a**) as well as frontal MIP display of the portal venous 3D data set (**b**) provide an excellent overview of the vascular anatomy in the abdomen. No anomalies are noted. The superior mesenteric artery is shown to be normal. Similarly, the portal venous system is shown to be normal. All tributaries to the portal venous system such as the splenic vein as well as the superior mesenteric vein are visualized to good advantage. Analysis of the portal venous system should be part of any MR-based evaluation of the liver. For most optimal results the portal venous phase data set should be collected immediately following the arterial phase acquisition. Both 3D data sets should be temporarily separated by a 5-10 sec break during which the patient is asked to breathe. Breath-holding during data acquisition is crucial for optimal image quality

lograft ischemia. Since blood supply to the liver is primarily via the portal vein, this is the most important vessel to evaluate. The most common site of obstruction is at the anastomosis. Usually, anastomoses are easy to identify because of the caliber change between donor and recipient portal veins [18]. Stenosis of the transplant arterial anastomosis may be seen on the arterial phase of a portal venous study, but its smaller size and often folded, tortuous course can make it difficult to assess. Occlusion of the transplant artery is important to detect because it results in ischemia to the donor common bile duct and can lead to biliary strictures and leaks. It is also important to assess the IVC since supra- and infrahepatic IVC anastomoses may also become narrowed and flow limiting.

Portal Vein Thrombosis and Cavernous Transformation

Portal vein thrombosis often occurs in liver cirrhosis, ascending portal thrombophlebitis, pancreatitis, and other conditions and after sclerotherapy of a gastroesophageal varix [19]. It is important to assess portal venous patency in these diseases. Con-

trast-enhanced 3D MR portography provides detailed information not only about the location and length of portal vein obstruction but also about portal collateral pathways. Over time, a network of small collateral vessels develops to bypass the portal venous occlusion. This network of collaterals, known as cavernous transformation, is identified by its characteristic enhancement pattern in the hepatic hilum during portal venous and equilibrium phases of 3D CE MRA.

Table 2 gives an overview of the accuracy of 3D MR portography. In potential candidates for liver transplantation, it is necessary to evaluate portal venous patency [20]. Color Doppler US may not allow portal venous patency to be established [21], but contrast-enhanced 3D MR portography provides accurate information.

Tumor Encasement

In patients with pancreatobiliary tumors, it is important to evaluate portal vein invasion before surgery. CT and DSA have been used for this purpose. 3D CE MR portography is also an accurate way to diagnose portal vein invasion [22, 23].

Table 2. Accuracy of 3D CE MR portography; # number of patients with angiography or surgical correlation

Author	Year	Journal	# Patients	Sensitivity	Specificity
Stafford-Johnson [29]	1998	Radiology	13	100%	100%
Wilson [35]	1998	Invest Radiol	27	86%	100%
Kopka [36]	1999	Radiology	140 (60*)	100%	100%
Kreft [30]	2000	Radiology	36	100%	98%
Glockner [37]	2000	AJR	34 (20*)	100%	94%
Ernst [38]	2000	AJR	33	100%	100%
Haliloglu [39]	2000	JMRI	3	100%	
Cheng [40]	2001	Transplantation	38	100%	100%
Squillaci [41]	2001	RadiolMed	28	100%	97, 3%

Invasion of the portal vein makes tumor resection with clear margins nearly impossible, thus, removing the patient as a surgical candidate. Tumors in the pancreatic head may encase the SMV, portal vein, and medial splenic vein. These tumors are usually detected early because they cause biliary obstruction, and thereby may be more likely to be resectable. Tumors in the body and tail of the pancreas may become larger before being detected and more commonly occlude the splenic vein. Splenic vein occlusion has a tendency to produce short gastric varices serving as venous collaterals and can be seen on delayed images.

Budd Chiari

Budd-Chiari syndrome is a rare disorder characterized by hepatic outflow occlusion and caused by various conditions including congenital or idiopathic obstruction, hepatic vein thrombosis due to hypercoagulative state, hepatic veno-occlusive disease after liver transplantation, and hepatic tumors [24]. The major symptoms include ascites, hepatomegaly, and abdominal pain. It has been classified into three types according to the location of the occlusion [25, 26]. Type 1 is defined as occlusion of the inferior vena cava with or without hepatic vein occlusion; type 2, occlusion of major hepatic veins; and type 3, obstruction of the small centrilobular venules (hepatic veno-occlusive disease). From the clinical point of view, Budd-Chiari syndrome should be classified according to whether it can be treated with anticoagulants, surgery, or interventional procedures. In planning treatment, it is important to determine the location and length of hepatic outflow obstruction [24], and contrast-enhanced 3D MR portography is an accurate means of doing this. No hepatic veins can be visualized in hepatic veno-occlusive disease, whereas narrowing of the intrahepatic portal vein may be seen with a delayed circulation time.

Pitfalls and Limitations

General contraindications to MR imaging also apply to 3D CE MR portography, which has several other limitations. First, there is a risk of allergic reactions to contrast media, although the incidence is low. Second, this technique is unable to demonstrate the flow direction of the portal venous system, unlike phase-contrast or time-of-flight MR angiography [27, 28]. Third, important portosystemic collateral vessels may be overlooked when they are too anterior or posterior to the imaging slab or when the slab is positioned inappropriately. Fourth, if the interval between injection of Gd-based contrast agent and the start of imaging is too prolonged, the arteries and portal vein may not be differentiated. Fifth, artifacts from respiratory motion and peristaltic bowel movement degrade image quality, especially in debilitated patients who are unable to hold their breath for 12–24 seconds. Sixth, when subtraction techniques are used, respiratory misregistration also degrades image quality.

Clip and Stent Artifacts

Metal clips used for cholecystectomy as well as wallstents (used in TIPS) can cause susceptibility artifacts which may hamper visualization of the portal vein and IVC. These artifacts can be minimized by using the shortest possible echo time. Newer stents made of non-magnetic material such as nitinol or platinum cause less artifacts.

Blurring

Many patients have limited breath-holding capabilities; therefore it might be difficult for those patients to suspend breathing twice in a row to image both the arterial and portal venous phase. Thus, it is crucial to minimize the examination time and to stress the importance of breath-holding to the patient. Oxygen, 2 liters by nasal connulae, can help.

Accuracy of MR Portography in the Literature

The value of MRA as a non-invasive imaging modality has been increasingly recognized for the assessment of the portal venous system. Time-of-flight (TOF) and phase contrast (PC) MR methods have been shown to be promising for the assessment of the portal venous system. Disadvantages include motion artifacts due to breathing, long acquisition times and incomplete coverage of the entire portal venous system [29]

3D CE MR portography accurately detects portal vein thrombosis (Table 2). Kreft et al. [30] reported that relevant thromboses of the portal venous system were identified in correlation to catheter arteriographic correlation in 32 of 36 patients with portal hypertension. In 4 patients there were discordant findings between 3D CE MR portography and DSA [30]. Further studies have confirmed the role of 3D CE MR portography in detection of thrombosis in the portal venous system and imaging collateral pathways [31]. The analysis of the portal venous system can be complemented by analyzing the flow characteristics with PC-MRA-techniques. The measurement accuracy of PC flow mapping with regard to quantification of portal venous flow is well documented [32]. MR portography in combination with ultrasound examination is a very useful tool in the diagnosis of Budd Chiari syndrome [33]. In addition 3D CE MRA accurately depicts vascular anastomoses after liver transplantation [34].

Okumura et al [1] used contrast-enhanced 3D MR portography and DSA to assess the portal venous system and determine surgical resectability in 20 patients with pancreatobiliary tumors (pancreatic cancer in 13, bile duct cancer in two, carcinoma of the papilla of Vater in two, gallbladder cancer in two, and duodenal tumor in one). These patients were being considered as candidates for surgical resection. Of the 20 patients, 16 underwent surgical exploration, whereas four did not because their tumors were deemed unresectable at CT, DSA, and 3D CE MR portography. Twelve tumors were surgically resected. Results of 3D CE MR portography and DSA agreed in 14 of 16 patients (88%). 3D CE MR portography allowed identification of 11 of 12 resectable tumors and three of four unresectable tumors with one false-negative and one false-positive reading. DSA allowed identification of all 12 resectable tumors and two of four

unresectable tumors with two false-negative readings. The accuracy of 3D CE MR portography was therefore the same as that of DSA.

Conclusion

MR angiography of the portal venous system has evolved from a research tool to a quick and robust clinical diagnostic modality and is in many center the technique of choice for evaluating the anatomy of the portal venous system and its pathologic conditions, such as portosystemic shunt, portal vein thrombosis, portal vein invasion by hepatic and pancreatobiliary tumors, portal vein aneurysm, and hepatic vein obstruction. Evolving indications include the assessment of liver transplant patients before and after transplantation and of living related liver transplant donors.

References

1. Okumura A, Watanabe Y, Dohke M et al (1999) Contrast-enhanced three-dimensional MR portography. Radiographics 19:973-987
2. Redvanly RD, Nelson RC, Stieber AC, Dodd GD 3rd. (1995). Imaging in the preoperative evaluation of adult liver-transplant candidates: goals, merits of various procedures, and recommendations. Am J Roentgenol 164:611-617
3. Hagspiel KD, Leung DA, Angle JF et al (2002) MR angiography of the mesenteric vasculature. Radiol Clin North Am 40:867-886
4. Michels NA (1955) Blood supply and anatomy of the upper abdominal organs. Philadelphia: J.B. Lipincott Co
5. Prince MR, Grist TM, Debatin JF (2003) Mesenteric Arteries. In: Prince MR, Grist TM, Debatin JF. 3D Contrast MR Angiography. Springer Berlin Heidelberg New York
6. Weinmann HJ, Laniado M, Muetzel W (1984) Pharmacokinetics of Gd-DTPA/dimeglumine after intravenous injection into healthy volunteers. Physiol Chem Phys Med NMR 16:167-172
7. Mclachlan SJ, Eaton S, DeSimone DN (1992) Pharmacokinetic behavior of gadoteridol injection Invest Radiol; 27(Suppl 1):S12-S15
8. Le Mignon M-M, Chambon C, Warrington S et al (1990) Gd-DOTA: pharmacokinetics and tolerability after intravenous injection into healthy volunteers Invest Radiol 25:933-937
9. Van Wagoner M, O'Toole M, Worah D et al (1991) A phase I clinical trial with Gd-DTPA-BMA injection, a non-ionic magnetic resonance imaging enhancement agent. Invest Radiol 26:980-986
10. Kirchin MA, Pirovano G, Spinazzi A (1998) Gd-BOPTA (Gd-BOPTA): an overview. Invest Radiol 33:798-809
11. Spinazzi A, Lorusso V, Pirovano G et al (1999) Safety, tolerance, biodistribution and MR imaging enhancement of the liver with Gd-BOPTA: results of clinical pharmacologic and pilot imaging studies in

non-patient and patient volunteers. Acad Radiol 6:282-291

12. Cavagna FM, Maggioni F, Castelli PM et al (1997) Gadolinium chelates with weak binding to serum proteins. Invest Radiol 32:780-796

13. de Haën C, Cabrini M, Akhnana L et al (1999) Gd-BOPTA 0.5M solution for injection (MultiHance®): pharmaceutical formulation and physicochemical properties of a new magnetic resonance imaging contrast medium. J Comput Assist Tomogr; 23 (Suppl 1):S161-S168

14. Goyen M, Debatin JF (2003) Gadobenate Dimeglumine (MultiHance®) for Magnetic Resonance Angiography: Review of the Literature. Eur Radiol Supplement 3

15. Vosshenrich R, Fischer U (2002) Contrast-enhanced MR angiography of abdominal vessels: is there still a role for angiography? Eur Radiol 12:218-230

16. Goyen M, Barkhausen J, Debatin JF et al (2002) Right-lobe living related liver transplantation: evaluation of a comprehensive magnetic resonance imaging protocol for assessing potential donors. Liver Transpl 8: 241-250

17. Lee VS, Morgan GR, Teperman LW et al (2001) MR imaging as the sole preoperative imaging modality for right hepatectomy: a prospective study of living adult-to-adult liver donor candidates. Am J Roentgenol 176:1475-1482

18. Pandharipande PV, Lee VS, Morgan GR et al (2001) Vascular and extravascular complications of liver transplantation: comprehensive evaluation with three-dimensional contrast-enhanced volumetric MR imaging and MR cholangiopancreatography. Am J Roentgenol 177:1101-1107

19. Abbitt PL (1992) Portal vein thrombosis: imaging features and associated etiologies. Curr Probl Diagn Radiol 21:115-147

20. Shaked A, Busuttil RW (1991) Liver transplantation in patients with portal vein thrombosis and central portocaval shunts. Ann Surg 214:696-702

21. Glassman MS, Klein SA, Spivak W (1993) Evaluation of cavernous transformation of the portal vein by magnetic resonance imaging. Clin Pediatr 32:77-80

22. Smedby O, Riesenfeld V, Karlson BM et al (1997) Magnetic resonance angiography in the resectability assessment of suspected pancreatic tumors. Eur Radiol 7:649-653

23. McFarland E, Kaufman JA, Saini S et al (1996) Preoperative staging of cancer of the pancreas: value of MR angiography versus conventional angiography in detecting portal venous invasion. Am J Roentgenol 166:37-43

24. Murphy FB, Steinberg HV, Shires GT et al (1986) The Budd-Chiari syndrome: a review. AM J Roentgenol 147:9-15

25. Spritzer CE (1997) Vascular disease and MR angiography of the liver. Magn Reson Imaging Clin N Am 5:377-396

26. Gore RM (1994) Vascular disorders of the liver and splanchnic circulation. In: Gore RM, Levine MS, Laufer I, eds. Textbook of gastrointestinal radiology. Philadelphia, Pa: Saunders 2018-2050

27. Edelman RR, Zhao B, Liu C et al (1989) MR angiography and dynamic flow evaluation of the portal venous system. Am J Roentgenol 1989; 153: 755-760

28. Applegate GR, Thaete FL, Meyers SP et al (1993) Blood flow in the portal vein: velocity quantitation with phase-contrast MR angiography. Radiology 187:253-256

29. Stafford-Johnson DB, Hamilton BH, Dong Q et al (1998) Vascular complications of liver transplantation: evaluation with gadolinium-enhanced MR angiography. Radiology 207:153-160

30. Kreft B, Strunk H, Flacke S et al (2000) Detection of thrombosis in the portal venous system: comparison of contrast-enhanced MR angiography with intraarterial digital subtraction angiography. Radiology 216:86-92

31. Leyendecker JR, Rivera E Jr, Washburn WK et al (1997) MR angiography of the portal venous system: techniques, interpretation, and clinical applications. Radiographics 17:1425-1243

32. Thomsen C, Stahlberg F, Henriksen O (1993) Quantification of portal venous blood flow during fasting and after a standardized meal: a MRI phase-mapping study. Eur Radiol 3:242-247

33. Kane R, Eustace S (1995) Diagnosis of Budd-Chiari syndrome: comparison between sonography and MR angiography. Radiology 195:117-121

34. Squillaci E, Crecco M, Apruzzese A (1995) Magnetic resonance angiography in liver transplant patients. Follow-up of vascular anastomoses Radiol Med (Torino) 89(1-2):65-71

35. Wilson MW, Hamilton BH, Dong Q et al (1998) Gadolinium-enhanced magnetic resonance venography of the portal venous system prior to transjugular intrahepatic portosystemic shunts and liver transplantation. Original investigation. Invest Radiol 33:644-652

36. Kopka L, Rodenwaldt J, Vosshenrich R (1999) Hepatic blood supply: comparison of optimized dual phase contrast-enhanced three-dimensional MR angiography and digital subtraction angiography. Radiology 211:51-58

37. Glockner JF, Forauer AR, Solomon H et al (2000) Three-dimensional gadolinium-enhanced MR angiography of vascular complications after liver transplantation. Am J Roentgenol 174:1447-1453

38. Ernst O, Asnar V, Sergent G et al (2000) Comparing contrast-enhanced breath-hold MR angiography and conventional angiography in the evaluation of mesenteric circulation. AJR Am J Roentgenol 174:433-439

39. Haliloglu M, Hoffer FA, Gronemeyer SA et al (2000) 3D gadolinium-enhanced MRA: evaluation of hepatic vasculature in children with hepatoblastoma. J Magn Reson Imaging 11:65-68

40. Cheng YF, Chen CL, Huang TL et al (2001) Single imaging modality evaluation of living donors in liver transplantation: magnetic resonance imaging. Transplantation 72:1527-1533

41. Squillaci E, Mazzoleni C, Sodani G et al (2001) Magnetic resonance angiography with three-dimensional dynamic technique after contrast media administration for the study of the portal system. Radiol Med (Torino) 102(4):238-244

SECTION VII

Peripheral Arteries

VII.1

MR Angiography of Peripheral Arteries: Upper Extremities

Martin N. Wasser

Introduction

Contrast-enhanced magnetic resonance angiography (CE MRA) has become a routine procedure for the non-invasive visualization of vessels in most radiology departments. Unlike older MRA techniques [i.e., phase contrast (PC) MRA and time-of-flight (TOF) MRA], CE MRA does not suffer from artifacts caused by turbulence and in-plane saturation. This usually makes CE MRA easier to interpret than PC MRA and TOF MRA. Also, the lack of in-plane saturation in CE MRA permits imaging in the coronal plane, allowing for coverage of much larger anatomic regions and much shorter examination times.

In conventional MRA of the peripheral arteries, cardiac triggering is required in order to prevent erroneous signal loss due to the triphasic flow pattern with diastolic flow-reversal [1]. However, this cardiac triggering causes additional lengthening of the conventional MRA studies.

Thus far, MRA studies of the legs far outnumber those of the arms; a situation comparable to that seen in conventional angiography. Although atherosclerosis affects both upper and lower limbs, arterial insufficiency of the upper extremity is less common than that of the lower extremity because of extensive collateral circulation. In this chapter an overview of the techniques and indications for CE MRA of the arteries in the upper extremities will be presented.

Normal Anatomy

The normal anatomy of the aortic arch is shown in Figure 1. The right brachiocephalic trunk gives rise to the common carotid artery, vertebral artery and the subclavian artery. The left subclavian artery originates from the aortic arch as the last major branch. The subclavian artery continues as the axillary artery after crossing the lateral margin of the first rib. The axillary artery then gives rise to the superior and lateral thoracic arteries and the arteries that supply the shoulder region. After coursing beyond the inferior lateral margin of the teres major muscle, the axillary artery becomes the brachial artery. The brachial artery courses along the medial aspect of the upper arm and gives rise to the deep brachial artery and arteries around the elbow joint (Fig. 2). Anteriorly in the antecubital fossa, the brachial artery divides into the radial

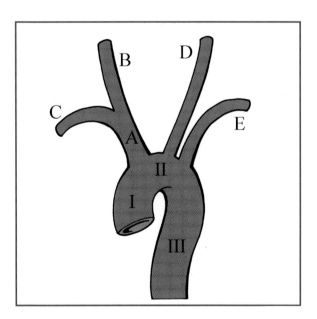

Fig. 1. Schematic drawing of the aortic arch
I   Ascending aorta
II Aortic arch
III Descending aorta

A Brachiocephalic trunk (innominate artery)
B Right common carotid artery
C Right subclavian artery
D Left common carotid artery
E Left subclavian artery

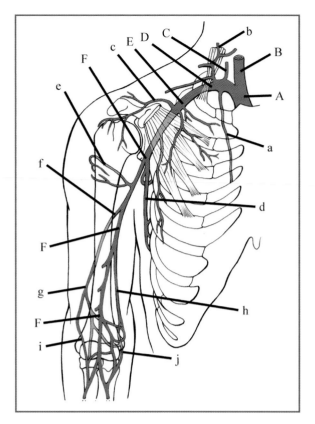

Fig. 2. Schematic drawing of the arterial anatomy of the right upper arm
A Brachiocephalic trunk (innominate artery)
B Right common carotid artery
C Right vertebral artery
D Right subclavian artery
E Right axillary artery
F Right brachial artery

a   Internal thoracic artery
b Thyreocervical trunk
c Thoracoacromeal artery
d Dorsal thoracic artery
e Anterior and posterior humeral circumflex artery
f Deep brachial artery
g Collateral radial artery
h Collateral ulnar artery
I Recurrent radial artery
j Recurrent ulnar artery

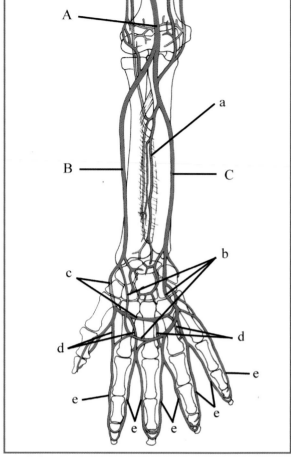

Fig. 3. Schematic drawing of the arterial anatomy of the right lower arm and the hand
A Brachial artery
B Radial artery
C Ulnar artery

a Interosseus artery
b Superficial arch
c Deep arch
d Metacarpal arteries
e Digital arteries

and ulnar arteries. The radial artery courses along the radial side of the forearm to the wrist, and then turns medially to give rise to the deep palmar arch. The ulnar artery is generally larger than the radial artery, and, at the level of the wrist, gives rise to the deep palmar arch and a superficial branch to the superficial arch. The superficial palmar arch is usually the more prominent and distal of the arches (Fig.3). Although many variants exist, the deep palmar arch is usually complete (97% of cases) with variations much less common than in the superficial arch [2]. The metacarpal and digital arteries arise from these palmar arches.

Techniques for CE MRA of the Upper Extremities

The basic principle behind CE MRA is that imaging is performed during the arterial first pass of a paramagnetic contrast agent in the vessel of interest after intravenous injection [3]. The delay between arterial and venous enhancement provides a time-window for preferential arterial imaging. This arterial-venous time-window depends on the rate of contrast agent injection, but also on the anatomical region being imaged. In the upper extremity, venous return is much faster than in the lower limbs, thereby conferring a markedly reduced period of time for preferential arterial enhancement (short arterial-venous time window). Since the technique depends on imaging of the first pass of the contrast agent, accurate timing of the start of image acquisition after contrast agent injection is essential. Various techniques have been developed to calculate this so-called scan-delay (see below).

The quality of the MRA images with regard to selective arterial visualization, resolution and volume of interest depends both on the sequence parameters used and on the geometry of the contrast agent bolus. Likewise, arterial enhancement depends not only on individual physiologic parameters such as cardiac output and blood volume, but also on contrast agent application parameters such as flow rate, dose and volume of saline flush, all of which can be manipulated. The T1-shortening of blood depends on the intravascular concentration of the contrast agent, which in turn depends on the rate of injection. In general, the faster the injection rate, the higher the arterial concentration of gadolinium contrast agent. However, injection rates exceeding 5 mL/sec do not result in any further increase in signal intensity. In fact, intravascular signal may become lower at rates higher than 6 mL/sec [4].

As with other CE MRA applications, one must always attain a balance between imaging time, resolution and arterial-venous time-window. The scan duration for imaging of the relatively large subclavian and brachial arteries can be relatively short since the spatial resolution does not have to be particularly high and the scan volume can be reasonably small. Therefore, in the upper arms, a flow rate of 2-3 mL/sec is usually adequate.

A heavily T1 weighted spoiled gradient echo sequence (short TR, short TE, flip angle 25-50°) is usually sufficient. The achievable field-of-view, matrix size, scan volume and number of partitions are determined by the arterial/venous time-interval. Subtraction of pre- and postcontrast images is performed to permit selective visualization of just the arteries. This facilitates a greater ease of image interpretation and reduces image artifacts [5]. The use of parallel imaging techniques (e.g. SMASH [simultaneous acquisition of spatial harmonics] or SENSE [sensitivity encoding]) permits a significant reduction in overall examination time, which can be used to improve spatial resolution.

The volumetric data set obtained (containing high signal intensity voxels corresponding to arteries) can be post processed using maximum intensity projection (MIP) or volume rendering algorithms. In many cases improved diagnostic performance can be achieved by reviewing the individual source images or by reformatting images in the transverse plane.

Imaging Protocols

To image the subclavian and brachial arteries a moderately thick slab of 80-90 mm is required. Pre- and post-contrast images are obtained during breath-hold to avoid image blurring of the intrathoracic portions of the vessels. When a conventional gadolinium contrast agent is used a bolus of 0.1-0.2 mmol/kg is typically injected at an injection rate of 2-3 mL/sec. Venous overlay can be avoided by injecting the contrast agent in the contralateral arm. Use of a body phased array coil results in higher signal-to-noise ratios.

MRA of the hand vessels is still a challenge due to the limited arterial/venous time window and the need for high spatial resolution imaging [6, 7]. The head coil or, preferably, a dedicated surface coil should be used to obtain images with as high a spatial resolution as possible. The arterio-venous transit time in the hands is short (approximately 12 seconds) and differs between the two hands in almost all cases (mean difference 4.5 seconds) [8]. Imaging of the arteries in the hand requires accurate timing of the start of image acquisition, preferably using a sequence with elliptically reordered k-space sampling. Wentz et al developed a promising technique for CE MRA of the hand vessels using timed arterial compression (tac-MRA) [9]. In this method, a blood-pressure cuff is placed around the upper arm and inflated after the first pass of contrast agent in order to arrest the flow in the arm. This lengthens the arterial-venous time window enabling a lengthening of the examination times in order to acquire images with higher spatial resolution than those obtained using standard first pass CE MRA without compression. Radial, ulnar and arch arteries also appear sharper with tac-MRA than with standard CE MRA.

Timing of Image Acquisition

In CE MRA, accurate timing of the start of data acquisition with the arrival of contrast agent in the vessels of interest is essential. It is crucial that arterial enhancement coincides with acquisition of central k-lines. For adequate arterial/venous differentiation, the central k-lines have to be sampled before venous return. Essentially three methods have been developed to ensure proper timing.

1. Test Bolus

Adequate timing can be performed by measuring the circulation time after the intravenous injection of a small test bolus (1-2 mL) of contrast agent using a rapid dynamic imaging sequence. With this dynamic series, the arrival time of the test bolus in the region of interest can be imaged and therefore the scan-delay can be calculated. In order to avoid pooling of the test bolus in veins, the tubing has to be flushed with saline. Both the test bolus and the final infusion should be injected at the same rate. This timing method is fairly robust and easy to perform. A disadvantage is that the test bolus method requires an additional administration of contrast agent although it lengthens the total procedure time by only 2-3 minutes. However in some cases as for example in patients with an irregular heart rate, the circulation time calculated from the test bolus may differ from the actual arrival time of the bolus during the CE MRA study.

2. Fluoroscopic Triggering

Fast imaging sequences can be used to visualize the influx of contrast agent into the region of interest. MRA data acquisition is then started automatically or manually (MR Smart-Prep [10] or "bolus track" [11]). A disadvantage of this method is the delay of 2-4 seconds that occurs between visualizing the arrival of the contrast bolus and the actual start of acquisition. Also the time available to give breathing instructions, if required, may be too short.

3. Time-resolved Imaging

With ongoing improvements in hardware and gradient technology the time required to image a large volume of interest with high resolution has been greatly reduced [12]. Therefore by acquiring a dynamic volumetric series of CE MRA datasets after intravenous injection of the contrast agent, the arterial phase will always be included in one of the datasets, thereby obviating the need for accurate bolus timing.

Image Presentation

To encourage acceptance of the technique by referring clinicians, one has to provide images in a format to which they are accustomed and which appear similar to what they are used to in conventional angiography. The number of images should be limited for ease of reference by vascular surgeons. The images should be large enough to be viewed from a distance, using a four- or six-on-one printing format. Also bony landmarks should be provided for better orientation, as occurs with images from conventional angiography.

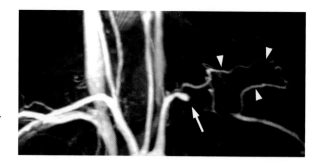

Fig. 4. The MIP reconstruction of a CE 3D MRA dataset obtained in a 54-year old patient (Gd-BOPTA, 0.1 mmol/kg) shows artherosclerotic occlusion of the left subclavian artery (*arrow*) distal to the origin of the vertebral artery with good regional collateral circulation (*arrowheads*) [Image courtesy of Dr. G. Schneider]

Clinical Applications

Atherosclerosis

Atherosclerosis frequently affects the proximal segments of the upper extremity vessels. Usually, these lesions remain clinically silent due to excellent regional collateral circulation (Fig. 4). Atherosclerosis in the forearm and hand vessels, although less frequent, leads to progressive stenoses and occlusions (Fig. 5). The slow progression induces development of multiple small, tortuous collateral vessels. Frequently, multiple severe stenoses may be present before symptoms occur.

Aneurysms

Aneurysms of the upper limbs occur less frequently than those of the legs. They are frequently secondary to arterial trauma. Other less frequent causes are atherosclerosis, mycotic aneurysm, postoperative pseudoaneurysm and aneurysms due to arteritis (Fig. 6).

Subclavian Steal Syndrome

Severe or complete stenosis of the subclavian artery proximal to the origin of the vertebral artery may lead to reversal of flow within the ipsilateral vertebral artery to supply the distal subclavian artery and ipsilateral upper extremity. This condition, referred to as subclavian steal syndrome, may lead to reduced vertebrobasillar blood flow which may be accentuated during exercise of the affected extremity. Clinical presentation and symptoms vary and depend on the anatomy of the circle of

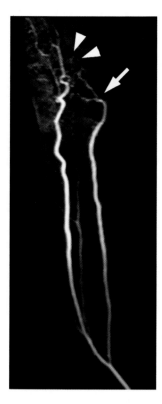

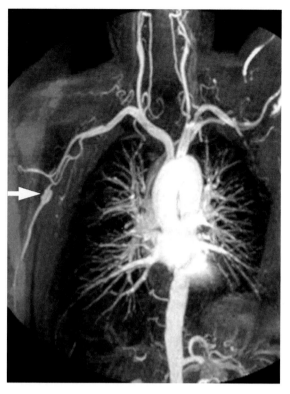

Fig. 5. The MIP reconstruction of a CE 3D MRA dataset (Gd-BOPTA, 0.1 mmol/kg) shows atherosclerotic stenosis and occlusion (*arrows*) of the radial deep and superficial arch as well as occlusion of several metacarpal arteries (*arrowheads*) [Image courtesy of Dr. G. Schneider]

Fig. 6. MRA in a patient with Takayasu arteritis and aneurysm formation (*arrow*) of the right brachial artery

Willis and the patency of the carotid system. Often collateral blood supply via the thyrocervical trunk, internal mammary artery, and branches of the external carotid and intercostal arteries may also be present.

Subclavian steal syndrome is most often an acquired condition, commonly due to atherosclerosis. Other potential causes are chest trauma, extrinsic compression by fibrosis or tumor, arteritis (Takayasu), radiation fibrosis, and fibrodysplasia. It can be congenital, such as in association with coarctation of the aorta, hypoplasia of the transverse aortic arch or proximal subclavian arteries, or coarctation of the aorta with aberrant branching of the subclavian artery. In 75% of patients, the left side is involved. With CE MRA stenosis or occlusion in the proximal subclavian artery can be demonstrated (Fig. 7). During the same exam, phase contrast velocity mapping can be used to document retrograde flow in the vertebral arteries (i.e. subclavian steal) [13].

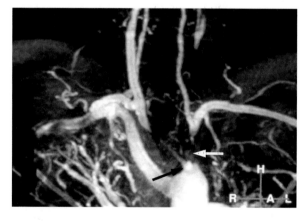

Fig. 7. MRA findings in a patient with severe atherosclerosis. The MIP image of the aortic arch reveals a common origin of both carotid arteries (*black arrow*) with severe stenosis of the right and occlusion of the left carotid artery. Furthermore, occlusion of the left brachiocephalic artery (*white arrow*) and steal in the left vertebral artery can be seen

Takayasu Arteritis

Takayasu disease is a primary arteritis of unknown etiology, usually afflicting younger patients, particularly Asian women. It affects the aorta and its major branches as well as the pulmonary
artery. Stenosis is the most common angiographic
finding in the aorta and its branches (Fig. 8), but
occlusion, aneurysm, and dilatation may also be
found (Fig. 6) [14]. Conventional angiography in
these patients is not without risk due to the increased frequency of ischemic complications,
probably related to the increased blood coagula-
tion activity in these patients [14].

In a study of 20 patients with Takayasu disease,
all 80 lesions in the aorta and its branch vessels
were detected with CE MRA [15]. However, seven
(2%) stenotic lesions in the branch vessels were
overestimated as occlusions. This may have been
related to a limitation in spatial resolution.

Early inflammation of the aortic wall can be
demonstrated on transverse images after contrast
agent injection [16].

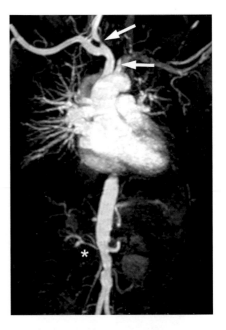

Fig. 8. MR angiogram of a 37-year old patient with Takayasu disease and stenosis of the right common carotid artery (*arrow*), occlusion of the left carotid and brachiocephalic arteries (*arrow*) and
stenosis of the right renal artery (*asterisk*)

Thoracic Outlet Syndrome

This syndrome refers to neurovascular complaints
caused by compression of the subclavian vessels or
the brachial plexus in the costoclavicular area. This
may arise due to anatomic variations in osseous
structures in this region (e.g., cervical ribs, but only in cases of completely developed anomalous
first rib) or to a broad insertion of the scalenus
muscle anteriorly on the clavicle. Other acquired
causes include fractures of the clavicle or first ribs
with imperfect alignment or excessive callus formation.

Patients may present with pain in the arm during elevation, loss of sensation during exercise, a
palpable thrill over the subclavian artery, diminished radial pulses and lowered brachial blood
pressure. Although neural compression is much
more common than vascular compression in this
syndrome, stenosis in the subclavian artery can be
demonstrated on CE MRA.

Dymarkowsky et al [17] found arterial compression in 3 of 5 patients suspected of having thoracic outlet syndrome. They performed time-resolved CE MRA of the subclavian arteries during
adduction and hyper-abduction of the arms. The
cause of the compression may be visible on T1-
weighted spin echo images.

Imaging of Extra-anatomic Bypasses

CE MRA also appears useful for surveillance of extra-anatomic bypass grafts. These grafts are typi-

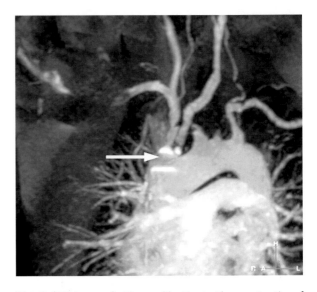

Fig. 9. MRA image of a 58 year old patient with reconstruction of
the right sublavian artery and the left common carotid artery (*arrow*) by means of an inverted small bifurcation prothesis

cally made of PTFE or Dacron since vein grafts are
not used in the upper extremity. Examples in the
upper limbs are carotid-subclavian bypass, reconstruction of innominate and subclavian arteries
(Fig. 9) and axilloaxillary bypass. Also, the axillary
artery is often used as a source of inflow in patients with lower extremity disease (axillofemoral
bypass), who are not candidates for direct aortic
reconstruction or in whom angioplasty or stenting
has failed (Fig. 10).

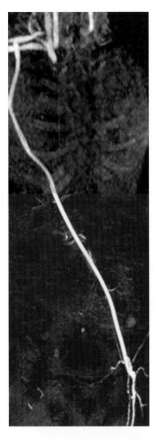

Fig. 10. Reconstruction of a double station MRA in a patient with an axillofemoral bypass

Imaging of Hemodialysis Access Fistulas

In general early and late complications in hemodialysis shunts have to be distinguished. Typically, early complications relate to surgical problems or atypical draining veins (Fig. 11). Late complications in hemodialysis shunts may occur in the feeding artery, the arterial anastomosis (Fig. 12), the fistula itself, the venous anastomosis and the draining vein (Fig. 13). Arterial complications are relatively infrequent; most common problems are due to stenoses at the venous anastomosis, most often due to intimal hyperplasia. Stenosis in hemodialysis arteriovenous fistulas is usually associated with thrombosis of the access. It is also important to visualize the draining veins, since stenoses of outflow veins remote from the fistula may occur. These are probably related to the unusual arterial pressure to which these veins are subjected (Fig. 14).

Recognition of the cause of impaired access function is important to prevent complete thrombosis of the dialysis fistula. The role of MRA in imaging of these fistulas has been evaluated in various studies [18-21]. Although CE MRA is less sensitive to disturbed flow compared to conventional nonenhanced techniques (PC and TOF MRA), flow

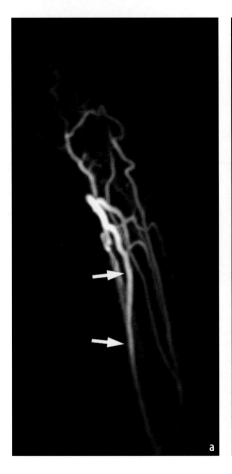

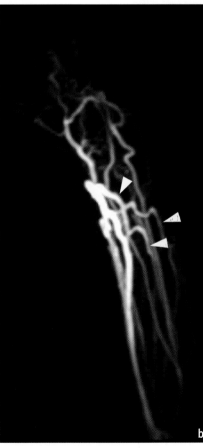

Fig. 11a. b. Postsurgical CE MRA study in a patient with dialysis access fistula of the lower arm in which insufficient flow was present for adequate dialysis. MIP reconstruction of two consecutive CE 3D MRA datasets (Gd-BOPTA, 0.1 mmol/kg; acquisition time per dataset 4 sec) demonstrates first (**a**) early enhancement of the fistula vein (*arrow* in **a**) and (**b**) increasing drainage into collateral veins (*arrowheads* in **b**). After surgical occlusion of the collateral veins sufficient flow was achieved [Images courtesy of Dr. G. Schneider]

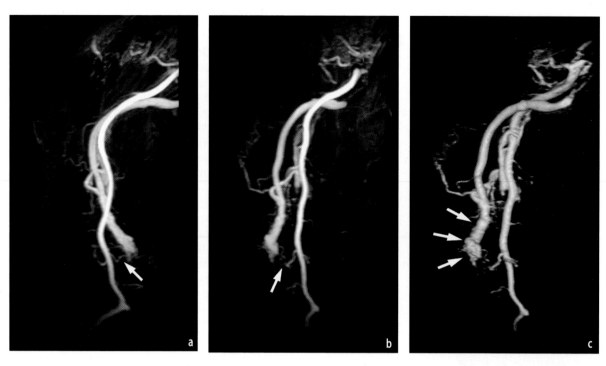

Fig. 12a-c. MIP reconstruction of a CE 3D MRA dataset (Gd-BOPTA, 0.1 mmol/kg) demonstrating artherosclerotic occlusion of the arterial anastomosis in a hemodialysis shunt (*arrows* in **a**, **b**). Note the irregular surface of the shunt (*arrows* in **c**) after 3-year access for hemodialysis [Images courtesy of Dr. G. Schneider]

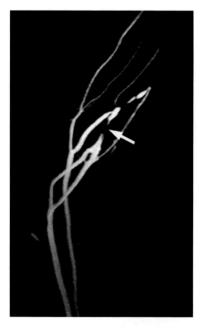

Fig. 13. High grade stenosis of the draining vein in a hemodialysis shunt (*arrow*) as demonstrated on CE MRA [Image courtesy of Dr. G. Schneider]

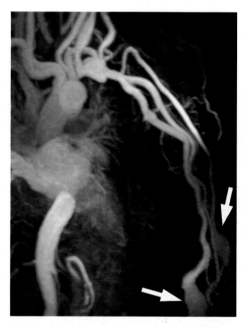

Fig. 14. Normal appearance of a hemodialysis shunt with two draining veins (*arrows*) which were both used for puncture [Image courtesy of Dr. G. Schneider]

related artifacts may still be present under the extreme flow conditions that can occur in dialysis fistulas (flow rates may range 100-3, 000 ml/min). Bos et al [22] eliminated these flow artifacts by temporal interruption of the flow by means of an inflated cuff placed around the upper arm. They

injected gadolinium contrast agent diluted 20:1 with saline directly into the fistula. On image evaluation, they found a slightly (3.7%) higher degree of stenosis on CE MRA compared to DSA which they concluded was due either to a real overestimation of stenosis on MRA because of limited res-

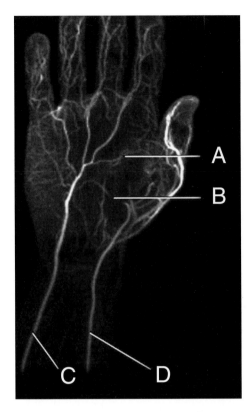

Fig. 15. CE MRA of the hand in a 28 year old volunteer. Both superficial (A) and deep (B) arches are visible and complete. (C = ulnar artery, D = radial artery)

olution, or to an underestimation of luminal diameter on DSA. They found low interobserver variation both with MRA (3.2%) and DSA (3.6%).

One advantage of CE MRA is that images are acquired in 3D, and can be reformatted to visualize the fistula in any desired plane. Also functional information on the hemodialysis access can be obtained by performing flow measurements [23]. However, an important disadvantage of MRA is that no interventions can be performed, at least using current commercial products.

Pathology of Hand Vessels

Atherosclerosis in the hand vessels is rare. Indications for imaging of the hand vessels in general may include arterial mapping prior to plastic surgery or radial artery bypass grafting (Fig. 15), hypothenar hammer syndrome [24], suspected emboli from cardiac disease or atherosclerotic lesions in the subclavian artery, Raynaud's syndrome, thrombangitis obliterans (Fig. 16) (Winiwarter-Buerger's disease), scleroderma, rheumatoid arthritis, vasculitis and repetitive trauma. Raynaud's syndrome or suspected distal emboli are particular indications for CE MRA, since DSA is generally not performed because of the risk of complications.

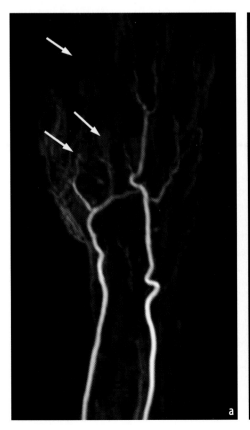
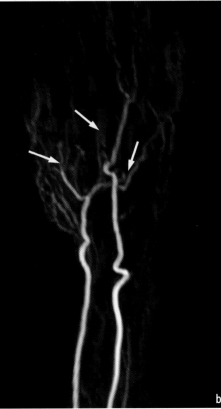

Fig. 16a, b. Thrombangitis obliterans (Winiwarter-Buerger's disease) in a 28-year old male patient. The MIP reconstructions of a CE 3D MRA dataset (Gd-BOPTA, 0.1 mmol/kg) demonstrate a missing deep arch together with occlusion of numerous metacarpal and digital arteries and interruption of the superficial arch [Images courtesy of Dr. G. Schneider]

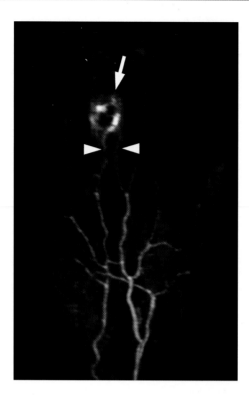

Fig. 17. CE 3D MRA dataset (Gd-BOPTA, 0.1 mmol/kg) in a patient with an angioma-like tumor of the finger. The MIP reconstruction demonstrates the tumor (*arrow*) as an early enhancing mass. Furthermore, an arterial supply of the lesion by the radial and ulnar digital artery (*arrowheads*) of the 3rd finger can be demonstrated. This is important for surgical planning [Image courtesy of Dr. G. Schneider]

Another indication would be for the pre-surgical evaluation of soft-tissue tumors of the hand and fingers since MRA can be combined noninvasively with imaging of the tumor in a one-stop shop procedure (Fig. 17).

In general, interpretation of hand MR angiograms can be considered difficult because of the numerous variations in hand vasculature.

Pitfalls

Although signal loss due to turbulence and in-plane saturation is usually not present in CE MRA, overestimation of the length of a stenosis can still occur especially at high velocity rates at the stenotic area and with a low concentration of contrast agent [25].

Other artifacts may also be encountered in CE MRA. For example, in the subclavian region susceptibility artifacts in the subclavian vein may result in signal void and thus an artificial stenosis of the adjacent artery [26]. Susceptibility artifacts may also occur due to signal voids arising from the presence of clips and metallic stents. Finally, as in all CE MRA procedures, subtraction misregistration artifact may also occur.

New Developments

MRI Technique

Ongoing improvements in hardware and gradient strength result in shorter scan times enabling improved time-resolved imaging at high resolution. Time-resolved imaging will continue to improve with higher spatial and temporal resolution, and faster real-time reconstruction. Besides obviating the need for contrast bolus timing, time-resolved imaging also adds an extra dimension to imaging of the peripheral arteries. Due to the dynamic nature of the acquired series it is possible to visualize differences in the influx of contrast agent in the two limbs, in a manner similar to that achievable with conventional angiography.

Further developments will see the more frequent use of dedicated coils for peripheral vascular imaging. These dedicated coils will not only permit acquisition of images with higher resolution and greater signal-to-noise ratio; but, in the case of the phased array coils, may also aid in reducing imaging times by allowing the acquisition of data in parallel. With the SMASH and SENSE techniques, combinations of coils can be used to compensate for omitted gradient steps. The increase in imaging speed can be used to reduce acquisition times or to increase the spatial resolution of the scan. Finally, widespread application of MR systems operating at higher field strengths (3T or even 7T) will probably lead to further improvements, especially for imaging of small blood vessels, such as hand arteries.

Contrast Agents

Although new intravascular MR contrast agents are currently being evaluated in clinical trials, their possible role in peripheral MRA is questionable. Because of the short arterio-venous window in the upper extremity, intravascular blood pool agents are at present not useful due to the rapid venous overlap. Probably only agents with higher relaxivity such as gadobenate dimeglumine (MultiHance, Gd-BOPTA; Bracco Imaging SpA) [8] or more highly concentrated agents such as gadobutrol (Gadovist, Schering AG), may be applied successfully to MR imaging of the small vessels in the hand [6].

Conclusion

CE MRA is now a routine procedure in many radiology departments. Although MRA of the upper extremities is less often performed than MRA of the lower extremities, there are clear indications for non-invasive imaging of the vessels of the arm and hand. Upper extremity MRA, however, is much more technically demanding than lower extremity MRA, since the arterio-venous time window is much shorter and the vessels (especially in the hand) are much smaller.

References

1. Ho KY, de Haan MW, Oei TK et al (1997) MR angiography of the iliac and upper femoral arteries using four different inflow techniques. Am J Roentgenol 169:45-53
2. Coleman SS, Anson BJ (1961) Arterial patterns in the hand based upon a study of 650 specimeens. Surg Gynecol Obstet 113:409-424
3. Prince MR, Yucel EK, Kaufman JA et al (1993) Dynamic gadolinium-enhanced three-dimensional abdominal MR arteriography. J Magn Reson Imaging 3:677-881
4. Kopka L, Vosshenrich R, Rodenwaldt J et al (1998) Differences in injecting rates on contrast-enhanced breath-hold three-dimensional MR angiography. Am J Roentgenol 170:345-348
5. Ho KY, de Haan MW, Kessels AG et al (1998) Peripheral vascular tree stenosis: detection with subtracted and nonsubtracted MR angiography. Radiology 206:673-681
6. Winterer JT, Ennker J, Scheffler K et al (2001) Gadolinium-enhanced elliptically reordered three-dimensional MR angiography in the assessment of hand vascularization before radial artery harvest for coronary artery bypass grafting: first experience. Invest Radiol 36:501-508
7. Krause U, Pabst T, Kenn W et al (2002) High resolution contrast enhanced MR-angiography of the hand arteries: preliminary experiences. Vasa 31:179-184
8. Winterer JT, Scheffler K, Paul G et al (2000) Optimization of contrast-enhanced MR angiography of the hands with a timing bolus and eliptically reordered 3D pulse sequence. J Comput Assist Tomogr 24:903-908
9. Wentz KU, Frohlich JM, von Weymarn C et al (2003) High-resolution magnetic resonance angiography of hands with timed arterial compression (tac-MRA). Lancet 361:49-50
10. Foo TKF, Saranathan M, Prince MR et al (1997) Automated detection of bolus arrival and initiation of data acquisition in fast, three-dimensional MR angiography image quality. Radiology 203:275-280
11. Leiner T, Ho KY, Nelemans PJ et al (2000) Three-dimensional contrast-enhanced moving-bed infusion-tracking (MoBi-track) peripheral MR angiography with flexible choice of imaging parameters for each field of view. J Magn Reson Imaging 11:368-377
12. Frayne R, Grist TM, Swan JS et al (2000) 3D MR DSA: effects of injection protocol and image masking. J Magn Reson Imaging 12:476-487
13. Yamada I, Numano F, Suzuki S. (1993) Takayasu arteritis: evaluation with MR imaging Radiology 188:89-94
14. Yamato M, Lecky JW, Hiramatsu K et al (1986) Takayasu arteritis: radiographic and angiographic findings in 59 patients. Radiology 161:329-334
15. Yamada I, Nakagawa T, Himeno Y et al (2000) Takayasu arteritis: diagnosis with breath-hold contrast-enhanced three-dimensional MR angiography. J Magn Reson Imaging 11:481-487
16. Choe YH, Han BK, Koh EM et al (2000) Takayasu's arteritis: assessment of disease activity with contrast-enhanced MR imaging. Am J Roengenol 175:505-511
17. Dymarkowski S, Bosmans H, Marchal G et al (1999) Three-dimensional MR angiography in the evaluation of thoracic outlet syndrome. Am J Roentgenol 173:1005-1008
18. Planken RN, Tordoir JH, Dammers R et al (2003) Stenosis detection in forearm hemodialysis arteriovenous fistulae by multiphase contrast-enhanced magnetic resonance angiography: preliminary experience. J Magn Reson Imaging 17:54-64
19. Cavagna E, D'Andrea P, Schiavon F et al (2000) Failing hemodialysis arteriovenous fistula and percutaneous treatment: imaging with CT, MRI and digital subtraction angiography. Cardiovasc Intervent Radiol 23:262-265
20. Laissy JP, Menegazzo D, Debray MP et al (1999) Failing arteriovenous hemodialysis fistulas: assessment with magnetic resonance angiography. Invest Radiol 34:218-24
21. Gehl HB, Bohndorf K, Gladziwa U et al (1991) Imaging of hemodialysis fistulas: limitations of MR angiography. J Comput Assist Tomogr 15:271-275
22. Bos C, Smits JH, Zijlstra JJ et al (2001) MRA of hemodialysis access grafts and fistulae using selective contrast injection and flow interruption. Magn Reson Med 45:557-561
23. Bakker CJ, Bosman PJ, Boereboom FT et al (1996) Measuring flow in hemodialysis grafts by non-triggered 2DPC magnetic resonance angiography. Kidney Int 49:903-905
24. Winterer JT, Ghanem N, Roth M et al (2002) Diagnosis of the hypothenar hammer syndrome by high-resolution contrast-enhanced MR angiography. Eur Radiol 12:2457-2462
25. Mitsuzaki K, Yamashita Y, Onomichi M et al (2000) Delineation of simulated vascular stenosis with Gd-DTPA-enhanced 3D gradient echo MR angiography: an experimental study. J Comput Assist Tomogr 24:77-82
26. Neimatallah MA, Chenevert TL, Carlos RC et al (2000) Subclavian MR arteriography: reduction of susceptibility artifact with short echo time and dilute gadopentetate dimeglumine. Radiology 217:581-586

VII.2

MR Angiography of Peripheral Arteries: Lower Extremities

James F.M. Meaney

Clinical Indications/Background

Although atherosclerotic narrowing can affect any artery in the body, by far the most common site is the lower extremity [1-4]. In the US, arteriosclerotic lower limb disease is responsible for approximately 60,000 percutaneous angioplasty procedures and 100,000 amputations [4]. Because of the widespread and systemic nature of the disorder and the multiplicity of lesions that typically occurs, accurate "mapping" of the arterial tree is essential to guide appropriate percutaneous or surgical intervention. Although this was traditionally only possible with conventional catheter arteriography [5-7], usually performed with a subtraction technique, recent developments in MRA now offer the potential for comprehensive non-invasive evaluation of the vasculature from above the aortic bifurcation to pedal arch. The limitation of poor spatial coverage in the cranio-caudal direction due to limited magnet bore length in relation to the large field-of-view requirement has been overcome by implementation of the "moving-table" technique. Other competing non-invasive modalities such as duplex ultrasound have failed to establish a widespread role in management of peripheral vascular disease [3, 8]. Multi-detector CT (MDCT) although promising shares with DSA the drawbacks of exposure of the patient to ionizing radiation and nephrotoxic contrast agents and has not undergone systematic review [9].

Clinical Presentation

Patients with peripheral vascular disease may present with one of the following two syndromes [1-4]:

1. Acute ischaemic syndrome (Rest pain or tissue necrosis):

Acute interruption of arterial supply almost always causes irreversible tissue amage and resultant tissue loss (gangrene). Two scenarios are encountered:

- Acute arterial embolism from a diseased heart valve, most often in a patient with atrial fibrillation. Many of these patients do not have a precedent history of intermittent claudication. These patients uncommonly present for MRA as patients are typically treated immediately by percutaneous catheter directed thrombolysis or surgical embolectomy.
- Patients with prior intermittent claudication, with "acute-on-chronic" symptoms.

2. Chronic ischaemic syndrome (Intermittent claudication):

Responsible atherosclerotic lesions occur anywhere from the infra-renal abdominal aorta to the feet and multiple distal lesions may mimic a single more proximally placed lesion. Multiple lesions are the rule. However, as the disease tends to affect the lower limbs asymmetrically, patients usually present with unilateral symptoms. However, pre-existing "asymptomatic" disease on one side may be "masked" by successful treatment of the symptomatic limb.

Fontaine has developed the following classification for clinical staging of peripheral artery occulusive disease PAOD (Table 1).

Table 1. Fontaine classification

Stage	Manifestation
I	Asymptomatic (Pulse deficit only on examination)
II	Arterial insufficiency with exercise (Pulse deficit + claudication)
III	Arterial insufficiency at rest (Pulse deficit + rest pain)
IV	Local tissue loss (Pulse deficit + gangrene)

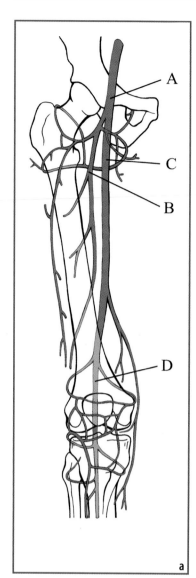

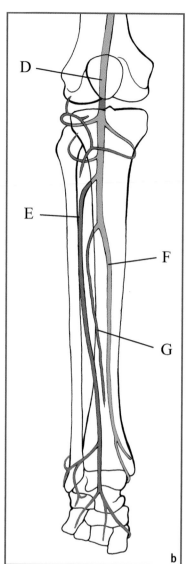

Fig. 1 a, b. Normal anatomy of the leg
A   Common femoral artery
B   Deep femoral artery
C   Superficial femoral artery
D   Popliteal artery
E   Anterior tibial artery
F   Posterior tibial artery
G   Peroneal artery

Normal Anatomy (Figs. 1, 2)

The abdominal aorta bifurcates at L4 level into the common iliac arteries. The common iliac artery bifurcates into internal iliac and external iliac arteries in front of the sacro-iliac joints at the level of L5/S1. The internal iliac artery travels inferiorly towards the sciatic foramen and divides into the anterior trunk (which supplies via numerous named arteries the pelvic viscera) and the posterior trunk (which supplies the muscles of the lateral pelvis). The external iliac artery becomes the common femoral artery where it crosses under the inguinal ligament, approximately half way between the anterior superior iliac spine and pubic tubercle. There are three branches of the external iliac artery, the superficial pudendal and superficial in-

ferior epigastric arteries which arise medially (rarely identified on moving table MRA), and the superficial circumflex epigastric artery which arises laterally, and which is usually identified on MRA especially in patients with PAOD as it forms one of the collateral pathways that typically enlarges in response to significant stenoses or occlusions of the iliac arteries. The common femoral artery, a short artery of 4-6 cms only, is the continuation of the external iliac artery but no identifiable anatomic landmark separates these structures on MRA. The common femoral artery divides into the profunda femoris artery, a medium sized artery arising from the lateral aspect and which typically gives 4 perforating muscular branches to the thigh in addition to the medial and lateral circumflex arteries, and the superficial femoral artery, the direct

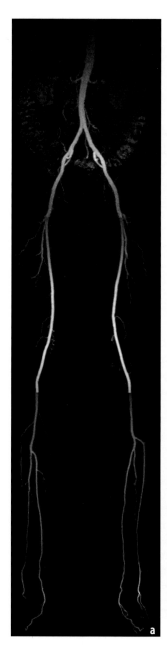

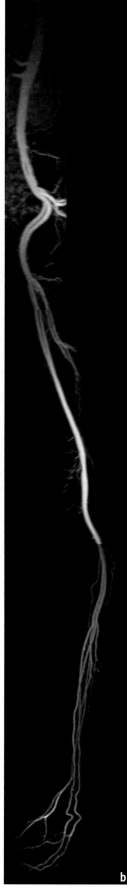

Fig. 2. Normal anatomy: Moving table CE-MRA of the lower extremity arteries gives adequate anatomic coverage of the relevant anatomy with three overlapping coronally oriented acquisitions. Note that different imaging volumes have been used for each of the three anatomic regions (demonstrated on lateral MIPs)

continuation of the CFA, which has no branches in the thigh. The SFA becomes the popliteal artery on passing through the adductor hiatus in the distal thigh, approximately at the junction of the upper two thirds and lower third of the femur. Upon entering the adductor canal the SFA gives rise to the medial and lateral genicular branches, which typically enlarge and form collateral channels in patients with severe stenosis or occlusion of the SFA.

Below the knee, the popliteal artery gives rise to the anterior tibial artery, usually the largest of the infrapopliteal arteries, and the peroneal (typically the smallest) and posterior tibial arteries, which arise from a common stem, the tibio-peroneal trunk. These arteries are collectively known as the "trifurcation" or "run-off" vessels.

The anatomy of the pedal arch and foot vessels will be described in the foot chapter.

Indications for MRA

There is currently no agreement on use of MRA for patients with PAOD. However, because MRA delivers similar information to DSA, without the associated risks of iodinated contrast material [10, 11] or arterial catheterization [5-7] it is appropriate to consider MRA in ANY patient referred for catheter arteriography, however, some patients deemed to be at high risk of complications of conventional arteriography may be particularly suited to assessment with MRA [12]. Table 2 lists the patients that may benefit from MRA.

Overview of Techniques

Time-of-Flight MRA

Prior to the introduction of CE-MRA, time-of-flight (TOF) MRA was used to evaluate the peripheral arteries. Because this technique is now rarely used (apart from niche indications, discussed later), the technique will not be described in detail and the reader is referred to Chapter I.1 on unenhanced MRA for a detailed description of the technique. However, in order to place the technique in historical context and to illustrate why CE-MRA has virtually replaced TOF MRA for the peripheral arteries, a short description of the limitations follows:

Limitations of TOF MRA

Despite the fact that "time-of-flight" MRA gave encouraging results compared to DSA (Tables 1-3) [13-22], it never became universally accepted as an acceptable alternative to arteriography primarily

Table 2. Indications for MRA

Potentially any patient in whom catheter angiography is requested
Patients in whom catheter angiography has failed to demonstrate all of the relevant arterial segments
Patients with poor or absent arterial access
Patients with prosthetic vascular grafts
Patients with impalpable femoral pulses
Patients with common-femoral, iliac or aortic occlusion which prevents appropriate placement of a catheter
Patients with any other contra-indication to arteriography
Patients with renal impairement
Patients with hypersensitivity to iodinated contrast material
Female patients of child-bearing age

because of the inherent limitations of an "inflow" based technique, as follows.

1. Studies, although non-invasive, were extremely time consuming. Long scan times were enforced by three limitations, all related to the need to maximize "inflow" as follows:
   - Mandatory use of the axial scan plane (gives "worst-fit" geometry for the lower extremity arteries which predominantly run in a head-foot direction)
   - A relatively long TR is essential (i.e. substantially greater than the shortest TR available and "long" in relation to that used for CE-MRA) because the "inflow" requirement mandates use of TR of 30msec or greater (adversely affects scan time compared to use of shortest available TR of 5msec or less on most systems)
   - Slow, absent, or in the case of severely diseased arteries, reversed diastolic flow mandates use of cardiac triggering with a further time penalty.
2. Images were prone to artefactual over-estimation of the degree and length of stenosis, because of intra-voxel dephasing secondary to turbulent, slow and pulsatile flow. This is one of the inherent drawbacks of the technique, however, it is particularly troublesome both in regions of stenoses and also in locations where the vessels follow an "in-plane" course (common iliac artery and horizontal initial part of the anterior tibial artery).
3. The length of occlusions was frequently over-estimated due to elimination of the retrograde component of flow in patients with distally reconstituted vessels by the trailing inferior saturation pulses designed to suppress venous flow.

Thus, TOF MRA has failed to offer a viable non-invasive screening test to conventional arteriography, and has not had a major impact on clinical practice.

Advantages of Contrast-Enhanced MRA Over Non-Contrast Techniques?

1. The technique is "flow-independent": CE-MRA relies on paramagnetic contrast agent induced T1 shortening for generation of intra-vascular signal [24, 25].
2. Therefore, lowest available TR's can be used which give shortest possible scan times.
3. The unique nature of the k-space domain exquisitely lends itself to some modifications that can be exploited to generate superior quality peripheral CE-MRA's [26]. For example, because central k-space data governs image contrast (and peripheral k-space governs resolution), images with unrivalled SNR are rapidly generated provided the contrast-defining central lines of k-space are synchronized with peak arterial enhancement. The fact that peripheral lines (determine resolution) are acquired during the venous phase does not adversely impact on image quality.
4. Optimized acquisition plane: As images are independent of "inflow-effects" 3D data-sets data be acquired in the **coronal plane** (which affords the greatest anatomical coverage for any combination of field-of-view, number of slices and slice thickness).
5. As selective arterial images are generated by appropriate timing of the 3D data-set in relation to the arterio-venous window, neither saturation bands (that may impair SNR in 2D TOF MRA) nor ECG triggering (that prolong scan time) are required.
6. The limitation of reduced spatial coverage in the cranio-caudal direction has been overcome by implementation of moving table technology [27, 28], which extends the FOV to encompass all of the relevant anatomy (and whole body if necessary – see Chapter VII.4 on Whole Body MRA)[29].

Table 3. Advantages and disadvantages of multi-station, multi-injection MRA

Advantages	Disadvantages
As the examination essentially consists of two discrete scans, scan parameters and image resolution can be optimized for each location	Because of background (venous and parenchymal) signal from the first injection, it is essential to perform image subtraction at 2nd ne 3rd locations
Dedicated moving-table software is not required	Although effective in removing venous signal, subtraction of intra-arterial signal persisting from the first injection will adversely affect the final subtracted image quality for locations subsequent to the first
	Clinical experience shows that elimination of venous signal in the legs (third station) is not reliably performed even with subtratction
	A three location study mandates use of a single dose (0.1mmol/kg) only at each location, if dosing regulations are not to be exceeded

Because of these combined advantages CE-MRA has largely replaced 2D TOF methods for evaluation of the peripheral arteries.

Contrast-Enhanced MRA of the Peripheral Vasculature

Three different approaches may be used, as follows:

1. Single-station MRA of the peripheral arteries [18,19,30]

This approach evaluates a single field-of-view only, and relies on prediction of the site of pathology by clinical or imaging (e.g. duplex) criteria. However, anatomical prediction of the location of occlusive lesion is difficult and multiple lesions occur at discrete sites, many of which lie outside a single-field-of-view in the majority of patients. Although of proven efficacy, this approach is mostly used for evaluating parts of the peripheral vasculature that have been "missed" by arteriography, especially the pedal arteries in patients in whom distal bypass grafting is an option. And, the approach plays an essential role in imaging patients with aortic or bilateral iliac occlusion where catheter arteriography is not possible. See Chapter VI.1 on aorto-iliac arteries as an example of "single-station" CE-MRA.

2. Multi-station, multi-injection MRA of the peripheral arteries [31]

This approach employs a single-station MRA at each of two or three consecutive locations, with a separate injection for each location. Although proven in clinical practice, this technique is now rarely employed since refinements in moving-table approach have been made (Table 3).

3. Moving Table Contrast-Enhanced MRA [27,28, 32-35]

By moving the patient rapidly through the iso-center of the magnet and acquiring 3D data-sets at three coronally-oriented overlapping FOV's, it is possible to image the arteries of the entire lower half of the body during a single contrast injection (Fig. 2-7). Initially, this approach employed manual movement of the table-top (detached from the drive mechanism) by the operator and "fixed" imaging parameters (scan volume, resolution, etc.) for all locations. Although successful, the requirement for higher resolution of the infra-popliteal vessels (due to their small size) and requirement to minimize acquisition time for the first two locations (to reduce venous enhancement within the legs) has fuelled advances in technology as follows:

- Automated table movement (a "floating" table)
- Resolution optimized individually for each location [36]
- Imaging volume optimized individually for each location [36]

Table 4 summarizes the advantages and disadvantages of moving-tabel CE-MRA.

The main challenge of MT CE-MRA is to eliminate or reduce to an acceptable level the degree of venous-enhancement in the 3rd location, which may degrade images of the infra-popliteal arteries.

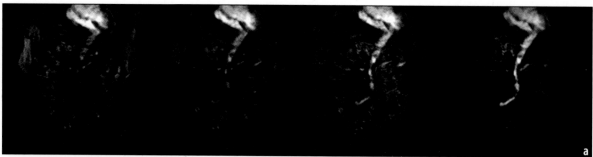

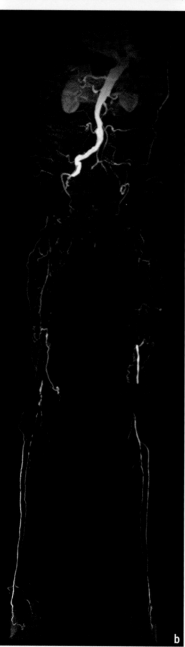

Fig. 3a, b. a Images from a time-resolved single thick slice MR fluoroscopic detection sequence (1 image/second) demonstrating arrival of contrast within the aorto-iliac arteries over 4 consecutive images. **b** There is occlusion of the right common and right superficial femoral arteries with reconstitution of flow into diffusely diseased popliteal artery. There is a good anterior tibial artery, a diffusely diseased but patent peroneal artery and occlusion of the posterior tibial artery. On the left side, there is occlusion of the common and external iliac arteries, and also of the superficial femoral artery throughout its length. The popliteal reconstitutes for a short distance, before occluding at the level of the joint with further reconstitution of popliteal flow more distally. There is a good left anterior tibial artery with a stenosis above the ankle joint, a diffusely diseased but patent peroneal artery, and occlusion of the left posterior tibial artery

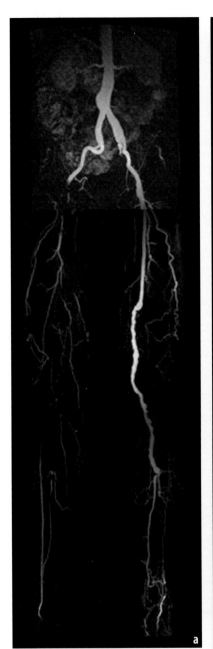

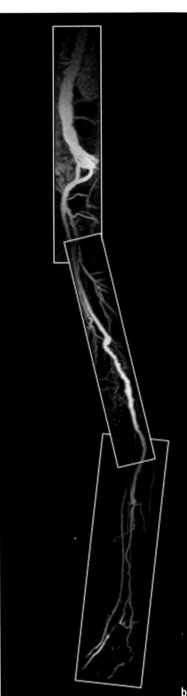

Fig. 4a, b. Frontal (**a**) and lateral (**b**) MIPs demonstrate occlusion of the right superficial femoral and popliteal arteries, with a single patent infrapopliteal artery (the anterior tibial which reconstitutes via collaterals). On the left side, note diffuse aneurysmal disease of the distal SFA and popliteal arteries. The posterior tibial artery is patent and enlarged, the peroneal artery is occluded and the left anterior tibial artery is of small caliber

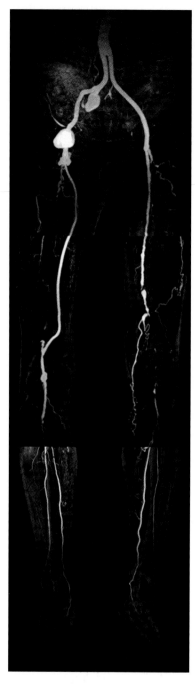

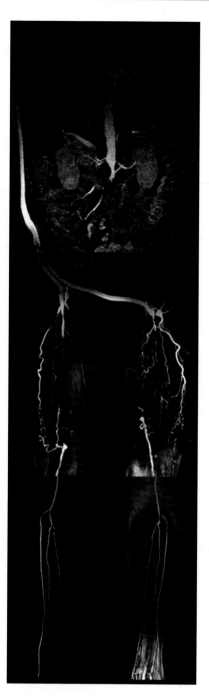

Fig. 5. Male patient with a previous history of aorto bi-femoral and right femoro-popliteal grafting. Note the typical appearance of the two limbs of the aorto bi-femoral graft. There is a 4cm aneurysm of the native right internal iliac artery. There is also an anastomotic pseudoaneurysm of the right common femoral artery in the right groin. The right femoro-popliteal graft is patent. The right anterior and posterior tibial arteries appear normal. On the left side, there is a tight stenosis in the distal superficial femoral artery just proximal to the point where the superficial femoral artery occludes within the adductor canal. Note the large collateral which runs medially and which conveys blood to the posterior tibial artery which appears normal throughout its length. Normal left peroneal artery, the anterior tibial artery is occluded

Fig. 6. 78 year old patient with Leriche syndrome in whom an axillo-femoral bypass graft has been constructed. There is occlusion of the aorta just below the level of the renal arteries and also occlusion of the iliac arteries bilaterally. Note the bifurcated right axillo-femoral graft which anastomoses with the profunda femoris arteries on both sides. Note occlusion of the superficial femoral artery on both sides, with reconstitution of flow into the popliteal artery on each side via well marked collaterals. Despite the severe proximal disease, three run-off arteries are identified on both sides

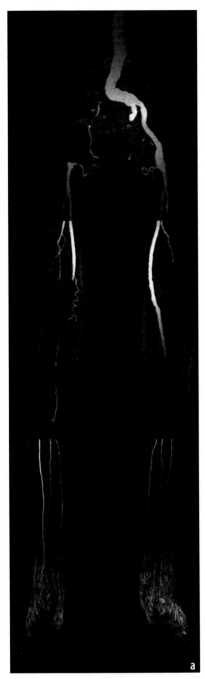

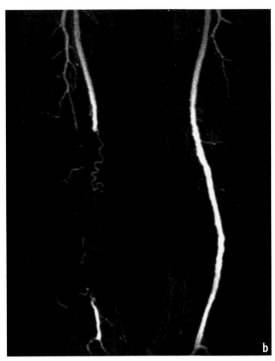

Fig. 7a, b. a Note fusiform aneurysmal disease of the infra-renal abdominal aorta, left common and left external iliac arteries. On the left side, there appears to be occlusion of the poplitreal artery, however, the appearance is somewhat unusual in that the signal intensity within the artery gradually drops of towards the "occlusion". A repeat single-station MRA of the thigh arteries alone 24 hours later (**b**) demonstrates a patent left popliteal artery, emphasizing the fact that the "pseudo-occlusion" was due to slow flow within the left SFA. Note occlusion of the right common and external iliac arteries and distal right superficial femoral arteries

Table 4. Advantages and disadvantages of moving table MRA of the peripheral arteries

Advantages	Disadvantages
It addresses the issue of extended anatomic coverage in the most time-efficient manner	It requires additional software and hardware
It makes the most efficient use of a single bolus	
In some instances results in less venous enhancement than other multi-station approaches	Although this approach offer a practical solution to the limitation of reduced spatial coverage, it is limited by the fact that, even using fast gradients, acquisition of high-resolution 3D MRA data at three consecutive locations takes substantially longer than the transit time from aorta to leg arteries, thus increasing the likelihood of venous enhancement within the legs which undoubtedly impairs image quality.

Venous Enhancement: Why Does it Occur at the 3rd but not the First two Stations? (Fig. 8)

Venous enhancement is virtually unknown in the aorto-iliac station, as commencement of imaging is signalled by contrast arrival in the region-of-interest (timing bolus/bolus detection, etc.). This is also true for the femoro-popliteal segment assuming a relatively short acquisition time for the 1st location (8-12seconds), rapid table movement (<4 seconds) and use of centric phase-encoding (i.e. sampling of central k-space data at the start of the scan) for the 2nd location. However, with MT-MRA, data collection at the 3rd location is delayed until scan data for the first two locations is completed. Venous enhancement occurs in the 3rd location when the combined imaging time for the first two locations (plus two table movements) is greater than the circulation time from aorta to calf *vein*. Although the transit time from aorta to calf artery varies widely, the transit time through the tissues gives additional time for arterial- phase imaging. Although superficial and mild enhancement within the deep veins is acceptable, substantial "problematic" venous enhancement is more common in patients with fast flow states (e.g. cellulitis/venous ulcers/diabetes). Because of the conflicting demands of higher resolution (lengthens scan time)

and elimination of venous enhancement (requires shorter scan time), each examination represents a challenge to trade-off one against the other. Therefore, careful optimization of MT peripheral MRA is required as follows:

1. Imaging at the first location (aorto-iliac) is commenced as soon as contrast arrives in the region-of-interest (timing bolus/bolus detection, etc.) to ensure that there is no "knock-on" delay for leg imaging. In our department we use 2D MR fluoroscopy which allows visualization of contrast arrival in real-time (Fig. 3a) [37-39].

2. Contrast infusion rate. The infusion must be tailored to the length of the first two scans + table movement x 2 + acquisition of the central lines of k-space for the 3rd location (the first few seconds only). In our institution we use a tailored biphasic injection rate (e.g. an initial injection rate of 1cc/sec x 10 secs, followed by 0.6-1.0cc/sec x 20cc) [40-42].

3. Use image subtraction. Superimposition of subcutaneous and marrow cavity fat on the lower extremity arteries in the AP plane might not be problem with faster infusion rates. However, the lower infusion rates mean that the enhancing arteries are not be clearly differentiated from fat on MIP images. Subtraction of a pre-contrast mask essentially eliminates fat-signal from the post-contrast image and gives dramatically improved image quality [43].

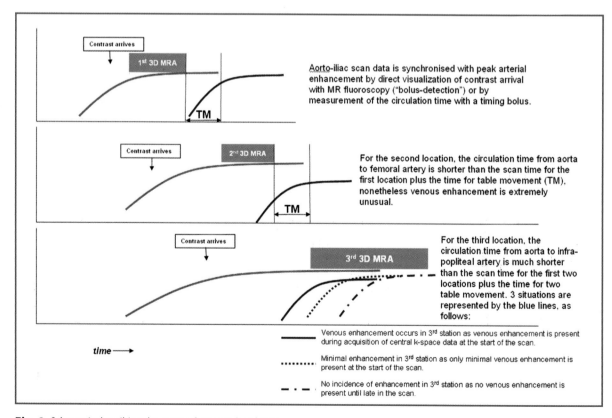

Fig. 8. Schematic describing the approach to peripheral MRA

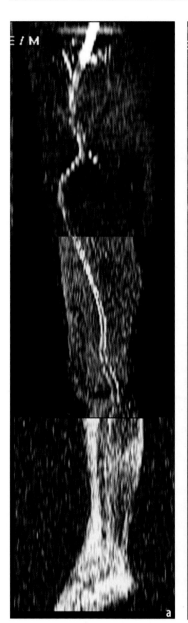 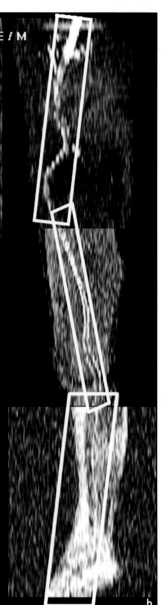

Fig 9. Lateral (**a**) MIP images generated from the low-resolution 2D time-of-flight localizer that allow appropriate positioning of the 3D volumes (*shown* in **b**)

4. Use optimized k-space filling strategies: Whilst "centric" k-space data acquisition reduces the likelihood of venous enhancement at all locations, it also facilitates higher resolution imaging of the (smaller) legs arteries by allowing acquisition of resolution-defining peripheral k-space mapping to continue regardless of venous enhancement.

5. Tailor the 3D scans to the anatomy and use individually tailored scan parameters for each ROI.

* **Localizer.** The localizer is more critical for MT-MRA than for any other CE-MRA application. The goal of arterial phase imaging over three consecutive locations can only be achieved if the smallest possible imaging volume per location can be prescribed. We use a low-resolution gradient-echo "time-of-flight" scan in the axial plane taking (approximately 1 minute per loca-

tion). Anterior and lateral MIP's generated from the axial data-set facilitate accurate 3D volume placement. Using manufacturer-specific moving-table software, localizers can now be acquired from the aorta to the level of the ankles, thus allowing accurate tailoring of the 3D volume for all three locations (Fig. 9).

* **Resolution.** 3D volumes with sufficient resolution to allow accurate grading of stenosis within the arteries of interest must be acquired at each of three successive locations. As the arteries progressively decrease in size from aorta to foot, it is advantageous to prescribe independent volumes at all three locations, with highest resolution reserved for the legs. Whilst isotropic voxels are ideal, in-plane spatial resolution and through-plane resolution must be sacrificed in

favour of shorter scan times. In-plane resolution for the aorto-iliac and thigh arteries of 1.2-1.6 mm (160-200 phase-encode steps) and through-plane resolution of 3-4mm (slices reconstructed to 1.5-2mm by interpolation or zero-padding) is sufficient. For the 3rd location, higher in-plane and through-plane resolution is required. It is essential to use centric phase-encoding to minimize venous enhancement at this station.

Patient Preparation

The patient is placed supine on the table top. In order to prevent change in patient position between the pre- and post-contrast images, the legs should be gently fixed in position using Velcro pads or some other suitable fixation device. Slight elevation of the heels on (rigid) foam pads often offers a comfortable position for the patient. If a dedicated peripheral coil is available, simply placing the patient within the coil usually gives sufficient immobilization. Supplemental oxygen may be used if appropriate, and may improve the patients breath-holding capability if examination of the renal arteries (requires breath-holding) is included in the evaluation. Headphones are placed on the patients head to allow communication with the operator.

An IV cannula is placed in an upper extremity vein. The connector tubing is attached to the mechanical injector if available.

Choice of Coil

- Best option: A dedicated peripheral MRA coil gives best results (the coil typically extends from pelvis to foot arteries) [46].
- Next best option: Use a "moving" coil that remains in the magnet bore by sliding over the patient as the patient is moved between locations.
- Acceptable option: Use the integral body coil for signal transmission/reception for the 1st and 2nd locations, and a flexible phase array coil (e.g. a torso phase array coil) for evaluation of the legs (where the arteries are smallest).
- Worst option: Use the integral body coil for signal transmission/reception for all locations. Although this was the approach initially used for moving table peripheral MRA with excellent results [27, 28] it is no longer recommended due to higher clinical expectation and refinements in technique that accept multi-channel coils.

Can I still do Moving Table Peripheral MRA even if I don't have a Dedicated Moving Table?

The answer is of course yes. However, there are several important drawbacks as follows:
1. 3D volumes independently tailored to the different anatomic locations is not possible (or at best extremely difficult). Therefore, lower resolution imaging must be accepted.
2. Registration of the pre-contrast mask and the post contrast images for subtraction is impossible without use of a home-made table position registration device.
3. The warranty on the MRI scanner may be voided if an un-approved method for moving the table is used.

Post-Processing (see Chapter I.4)

The MIP forms the basis of image display. Although other reconstruction algorithms such as surface-shaded display and video "angioscopy" (fly-through) are available, the MIP gives a satisfactory overview of the affected arteries and is the format closest to image display for conventional arteriography [48]. There is no universally accepted format for display of reconstructed images; however, the following format is widely accepted:
1. All data-sets should be interrogated using multi-planar reformatting, whole volume and sub-volume MIP, to optimally demonstrate the arterial tree.
2. For the pelvis, at least three projections, corresponding to "standard" angiographic projections should be generated.
3. For the thighs, AP MIP's corresponding to "standard" angiographic projections should be generated.
4. For the legs, AP MIP's corresponding to "standard" angiographic projections should be generated in addition to
5. A lateral view of the ankle is essential in cases where vessels are identified to the level of the ankle joint.
6. Sub-volume MIP's of each renal artery and the visceral arteries where appropriate.

Novel Methods for Increasing Acquisition Speed and Reducing Venous Enhancement

Two methods offer promise for increasing acquisition speed overall, as follows:

1. Hybrid techniques combining both 2D and 3D acquisitions

2D images offer much shorter scan times compared to 3D imaging. For the arteries of the thighs and legs, due to the fact that the arteries course between muscle groups, there is no potential for increased tortuosity with increasing age. Therefore, thick 2D images (with a slice thickness appropriate to the anatomy – typically 6-8 cms) with complex subtraction and high in-plane spatial resolution can be achieved in a short scan time (<3secs), however, there is no through-plane resolution (52, 53). Because of the tortuosity of the arteries of the pelvis, and the fact that the renal artery origins overlap the aorta on single frontal images, 2D imaging is not appropriate for this location (theoretically multiple oblique 2D images could be acquired although this has not yet been validated), and therefore 3D imaging must be used for the first locations. The advantage of 2D imaging therefore is probably as part of a hybrid technique that uses 3D acquisitions for the aorto-iliac location, 2D for the thighs, and 2D or 3D for the legs and feet [49-51].

2. Parallel Imaging

This approach gives increased acquisition speed by utilization of multiple phase-array coils with known sensitivities. Scan time is typically reduced by a factor of two, although higher SENSE factors may be used which give greater time savings. There is an SNR penalty proportional to the square root of the time saving (i.e. halving the scan time gives an SNR penalty of $\sqrt{1/2}$ = 30% penalty). For any SENSE factor, all of the savings can be exploited in the interests of more rapid imaging, the resolution can be doubled for any scan time, or a combination of the two can be used. SENSE is particularly attractive for the peripheral vasculature, where most of the time savings can be invested in more rapid imaging for the first two locations, with use of much higher resolution for the legs [44, 45].

3. Slow down the circulation

Use tourniquets to slow down the flow rate and therefore diminish the chance of venous enhancement within the legs [47]. Compression of the veins at mid thigh level by means of an inflatable cuff is a simple method for reducing venous enhancement within the legs that can be implemented without costly hardware or software upgrades. It is ideally suited to and facilitates high-spatial-resolution imaging of the lower extremity arterial system using a moving table approach with a single injection of contrast material. This is a modification of the "tac" (timed arterial compression technique) used for upper extremity. However, for upper extremity MRA a cuff is inflated to supra-arterial pressures(e.g. 200 mm Hg) but this approach would almost certainly not be tolerated by patients with lower extremity arterial disease. Standard lower extremity blood pressure cuffs can be used, however, dual cuffs which provide bilateral thigh compression are currently being evaluated.

Summary of Clinical Results

Numerous studies attest to the applicability and clinical success of both TOF MRA (Table 5) and moving-table CE-MRA (Table 6). Of importance is

Table 5. Accuracy of 2D TOF MRA for significant (>50%) stenosis or occlusion by territory

Author	Year	# Patients	# Segments	Sens (%)	Spec (%)
Aorto-iliac arteries:					
Baumgartner	1993	15	15	82	100
Glickerman	1996	23	161	89	98
Snidow	1996	42	68	100	23
Quinn	1993	30	118	94	91
Yucel	1993	25	93	93	83
Poon	1997	15	90	100	86
Femoro-popliteal arteries:					
Baumgartner	1993	15	26	88	100
Glickerman	1996	23	324	88	98
Snidow	1996	42	170	92	82
Yucel	1993	25	82	93	92
Infra-popliteal arteries:					
Glickerman	1996	23	384	86	91
Snidow	1996	42	88	92	91
McDermott	1995	24	216	89	91

Table 6. Accuracy of 2D TOF MRA for significant (>50%) stenosis or occlusion by territory

Author	Year	# Patients	# Segments	Sens (%)	Spec (%)
Ho	1997	28	242	92	93
Yamashita	1998	20	140	96	83
Meaney	1999	20	620	85	93
Ruehm	2001	61	1739	92	98
Rofsky	2000	15	150	97	96

Table 7. Summary of results of three recent meta-analyses

	Technique studies	# Patients	# Segments	Sens (%)	Spec (%)	DOR*
Nelemans[52]	2D TOF	13	344	64-100	68-96	1.0
	3D CE-MRA	10	253	92-100	91-99	7.46
Koelemay[53]	2D TOF	18	474	69-100	73-97	1.0
	3D CE-MRA		482	85-97	83-98	2.8
Visser & Hunink [54]	3D CE-MRA	9	216	97.5	96.2	
	Duplex US	18	1059	87.6	94.7	

*The diagnostic odds ratio (DOR) a powerful method for comparing techniques and gives the odds of a positive test in a diseased person compared to the odds if a diseased test in a non-diseased person

the fact that peripheral MRA has been subjected to three meta-analyses of the reported literature (Table 7) [52-54].

Future Developments

Currently, examination of the entire "run-off" arteries relies on acquisition of three "static" acquisitions in rapid exploiting three coronal oriented overlapping acquisitions. However, researchers recently devised a method for data acquisition using continuous table motion [54, 55]. Although in its infancy, this technique offers promise for the future as another novel and potentially useful method for peripheral MRA. Newer contrast agents, including "blood-pool" agents and those with higher relaxivity potentially offer significant advantage over existing agents [56-58]. Continuous refinements in pulse sequence methodology and the potential for functional assessment in the future offer further promise for improved peripheral MRA techniques.

Conclusion

Moving-table contrast-enhanced MRA offers substantial advantages over other techniques for evaluating the lower extremities, and, if successful, results in comprehensive non-invasive evaluation of all of the relevant vascular territory.

References

1. Fowkes FG, Housley E, Cawood EH et al (1991) Edinburgh Artery Study: prevalence of asymptomatic and symptomatic peripheral arterial disease in the general population. Int J Epidemiol. 20:384-92
2. Voyt NT, Wolfson SK, Kuller LH (1992) Lower extremity arterial disease and the ageing process: a review. J Clin Epidemiol 45:529-542
3. Dormandy JA, Rutherford RB, Kalra M et al (2000) Management of peripheral arterial disease (PAD). TASC Working Group. Trans Atlantic Inter-Society Concensus (TASC). J Vasc Surg 31:S192-274
4. Jenkins GD, Stanson AW, Toomey BJ et al (2001) Limb salvage after successful pedal bypass grafting is associated with improved long-term survival. J Vasc Surg 33:6-16
5. Bron KM (1983) Femoral arteriography. In: Abrams HL, Ed. Abrams Angiography: Vascular and Interventional Radiology. Boston: Little, Brown 1835-1876
6. Waugh JR, Sacharias N (1992) Arteriographic complications in the DSA era. Radiology 182:243-246
7. Reidy JF, Ludman C (1996) Technical note: safety of outpatient arteriography using 3F catheters. Br J Radiol 66:1048-52
8. Wilson YG, George JK, Wilkins DC et al (1997) Duplex assessment of run-off before femorocrural reconstruction. Br J Surg 84:1360-3
9. Ota H, Takase K, Igarashi K et al (2004) MDCT compared with digital subtraction angiography for assessment of lower extremity arterial occlusive disease: importance of reviewing cross-sectional images. AJR Am J Roentgenol 182(1):201-9
10. Tepel M, avn Der Giet M, Schwarzfeld C et al (2000)

Prevention of radiographic contrast agent induced reductions in renal function by acetylcysteine. N Engl J Med 343:180-4

11. Conlon PJ, O'Riordan E, Kaldra PA (2000) New insights into the epidemiological anda clinical manifestations of atherosclerotic renovascular disease. Am J Kidney Dis 35:573-587

12. Brillet PY, Vayssairat M, Tassart M et al (2003) Gadolinium-enhanced MR angiography as first-line preoperative imaging in high-risk patients with lower limb ischemia. J Vasc Interv Radiol Sep; 14(9 Pt 1):1139-45

13. Owen RS, Carpenter JP, Baum RA et al (1992) Magnetic Resonance Imaging of angiographically occult runoff vessels in peripheral arterial occlusive disease. N Engl J Med 326:157-1581

14. Baumgartner I, Maier SE, Koch M et al (1993) Magnetresonanzarteriographie, Duplexsonographie und konventionelle Arteriographie zur Beurteilung der peripheren arteriellen Vers-chlusskrankheit. Rofo Fortschr Geb Rontgenstr Neuen Bildgeb Verfahr 159:167-173

15. Quinn SF, Demlow TA, Hallin RW et al (1993) Femoral MR angiography versus conventional angiography: preliminary results. Radiology 189:181-184

16. Yucel EK, Kaufman JA, Geller SC et al (1993) Atherosclerotic occlusive disease of the lower extremity: prospective evaluation with two-dimensional time-of-flight MR angiography. Radiology 187:635-641

17. Glickerman DJ, Obregon RG, Schmiedl UP et al (1996) Cardiac-gated MR angiography of the entire lower extremity. A prospective comparison with conventional angiography. Am J Roentgenol. 167:445-451

18. Snidow JJ, Johnson MS, Harris VJ et al (1996). Three-dimensional gadolinium-enhanced MR angiography for aorto-iliac inflow assessment plus renal artery screening in a single breath hold. Radiology 198:725-729

19. Poon E, Yucel EK, Pagan-Marin H et al (1997) Iliac artery stenosis measurements: comparison of two-dimensional time-of-flight and three-dimensional dynamic gadolinium-enhanced MR angiography. Am J Roentgenol 169:1139-1144

20. Ho KY, de Haan MW, Oei TK et al (1997) MR angiography of the iliac and upper femoral arteries using four different inflow techniques. Am J Roentgenol 169:45-53

21. McDermott VG, Meakem TJ, Carpenter JP et al (1995) Magnetic resonance angiography of the distal lower extremity. Clin Radiol 50:741-746

22. Carpenter JP, Golden MA, Barker CF et al (1996) The fate of bypass grafts to angiographically occult runoff vessels detected by magnetic resonance angiography. J Vasc Surg 23: 483

23. Cortell ED, Kaufmann JA, Geller SC et al (1996) MR angiography of tibial run-off vessels: imaging with the head coil compared with conventional arteriography. Am J Roentgenol 167:147-151

24. Prince MR (1994) Gadolinium-enhanced MR aortography. Radiology 191:325

25. Prince MR, Narasimham DL, Stanley JC et al (1995)

Breath-hold gadolinium-enhanced MR angiography of the abdominal aorta and its major branches. Radiology 197:785-671

26. Mezrich R (1995) A perspective on k-space. Radiology 195: 297-315

27. Ho KY, Leiner T, de Haan MW et al (1998) Peripheral vascular tree stenoses: evaluation with moving-bed infusion-tracking MR angiography. Radiology 206:683-92

28. Meaney FM, Ridgway JP, Chakraverty S et al (1999). Stepping-Table Gadolinium-enhanced Digital Substraction MR Angiography of the Aorta and lower extremity Arteries: Preliminary Experience. Radiology 211:59-67

29. Ruehm SG, Goyen M, Barkhausen J et al (2001) Rapid magnetic resonance angiography for detection of atherosclerosis. Lancet 357:1086-91

30. Kreitner KF, Kalden P, Neufang A et al (2000). Diabetes and peripheral arterial occlusive disease: prospective comparison of contrast-enhanced three-dimensional MR angiography with conventional digital subtraction angiography. AJR Am J Roentgenol 174:171-9

31. Rofsky NM, Johnson G, Edelman MA et al (1997) Peripheral vascular disease evaluated with reduced-dose gadolinium-enhanced MR angiography. Radiology 205:163-169

32. Sueyoshi E, Sakamoro I, Matsuoko Y (1999) Aortoiliac and lower extremity arteries: comparison of three-dimensional dynamic contrast-enhanced subtraction MR angiography and conventional angiography. Radiology 210:683-8

33. Ruehm SG, Hany TF, Pfammater T et al (2000) Pelvic and lower extremity arterial imaging: diagnostic performance of three-dimensional contrast-enhanced MR angiography. AJR Am J Roentgenol 174:1127-35

34. Yamashita Y, Mitsuzaki K, Ogata I et al (1998) Three-dimensional high resolution dynamic contrast-enhanced MR angiography of the pelvis and lower extremities with use of a phased array coil and subtraction. J Magn Reson Imaging 8:1066-1072

35. .Ho VB, Choyke PL, Foo TK et al (1999) Automated bolus chase peripheral MR angiography: initial practical experiences and future directions of this work-in-progress. J Magn Reson Imaging 10:376-88

36. Leiner T, Ho KYJAM, Nelemans PJ et al (2000) Three-Dimensional Contrast-Enhanced Moving-Bed Infusion-Tracking (MoBI-Track) Peripheral MR Angiography With Flexible Choice of Imaging Parameters for Each Field of View. JMRI 11:368–377

37. Prince MR, Chenevert TL, Foo TK et al (1997) Contrast-enhanced abdominal MR angiography: Optimization of imaging delay time by automating the detection of contrast material arrival in the aorta. Radiology 203:109-114

38. JFM Meaney, RC Fowler, M Saysell et al (1999) Visualisation of Bolus arrival for 3D contrast enhanced renal MRA: Use of large field of view dynamic single slice 2-D fluoroscopic acquisition with complex subtraction, real-time reconstruction and real-time display (BolusTrak). Radiology 213(P): 271

39. Riederer SJ, Bernstein MA, Breen JF et al (2000)

Three-dimensional contrast-enhanced MR angiography with real-time fluoroscopic triggering: design specifications and technical reliability in 330 patient studies. Radiology 215:584-93

40. Kopka L, Vosshenrich R, Rodenwaldt J et al (1998) Differences in injection rates on contrast-enhanced breath-hold three-dimensional MR angiography. AJR Am J Roentgenol 170:345

41. Maki J (1997) The effect of time-varying intravascular signal intensity and k-space acquisition order on three-dimensional MR angiographic image quality. J Magn Reson Imaging 6:642-651

42. Earls JP, Rofsky NM, DeCorato DR et al (1996) Breath-hold single-dose gadolinium-enhanced three-dimensional MR aortography: usefulness of a timing examination and MR power injector. Radiology 201:705-710

43. Ho KY, de Haan MW, Kessels AG et al (1998) Peripheral vascular tree stenoses: detection with subtracted and nonsubtracted MR angiography. Radiology 206:673-81

44. Weiger M, Pruessmann KP, Kassner A et al (2000) Contrast-enhanced 3D MRA using SENSE. J Magn Reson Imaging 12:671-7

45. Maki JH, Wilson GJ, Eubank WB (2002) 3D Gd-Enhanced moving table peripheral MR angiography using multi-station SENSE to include the pedal vasculature. Book of abstracts, p 1743. Presented at the ISMRM annual meeting, May 2002, Honolulu

46. FM Vogt, Ajaj W, Hunold P et al (2004) Quick, Jörg F. Debatin, and Stefan G. Ruehm. Venous Compression at High-Spatial-Resolution Three-dimensional MR Angiography of Peripheral Arteries Radiology Oct. (ePub ahead of print)

47. Goyen M, Ruehm SG, Barkhausen J et al (2001) Improved multi-station peripheral MR angiography with a dedicated vascular coil. J Magn Reson Imaging 13:475-480

48. Hany TF, Schmidt M, Davis CP et al (1998) Diagnostic impact of four post-processing techniques in evaluating contrast-enhanced Three-dimensional MR Angiography AJR Am J Roentgenol 170: 907-912

49. Lee HM, Wang Y et al (1998) Distal Lower Extremity arteries: Evaluation with two-dimensional MR digital subtraction angiography. Radiology 207:505-512

50. Maki JH, Ephron JH, Glickerman DJe et al (2000) Moving Table Gd-Enhanced MR Angiography of the Lower Extremities: A Combination 3D and 2D Technique – Preliminary Results (abstr.) Proceedings of the Eighth Scientific Meeting and Exhibition of the International Society for Magnetic Resonance in Medicine p 1810

51. Wang Y, Winchester PA, Khilnani NM et al (2001) Contrast-enhanced peripheral MR Angiography from abdominal Aorta to the pedal arteries. Combined dynamic two-dimensional and bolus-chase three-dimensional acquisition. Invest Radiol 36:170-177

52. Nelemans PJ, Leiner T, de Vet HCWet al (2000) Peripheral arterial disease: Meta-analysis of the diagnostic performance of MR Angiography. Radiology 217: 105-114

53. Visser K, Hunick MG (2000) Peripheral arterial disease: gadolinium-enhanced MR angiography versus color-guided duplex US - a meta-analysis. Radiology 216:67-77

54. Koelemay MJ, Lijmer JG, Stoker J et al (2001) Magnetic resonance angiography for the evaluation of lower extremity arterial disease: a meta-analysis. JAMA 285:1338-45

55. Kruger DG, Riederer SJ, Grimm RC, Rossman PJ (2002) Continuously moving table data acquisition method for long FOV contrast-enhanced MRA and whole-body MRI. Magn Reson Med 47(2):224-231

56. Knopp MV, Tengg-Kobligk H von, Froemer F, Schonberg SO (1999) Contrast agents for MRA: future directions. J Magn Reson Imaging 10:314-316

57. Tombach B, Heindel W (2002) Value of 1.0-M gadolinium chelates: review of preclinical and clinical data on gadobutrol. European Radiology 12:1550-6

58. Perreault P, Edelman MA, Baum RAeta l (2003) MR angiography with gadofosveset trisodium for peripheral vascular disease:phase II trial. Radiology 229:811-20

VII.3

Pedal MR Angiography

Jeffrey H. Maki

Clinical Indications/Background

Ischemic disease of the foot remains an important complication of atherosclerotic vascular disease, particularly in the diabetic population, who have a 15-46 times higher incidence of lower extremity amputation than do nondiabetics [1]. In fact, a large surgical review of patients undergoing venous grafting to the pedal arteries for limb salvage recorded a 95% incidence of diabetes [2]. Furthermore, 55% of these cases were complicated by infection. Other factors contributing to diabetic pedal disease include peripheral neuropathy, structural foot deformities, and soft tissue ulceration [1]. The ultimate therapeutic goal under these circumstances, as with all ischemic disease, is the restoration of pulsatile blood flow to the affected region. Thus evaluation of the ischemic foot, typically diabetic and often infected, is the most common indication for pedal angiography.

Recent surgical thinking and techniques have moved away from primary amputation toward revascularization for limb salvage in pedal ischemic disease [2-8]. This is in part because the pedal arteries (particularly the dorsalis pedis) often remain patent despite severe multilevel proximal disease, which in diabetics is most often in the infra-popliteal arteries [2, 9]. A recent study following two subgroups with limb-threatening pedal ischemia (108 patients), demonstrated that the subgroup treated with bypass grafting had a much more favorable limb preservation rate than those treated non-surgically (limb salvage rates at 1 and 24 months of 95/85% vs. 35/17% respectively) [7]. A separate ten year review of 1032 patients (92% with diabetes) undergoing dorsalis pedis grafting for limb-threatening ischemia demonstrated five year primary patency, secondary patency, and limb salvage rates of 57%, 63%, 78% respectively [3] . In this study, the inflow portion of the graft was most often the below knee popliteal artery (41%), consistent with the majority of disease being in the infrapopliteal vessels.

In order to achieve results such as these, accurate mapping and understanding of the vascular anatomy is required to optimally choose the distal anastomotic site, as outcome has been shown to be directly related to the adequacy of pedal outflow [10-12]. Thus a complete preoperative evaluation must sufficiently depict the pedal vasculature to allow for the management decision of revascularization vs. amputation vs. medical therapy. Until recently, conventional x-ray digital subtraction angiography (DSA) was considered the gold standard for evaluating peripheral vascular anatomy [10, 13]. Recent experience with peripheral magnetic resonance angiography (MRA), however, suggests MRA is superior to DSA in terms of visualizing infrapopliteal runoff vessels, and thus the term angiographically "occult" vessel emerged [9, 14-18]. Regardless of modality, pedal arterial imaging must adequately depict the arterial anatomy (see paragraph "Normal Anatomy" below). Luminal enhancement must be sufficient to define vessels to at least the distal metatarsal level, and resolution must be adequate to assess the patency of main pedal branch vessels as well as define any stenoses distal to a planned site of graft anastomosis [10]. In addition, the primary and secondary pedal arches must be evaluated for patency, as limb salvage has been shown to be related to patency of the pedal arch [10, 11, 19].

Normal Anatomy

Pedal arterial anatomy can be divided into the anterior circulation, the posterior circulation, and the pedal arches, which connect the two circulations (Figs. 1-3). The anterior circulation consists of the

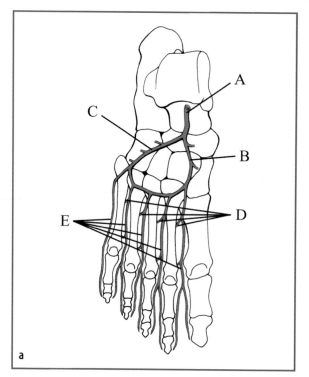

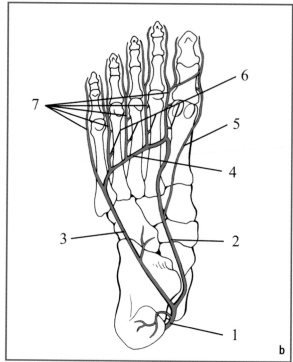

Fig. 1. Pedal arteries. Frontal (**a**) and plantar (**b**) views

a
A Anterior tibial artery
B Dorsalis pedis artery
C Lateral tarsal artery
D Perforating arteries
E Dorsal metatarsal arteries

b
1 Posterior tibial artery
2 Medial plantar artery
3 Lateral plantar artery
4 Plantar arch
5 Superficial branch
6 Perforating arteries
7 Plantar metatarsal arteries

dorsalis pedis artery, the medial and lateral tarsal arteries, the arcuate artery, and the deep plantar (or perforating) artery. These vessels are all quite small, with the dorsalis pedis artery being 2.0 – 3.0 mm in diameter [20]. The posterior circulation begins as the distal posterior tibial (or common plantar) artery, bifurcating into the medial and lateral plantar arteries. The lateral plantar artery continues as the plantar arch, which anastomoses to the deep plantar artery, thereby forming the primary pedal arch. The first dorsal metatarsal artery is the largest artery off of the primary arch, being 1.0 to 1.5 mm in diameter [20]. Secondary arches may form via

(a) the dorsalis pedis, lateral tarsal, lateral plantar, and common plantar arteries,

(b) the dorsalis pedis, the medial tarsal, the medial plantar, and common plantar arteries, or

(c) dorsalis pedis, arcuate artery, lateral plantar, and common plantar arteries (Figs. 2, 3).

In imaging, non-filling of one of these named segments cannot be considered definitive occlusion unless clearly opacified unnamed pedal vessels and collaterals are seen along its course [10].

Technique

Pedal MRA is most commonly performed as 2D TOF or 3D CE-MRA. In general, 3D CE-MRA is less prone to artifacts and of better diagnostic quality [21, 22], but we believe both should be performed, as shortcomings with either sequence may be overcome by evaluating the two exams simultaneously (Fig. 4) [23]. Other authors advocate 2D CE-MRA as an alternative to 3D-CE MRA. (24, 25) Pedal MRA can be performed as a targeted pedal only exam, as part of a multi-station complete peripheral MRA study, or as part of an entire below knee lower extremity MRA [9, 21, 23, 26]. Regardless of the context, several basic principles apply, and these will be discussed in detail.

Coils

High quality pedal MRA, like MR of any small region, requires an appropriately sized birdcage or surface phased array coil. For cases of targeted pedal only MRA, most investigators use a birdcage

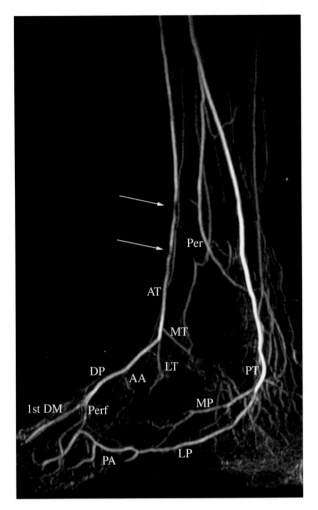

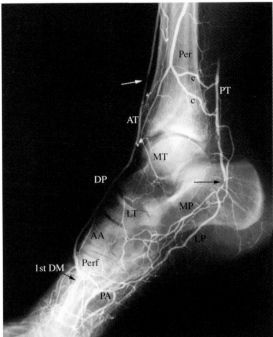

Fig. 3. Lateral DSA. AT = anterior tibial artery, PT = posterior tibial artery, Per = peroneal artery, MT = medial tarsal artery, LT = lateral tarsal artery, AA = arcuate artery, DP = dorsalis pedis artery, Perf = perforating artery, PA = plantar arch, LP = lateral plantar artery, MP = Medial plantar artery, 1st DM = first dorsal metatarsal artery. The PT is occluded proximally and reconstitutes just above the ankle via collaterals from the Per (c). There is significant disease of the PT just proximal the bifurcation into MT/LT (black arrow) and the distal PT (*white arrow*). Note the significantly better depiction of tiny vessels compared to MRA (Fig 2)

Fig. 2. Pedal MRA demonstrating anatomy of the pedal vasculature (lateral view MIP). AT = anterior tibial artery, PT = posterior tibial artery, Per = peroneal artery, MT = medial tarsal artery, LT = lateral tarsal artery, AA = arcuate artery, DP = dorsalis pedis artery, Perf = perforating artery, PA = plantar arch, LP = lateral plantar artery, MP = Medial plantar artery, 1st DM = first dorsal metatarsal artery. Note complete primary arch formed by AT, DP, Perf, PA, LP, PT. Portions of the secondary arches can be visualized. Disease is seen in the distal AT (*arrows*). This study was performed using the gadolinium blood pool agent MS-325 (EPIX Medical, Cambridge, MA) in the arterial phase

quadrature head or knee coil, although new dedicated phased array ankle coils are becoming available [9, 14, 15]. In cases where the pedal arteries are included as a part of the entire lower leg (single or multi-station), a larger field of view phased array coil is typically used [27, 29]. These can be independent one station coils (e.g. torso array), or larger arrays designed to cover the entire body from the abdominal aorta to the feet (e.g. peripheral vascular). Such coils have the advantage of being capable of imaging both feet simultaneously. Another important advantage to the phased array approach is that parallel imaging techniques such as SENSE become possible [26, 30, 31]. These tech-

niques can be used to accelerate data acquisition, accelerate volume coverage, or improve resolution.

Patient Preparation

As with all CE-MRA techniques, an intravenous line (22 g. or better) should be placed in the arm before the patient enters the magnet. The shoes should be removed, and care should be taken to ensure any metallic objects such as clips holding stretchable bandage material have been removed from the foot. When the foot is placed in the coil, a combination of padding and/or straps should be used to immobilize the foot as much as practical. Multi-element phased array coils, if used, can have decreased signal to noise secondary to cross talk if the coil elements are too close to one another, and some padding to ensure the coils remain symmetrically spaced from each other can be helpful. The foot should be in a relatively neutral position, as even moderate plantar flexion is known to cause an artifactual stenosis of the proximal dorsalis pedis artery due to compression by the inferior extensor retinaculum [32]. Care should be taken to ensure the patient is as comfortable as possible (pillows, bolster under knees, etc.) to minimize restlessness and subsequent motion.

Imaging Protocol

Sample protocols for both 2D TOF and 3D CE-MRA are shown below (Tables 1, 2). These assume unilateral pedal only imaging, and can be modified accordingly if planned as part of a peripheral study. Some general considerations follow. First, in order to accurately characterize a stenosis, true spatial resolution (in all three planes) must be such that the vessel is spanned by three pixels – i.e. resolution equals (vessel diameter)/3 [33, 34]. For pedal arteries with diameters of 2-3 mm (or even smaller), an absolute minimum resolution is 1 mm isotropic. This is not typically achievable with 2D TOF. Sec-

Table 1. Suggested parameters for 2D Time-of-Flight MRA of the pedal arteries

2D TOF MRA	
Coil	Head, knee, or phased array
Patient Positioning	Supine – feet first
CM dose/flow rate	N/A – must do pre contrast
Saturation band	Inferior
Bolus Timing	N/A
Breath-hold/free breathing	Free breathing
Sequences	2D TOF GRE
Sequence orientation	Oblique axial – angle with dorsalis pedis(23)
TR, TE, flip angle	20 ms, ~7 ms (flow comp), 60
Matrix	256 x 256, phase direction AP
FOV, # slices, st	260 x 260 mm^2, 150-200, 1.5-2.0 mm (contiguous)
Voxel size	1.0 x 1.0 x 1.5-2.0 mm^3
Acquisition time	6-8 minutes
Landmarks for slab position	Use scouts to cover anatomy
Image subtraction	N/A
Evaluation of images	Source, MIP, MPR

Table 2. Suggested parameters for 3D Contrast-Enhanced MRA of the pedal arteries

3D CE-MRA	
Coil	Head, knee, or phased array
Patient Positioning	Supine – feet first
CM dose/flow rate	20 ml, 1.5 – 2.0 cc/sec. Flush 25 ml NS
Saturation band	N/A
Bolus Timing	Axial timing bolus ankle – 2cc contrast
Breath-hold free breathing	Free breathing
Sequences	3D GRE, centric
Sequence orientation	Sagittal – phase direction AP
TR, TE, flip angle	<6.0 ms, < 2.0 ms, 35-45
Matrix	320 x 320
FOV, # slices (true/recon), st (true/recon)	280 x 182 x 65 mm^3, 54/108, 1.2/0.6 mm
Voxel size(true/recon)	0.9 x 0.9 x 1.2/0.55 x 0.55 x 0.6 mm^3
Acquisition time	~ 60 sec
Landmarks for slab position	Use TOF MIP's to show vascular anatomy
Image subtraction	Yes
Evaluation of images	MIP, MPR

ond, mask subtraction is mandatory for CE-MRA, as small pedal vessels quickly become obscured by bright signal from the fatty bone marrow. This means a pre-contrast "mask" must be obtained, and the patient must hold the foot still from that point until the contrast examination. Finally, venous contamination is particularly problematic with CE-MRA, especially in diabetic patients with ischemic soft tissue disease, where there is rapid AV shunting. Avoiding venous contamination requires precise timing with respect to contrast administration (timing bolus), or a time resolved acquisition [21, 24, 35]. Because 2D TOF MRA can saturate venous inflow using an inferior saturation band, venous enhancement is much less problematic, and TOF images can often be used to help interpret a CE-MRA otherwise clouded by venous enhancement (Fig. 4).

For the timing bolus, we suggest a single axial 1 cm thick dynamic 2D slice through the ankle using 2 cc of contrast agent injected via power injector at the anticipated contrast flow rate (Fig. 5a). Both this timing dose as well as the diagnostic dose should be flushed with at least 25 cc of saline. Acquisition should be at least 1 image every 2 sec (for a total duration of approximately 120 sec), with simultaneous initiation of timing dose injection and scanning to make timekeeping simple. Both superior and inferior saturation bands should be used. The resultant data can either be quantitatively plotted from ROI data (as shown in Fig. 5b), or can be examined visually to find the peak. Proper interpretation and application of the timing bolus data is critical to success, and requires an at least basic understanding of *k*-space acquisition order. The key is to allow contrast to fill the arteries as long as possible before acquiring the center of *k*-space, with the limiting factor of course being onset of venous enhancement. Experience has demonstrated that venous enhancement (when it occurs) is readily seen on the timing bolus images (Fig. 5a) [36]. Hence using the timing bolus data, an arteriovenous transit time or "AV window" can be determined. The optimum position for the center of k-space (i.e. start time for an elliptical centric sequence) is as far into this window as possible without obtaining overwhelming venous enhancement, thus allowing for maximal arterial opacification. Computer modeling, corroborated by data from peripheral MRA studies, strongly suggests that venous enhancement will be acceptable (50% or less signal intensity relative to artery) provided the center of k-space occurs at least 3-4 seconds before onset of venous enhancement [36]. This window varies depending on vessel size and pulse sequence parameters, and the 3-4 sec given here is for the parameters in Table 2 and a 2.5 mm vein. Thus if venous is seen relatively rapidly on the timing bolus, we recommend timing a centric acquisition such that acqui-

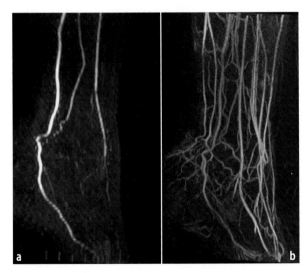

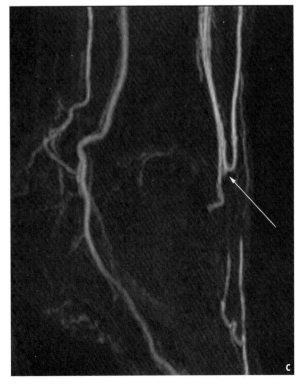

Fig. 4. Sagittal TOF-MRA (**a**) and CE-MRA (**b**) MIP's of the right foot in a patient with foot ulcers. Severe venous enhancement on the CE-MRA (**b**) makes interpretation extremely difficult, however the TOF study (**a**) clearly defines patent posterior tibial and lateral plantar arteries, and an abrupt occlusion of the mid dorsalis pedis artery. Using this TOF information, the anatomy can be better defined on the sagittal subvolume CE-MRA MIP (**c**), where the *arrow* marks the dorsalis pedis occlusion

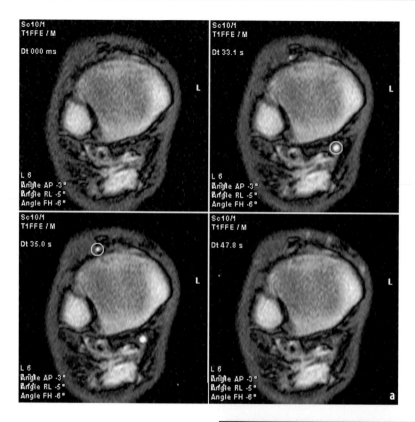

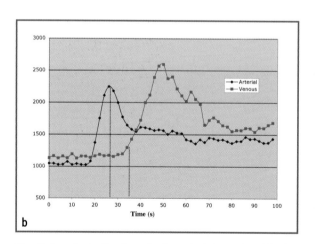

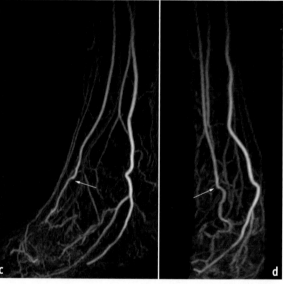

Fig. 5. Four single slices from the dynamic timing series with ROI's around the posterior tibial artery and an anterior vein (**a**). The signal intensity for artery and vein is plotted (**b**). Arterio-venous separation should be possible, as the time from arterial peak to onset of venous (dashed lines in (**b**)) is 7-8 sec. Resultant pedal sagittal and coronal MIP's are seen in (**c**) and (**d**). The dorsalis pedis is occluded proximally (arrows) and continues via collaterals. The lateral plantar artery is mildly diseased, and there is no complete plantar arch. Some mild venous contamination in seen

sition begins approximately 3-4 sec before venous onset. If on the other hand, no venous is seen or venous delay is more than 9-10 sec beyond the arterial peak, we recommend acquisition begin approximately 6 sec after arterial peak (allows for improved small vessel filling without missing the bolus). For the example in Figure 5b, we would begin acquisition of the CE-MRA sequence at approximately 31 sec, which is approximately 5 sec after the arterial peak.

Anatomic Variations

Anatomic variations abound within the pedal vasculature, particularly in relation to the origins of the different plantar and dorsal metatarsal arteries [37, 38].

As these smaller vessels off the plantar arch are typically beyond the resolution of MRA, perhaps the most relevant of the many variants to MR angiographers are the four variants of the dorsalis pedis artery (DP – Figs. 2 and 3):
• Type A – the DP begins as a continuation of the perforating peroneal artery (3%),
• Type B – the anterior tibial artery courses medially to be in the position of the perforating peroneal artery before becoming the DP (1.5%),
• Type C – the DP arises equally from both the anterior tibial and perforating peroneal artery (0.5%), and the most common,
• Type D – the DP is very reduced in size to be considered essentially absent (12%) [20].

Clinical Examples

As discussed, the main indication for pedal MRA is work-up of ischemic pedal disease, typically in diabetic patients, and typically to determine whether limb salvage is possible. In general, some other imaging of the aorto-iliac and outflow vessels (either DSA or moving table CE-MRA) will have already been performed, and information regarding the pedal vasculature is sub-optimal, incomplete, or angiographically occult vessels are being sought in attempt to avoid amputation.

Figure 5c, d demonstrates the case of a 68 year old male with diabetes and a right Charcot foot. There was no tissue loss, and he underwent the pedal MRA as part of an evaluation for a pedal fluid collection eventually determined to be a hematoma. The MRA demonstrates normal appearing distal peroneal as well as anterior and posterior tibial arteries, a relatively intact lateral plantar (some mild disease), and an occluded dorsalis pedis artery. There are good collaterals, and portions of the primary as well some probable secondary arches are seen.

Figure 6 demonstrates a right pedal MRA for a 58 year old male with diabetes, vascular disease, and a history of a prior left below-knee and right trans-metatarsal amputations. He presented with ulcerations and osteomyelitis at the metatarsal amputation site. Pedal MRA demonstrates relatively good outflow in the peroneal, anterior and posterior tibial, and dorsalis pedis arteries. Although the medial and lateral plantar arteries are

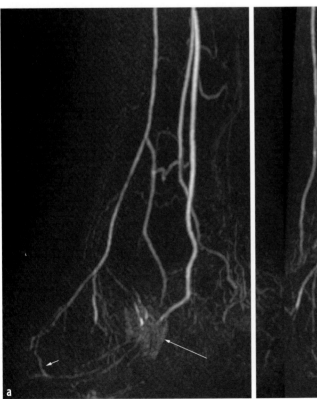
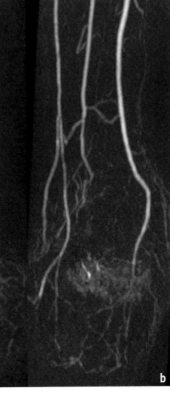

Fig. 6. Right foot sagittal (**a**) and coronal (**b**) MIP's from a 58 year old male diabetic status post trans-metatarsal amputations with amputation site ulcers and osteomyelitis. The pedal inflow is relatively normal (peroneal, anterior and posterior tibial arteries). The dorsalis pedis is somewhat attenuated distally, and there is a severely diseased primary plantar arch (*short arrow*). The lateral plantar terminates proximally into a region of ulcer blush (*long arrows*)

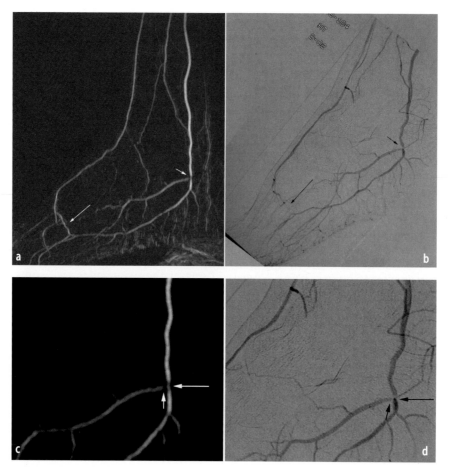

Fig. 7. Right foot sagittal MIP from a CE-MRA (**a**) and a sagittal frame from a DSA (**b**) in a non-diabetic 82 year old male with right 5th toe necrosis. Both modalities demonstrate the pedal arterial anatomy well, but the pedal arch is better visualized with MRA (*long arrows*) - an example of the "angiographically occult" vessel. Stenoses in the distal posterior tibial artery (*short arrows* in (**a**) and (**b**)) are visualized with both techniques, but an oblique subvolume MIP (**c**) shows this stenosis (*long arrow*) and a stenosis of the proximal medial tarsal artery (*short arrow*) to better advantage as compared to the single view planar DSA (**d**). This study was performed in arterial phase using the gadolinium blood pool agent MS-325 (EPIX Medical, Cambridge, MA)

occluded, significant ulcer blush is seen in the arch region, and this was not felt to be an outflow problem that could be remedied with a graft. The patient received a below-knee amputation.

A non-diabetic 82 year old male with right fifth toe necrosis is demonstrated in Figures 7a and 7b, showing a sagittal CE-MRA MIP and DSA, respectively. Note both modalities demonstrate the pedal arterial anatomy well, but the pedal arch is better visualized with MRA – an example of the "angio-

graphically occult" vessel. Also seen with both modalities is a stenosis of the distal posterior tibial artery. Figure 7c, however, demonstrates a significant advantage of 3D MRA – subvolume MIP's allow for viewing different projections, better defining the distal posterior tibial and proximal medial plantar artery stenoses as compared to DSA (7d). This patient had significant proximal disease (not shown – an occluded right superficial femoral artery), and underwent a right fem-pop bypass and amputation of the fifth toe.

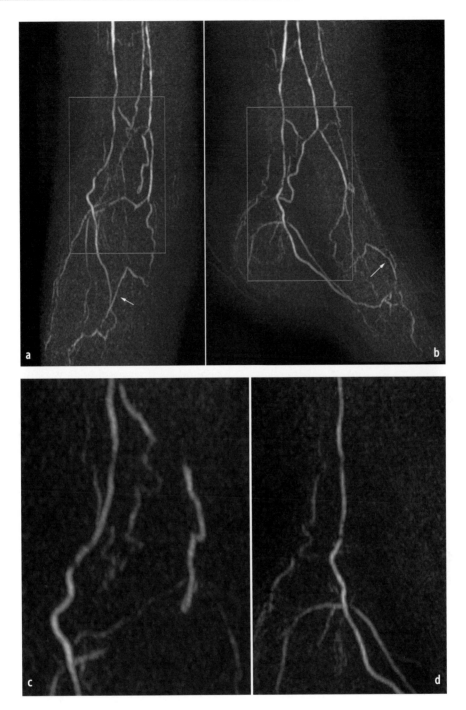

Fig. 8. Coronal (**a**) and sagittal (**b**) left foot CE-MRA MIP's from a 77 year old diabetic male with non-healing foot ulcers. The dorsalis pedis artery is occluded, with a short distal segment reconstituting (*arrow*), but no patent pedal arch. Diffuse multivessel disease is seen, particularly involving the posterior tibial artery, which is better seen on the coronal (**c**) and sagittal (**d**) zoomed subvolume MIP's

Figure 8 shows a coronal (a) and sagittal (b) left foot CE-MRA MIP from a 77 year old diabetic male with non-healing foot ulcers. Note the dorsalis pedis is occluded, with some focal distal reconstitution but no patent pedal arch, and there is diffuse multivessel disease, particularly involving the posterior tibial artery (better seen on the zoomed views (c) and (d)). Because of the diffuse disease and lack of a good target vessel, the patient was treated medically.

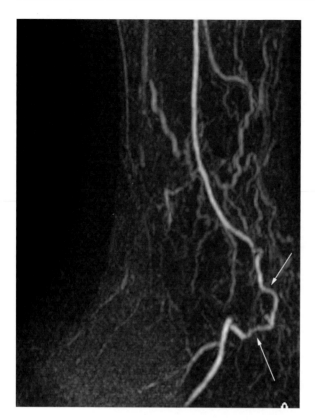

Fig. 9. Sagittal MIP from a right foot CE-MRA in an 85 year old male with multiple foot ulcers. The anterior tibial and dorsalis pedis arteries are occluded. The distal posterior tibial artery has a short segmental occlusion circumvented by well-formed collaterals (*arrows*) reconstituting just proximal to the bifurcation into the plantar arteries

Figure 9 demonstrates another patient with foot ulcers. This study shows occlusion of the anterior tibial and dorsalis pedis arteries, with an occlusion of the distal posterior tibial artery circumvented by well-formed collaterals reconstituting the posterior tibial just proximal to the bifurcation into the plantar arteries. As there were no major functional obstructions suitable for bypass, and the circulation was deemed adequate for healing, the patient was treated medically.

Pitfalls and Limitations

While pedal MRA is relatively straightforward to perform, several pitfalls await the unwary practitioner. The two most troublesome are venous enhancement and inadequate vessel visualization, both of which are related to timing (see discussion in *Imaging Protocol* above). While venous enhancement is not typically a concern with TOF, it can easily render CE-MRA uninterpretable (Fig. 4b). Venous enhancement tends to be much more problematic in patients with ischemic soft tissue

disease – i.e. the exact patient population in need of pedal imaging [9]. Nonetheless, if a careful timing bolus is performed, significant venous enhancement can usually be avoided. Luckily, in cases where venous enhancement is most problematic (diabetics, soft tissue disease), we find the TOF images are of generally good quality, likely a reflection of the fast arterial flow. Thus we are, among others, proponents of always performing both TOF and CE-MRA for the pedal arteries [23].

Another pitfall lies with spatial resolution. Even with the ~1 mm isotropic resolution advocated here (and all published pedal MRA to date falls short of this), this remains much inferior to the 0.3-0.4 mm resolution routinely obtained with DSA (compare fine vessel detail between Fig. 2 and 3) [9, 14, 21]. As previously stated, resolution requirements are a minimum of 1/3 the size of the vessel of interest in order to accurately characterize a stenosis [33, 34]. This assumes adequate SNR and CNR, and likely explains the poor inter-observer agreement in interpreting MRA studies in general, as if a vessel edge is poorly defined, it is extremely subjective where to place an electronic caliper to measure lumen size. Zero filling to as high a factor as possible (minimum of 512 in both frequency and phase and a factor of 2 in slice) helps to smooth out the vessel edges, and is particularly helpful for reformats, but is not a substitute for true spatial resolution [39]. Very often, MRA practitioners sacrifice resolution in the slice (z) direction as compared to the frequency and phase direction, the extreme example being true 2D MR DSA as advocated by Wang et al [24]. Sacrificing z spatial resolution becomes a problem when examining a vessel in a plane other than the acquired sagittal plane, something often required to sort out complicated pedal anatomy, and certainly one of the biggest advantages that 3D MRA has over planar DSA (Fig. 7c, 7d)

Accuracy of Technique published in Literature (Review of Papers)

The earliest of the MRA vs. DSA studies utilized 2D time of flight (TOF) MRA. In one early TOF study, coming as somewhat of a surprise to the MR community, TOF MRA was able to visualize 22% of the arterial lower extremity arterial segments that were not seen with DSA; vessels that may be suitable for distal bypass grafting [18]. Thus originated the so called angiographically "occult" vessel. This phenomenon is felt to be a combination of MRA's sensitivity to slow flow, and inadequate DSA vessel opacification due to contrast dilution as contrast passes through multisegmental occlusions. A follow up study focusing on the ankle and

Table 3. Accuracy of MRA versus conventional DSA for diagnostic pedal imaging

Author	MRA Technique	# Pts	Arteries	Sensitivity	Specificity
Cronberg [21]	3D CE-MRA	35	Pop-Foot	92	64
Kreitner [15]	3D CE-MRA	24	Foot	71	92
Cambria [44]	2D TOF	79	Pelvis-Foot	69% agreement w/DSA, 20% major discrepancy	
Hoch [41]	2D TOF	45	DP only	Exact match w/DSA 94%, mismatch 6%	
McDermott [16]	2D TOF	10	Foot	88	95

Table 4. Value of pedal MRA versus conventional DSA for treatment planning and intervention

Author	MRA Technique	# Pts	Results
Dorweiler [14]	3D CE-MRA	15	Grafts performed to angiographically occult pedal vessels. Limb salvage 90%, secondary patency 93% @ 3 years
Hofmann [9]	3D CE-MRA	37	MRA depicted more segments than DSA (p=0.0001). MRA superior to DSA in predicting distal site of graft anastomosis (CE-MRA kappa 0.82 vs. DSA kappa 0.6).
Kreitner [45]	3D CE-MRA	24	In 9/24 pts, angiographically occult pedal vessels by MRA. (No arteries seen with DSA only – 30/168 segments seen w/ MRA only). MRA altered treatment plan in 7 pts (29%).
Baum [17]	2D TOF	155	Odds of correctly distinguishing patent segments 1.6 greater for MRA than DSA (p<0.01). MRA changed treatment plan in 13%. In 87% of those with altered plans, MRA-inclusive plan superior.

foot in 24 limbs showed 2D TOF MRA visualized 120 arterial segments, whereas DSA visualized only 100 [16]. Further follow-up studies looking at surgical planning and outcomes suggested MRA was equivalent or even superior to DSA in terms of proper surgical management for lower extremity ischemic disease, with Owen et al. reporting MRA altering surgical management in 17% of cases, and Carpenter et al. reporting similar limb salvage rates for grafting to angiographically occult vs. angiographically visible lower extremity vessels [17, 18, 40-42]. More recent work with contrast enhanced MRA (CE-MRA), which is generally considered superior to TOF, corroborates these early findings. Kreitner et al. showed that dedicated pedal CE-MRA demonstrated patent pedal vessels not revealed by DSA in nine of twenty four patients (38%) [15]. A more recent study comparing CE-MRA, DSA, and duplex ultrasound for preoperative evaluation of the pedal vasculature showed both CE-MRA and duplex ultrasound to be superior to DSA in predicting the distal site of graft anastomosis, and furthermore suggests DSA is questionable as the "gold standard" [9]. Thus MRA is poised to substantially contribute to the important diagnostic area of pedal arterial imaging, perhaps even replacing DSA as an improved "gold standard" for non-invasive diagnostic pedal imaging.

Tables 3 and 4 summarize the sparse literature on Pedal MRA vs. DSA. As can be seen from Table 3, very few studies have been performed specifically comparing MRA and DSA in the foot, and more comparative studies are needed, particularly now that 3D CE-MRA techniques are more refined (for a more thorough synopsis of the current literature for generalized peripheral arterial disease, the reader is referred to the chapter on **"MRA of the peripheral arteries"** and the excellent meta-analysis by Nelemans et. al [43]). Keep in mind that what few pedal MRA studies are available do not always report findings as sensitivity and specificity. This is due in part to the widely held belief that DSA does not necessarily represent the "gold standard" for pedal arteriography, and therefore the sensitivity and specificity numbers listed in Table 3 must be approached cautiously [9, 14]. Most authors agree that intraoperative contrast angiography is the best gold standard [17], but this is difficult to achieve in large numbers of patients. Thus, several authors have posed the following questions:

(1) how many arterial segments can be seen with MRA that are not seen with DSA;
(2) is surgical intervention modified by MRA, and
(3) if so, how does this affect outcome?

Table 4 summarizes the studies addressing these questions. Although the total number of study patients remains small to date, these data uniformly suggest that:

(a) MRA depicts more pedal arteries than does DSA,

(b) the improved arterial visualization afforded by MRA improves the treatment plan, and

(c) surgical outcome with the MRA inclusive plan is superior to DSA alone.

Thus pedal MRA should be considered as an important diagnostic component in the complete work-up of the ischemic foot, particularly if revascularization or amputation is contemplated.

Critical Review of Clinical Applications

Despite some shortcomings [9] , DSA remains the present day gold standard for evaluating the peripheral arteries. It must also be stated that selective angiography (unilateral injection into iliac, femoral, or popliteal artery) is vastly superior to a non-selective exam where the contrast is injected into the distal aorta. [10, 46]. Most peripheral vascular studies are for one of two generalized indications. The first is claudication, in which case most emphasis is on the aortoiliac and femoral arteries, with the infrapopliteal arteries much less important to patient management. The second is for peripheral ischemic disease – non-healing ulcers, gangrene, rest pain, chronic osteomyelitis etc. In these circumstances, the below-knee arteries, including the pedal arteries, are extremely important to determining optimum patient therapy. Peripheral MRA has become quite reliable for work up of the claudication patient, but is in general somewhat lacking for the peripheral ischemic patient, as below-knee resolution limitations and problems with obscuring venous enhancement hinder peripheral MRA [28, 47-50]. Until recently, many investigators have been satisfied with MRA examinations that extend from the aorta to the ankle, yet exclude the pedal arteries. While this is striking as an advance for MRA, in the case of an ischemic patient, a vascular surgeon or angiographer will not consider the study complete until the pedal arch is depicted.

Thus pedal MRA, while presently not typically performed as a stand alone exam, is increasingly recognized as an important component of the complete peripheral MRA exam, and MR angiographers are attempting to include high quality pedal imaging as part of the peripheral MRA examination [24, 26]. In addition, with the recognition that even selective DSA does not visualize all lower extremity and pedal arteries, including pedal arteries that have been proven capable of receiving grafts [14], there is heightened interest in MRA being the examination of choice for lower extremity ischemic disease. In fact, Velazquez et al. believe that for patients in whom conventional contrast angiography fails to show suitable runoff vessels for use in a limb-salvage procedure, MRA should always be performed [51]. With regard to pedal vascular imaging, we can perhaps extend this logic to state that when considering a patient for possible limb salvage, if a pedal bypass is felt to be viable surgical option but DSA or a non pedal-focused peripheral MRA fails to demonstrate a suitable pedal bypass artery, dedicated pedal MRA as described in this chapter should be performed before proceeding with amputation.

Finally, this section would not be complete without a brief mention of Doppler Ultrasound (DUS) and Multi-Detector CT Angiography (MD-CTA). A recent large series (n=485) of patients with peripheral vascular disease evaluated with DUS showed that ultrasound alone was adequate for surgical planning in all but 36 patients (7%) [52]. The author goes on to state that such ultrasound examinations demand the sonographer have a high level of technical proficiency, anatomic understanding, and advanced training. This is another way of saying that the quality of DUS is highly operator dependant. Another study comparing pedal DUS, CE-MRA, and selective DSA in 37 patients concluded that DSA is questionable as a gold standard, showing both DUS and CE-MRA superior to DSA in predicting the ultimate distal anastomotic site [9]. Furthermore, the probability that a vessel was either faintly or not visualized was greater for DSA than for DUS or MRA, with no significant difference between DUS and MRA. Thus with a well-trained technician, DUS shares many advantages of MRA in terms of surgical planning and finding DSA occult arteries for bypass. One advantage of DUS is the relative availability of the modality compared to MRI. On the downside, however, DUS is only as good as the technologist, and results are provided in a tabular or chart form rather than a true anatomic roadmap image.

Multi-Detector CTA is appealing, primarily because of its relative simplicity, with preliminary studies suggesting peripheral MD-CTA performs quite well (although no dedicated pedal CTA studies have been published to date) [53-55]. Spatial resolution is quite similar to pedal MRA, at ~0.7 x 0.7 x 1.25 mm [55], and agreement between MD-CTA (peripheral studies that include the dorsalis pedis) and DSA is quite good, particularly for the

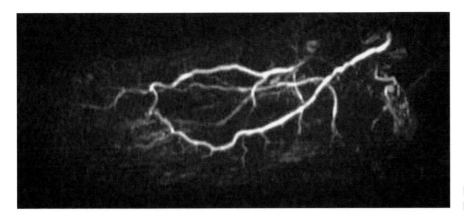

Fig. 10. Lateral MIP view of the pedal arch with MultiHance

above-knee arteries (sensitivity and specificity 91% and 92% in one study [53], 87% agreement with DSA above the knee vs. 80% agreement below in another [54]). CTA, however, suffers several drawbacks [55]. First, data is acquired in a transverse plane, meaning very large datasets are collected. Second, venous enhancement can be a problem, as it can with MRA. Third, bony segmentation is mandatory, and this is difficult, particularly in the lower extremities when there is venous enhancement and opacified arteries in near proximity to bones. And finally, calcified vascular plaques can confuse image interpretation, being a main reason for misinterpretation [53]. Of course, the nephrotoxic effects of iodinated contrast must be considered as well. All said, MRA remains the preferred modality over CTA at this time, although more work remains to be done [55].

Future Perspectives

In the future, pedal MRA will likely become recognized as an integral part of the complete peripheral MRA exam, and techniques, coils, and contrast agents that allow for optimal inclusion of the pedal vasculature will be refined. As pedal MRA is not in general performed or interpreted without the remainder of the peripheral exam (abdominal aorta down), new techniques will focus on ways of incorporating high-resolution pedal arterial images into complete peripheral MRA studies. Whether these exams will be single injection moving table vs. multiple injection multi-station examinations vs. time-resolved acquisitions remains to be seen.

A significant part of future advances will likely come from new coil technology [27, 56]. Improved coils not only increase SNR and field of view, but allow for higher parallel imaging factors with techniques such as SENSE [26, 28, 57]. This can speed up acquisition time and improve spatial resolution at each station of a moving table peripheral MRA,

thereby decreasing chances of venous enhancement and providing improved pedal coverage and spatial resolution.

Another recent advance in peripheral MRA designed to decrease venous enhancement and prolong the arteriovenous window (which can in turn allow for better pedal imaging) uses venous compression. By inflating thigh or calf blood pressure cuffs to sub-systolic pressures, several preliminary studies demonstrate a substantial decrease in venous enhancement (58, 59) While this technique is in its infancy, it may prove extremely useful for pedal imaging in certain cases, although caution must be used, as many patients with critical ischemia cannot tolerate venous compression.

Contrast agents will likely also play a role in the future of pedal MRA. Several new gadolinium chelates have been developed, including conventional extracellular agents at higher concentrations (1.0 Molar vs. 0.5 Molar – gadobutrol – Schering AG, Berlin, Germany), agents with higher relaxivities due to weak protein interaction (Gd-BOPTA – MultiHance – Bracco Imaging, Milan, Italy), and blood pool agents such as MS-325 (EPIX Medical, Cambridge, MA) and B-22956 (Bracco Imaging, Milan, Italy) [60]. None of these agents has, at the time of this writing, been approved for clinical use in the United States, but near future approval is likely in several cases. Early trials (non-pedal) with both the higher concentration and weak protein interaction contrast agents suggest they may be advantageous compared to conventional contrast agents, particularly for imaging of smaller arteries, as would be the case in the foot (Fig. 10) [61-64]. Blood pool agents can be used for first pass MRA in a fashion identical to conventional contrast agents, but then open up the possibility of steady state vascular imaging at very high resolution (Figs. 7, 11) [65, 66]. How well AV segmentation algorithms [67, 68] can eventually strip away the veins in a study such as Figure 11 remains to be seen.

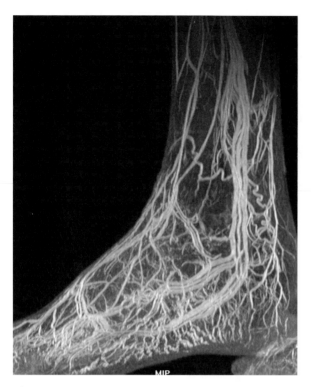

Fig. 11. Sagittal MIP in the steady state phase using MS-325 (EPIX Medical, Cambridge, MA). This is the same foot as in Fig. 7. Note the superb spatial resolution (0.9 x 0.9 x 0.8 mm) but extremely large number of confounding veins, making AV segmentation mandatory for arterial interpretation

One significant advantage of MRI has always been that it does more than purely anatomic imaging. A recent study by Zhang et al. evaluated soft tissue enhancement in the feet of diabetic patients undergoing time-resolved pedal CE-MRA [69]. They found enhancing lesions in 92% of diabetic patients (vs. 51% in non-diabetics, diabetics had greater intensity of enhancement). These regions of soft tissue enhancement occurred in regions where diabetics tend to get ulceration, and the authors suggest these represent precursor lesions to diabetic ulceration. If true, this could add an entirely new dimension to pedal MRA – not only the ability to evaluate the pre-operative diabetic foot, but also help screen for and predict potential sites of ulceration, thereby allowing for pre-emptive preventative treatment.

References

1. Armstrong D, Lavery L (1998) Diabetic foot ulcers: prevention, diagnosis and classification. Am Fam Physician 15 57(6):1325-1332, 1337-1328
2. Pomposelli FJ, Marcaccio E, Gibbons G et al (1995) Dorsalis pedis arterial bypass: durable limb salvage for foot ischemia in patients with diabetes mellitus. J Vasc Surg 21(3):375-384
3. Pomposelli F, Kansal N, Hamdan A et al (2003) A decade of experience with dorsalis pedis artery bypass: analysis of outcome in more than 1000 cases. J Vasc Surg 37(2):307-315
4. Saltzberg S, Pomposelli FJ, Belfield A et al (2003) Outcome of lower-extremity revascularization in patients younger than 40 years in a predominantly diabetic population. J Vasc Surg 38(5):1056-1059
5. Marks J, King T, Baele H et al (1992) Popliteal-to-distal bypass for limb-threatening ischemia. J Vasc Surg 15(5:755-759
6. Taylor LJ, Hamre D, Dalman R et al (1991) Limb salvage vs amputation for critical ischemia. The role of vascular surgery. Arch Surg 126(10):1251-1257
7. Holstein P, Sorensen S (1999) Limb salvage experience in a multidisciplinary diabetic foot unit. Diabetes Care 22 Suppl 2:B97-103
8. Ascer E, Veith F, Gupta S (1988) Bypasses to plantar arteries and other tibial branches: an extended approach to limb salvage. J Vasc Surg 8(4):434-441
9. Hofmann W, Forstner R, Kofler B et al (2002) Pedal artery imaging–a comparison of selective digital subtraction angiography, contrast enhanced magnetic resonance angiography and duplex ultrasound. Eur J Vasc Endovasc Surg 24(4):287-292
10. Alson M, Lang E, Kaufman J (1997) Pedal arterial imaging. J Vasc Interv Radiol 8(1 Pt 1):9-18
11. Bartos J, Mayzlik J, Puchmayer V et al (1991) Significance of pedal arch for femoropopliteal vein bypass patency. Int Angiol 10(1):25-28
12. Imparato A, Kim G, Madayag M et al (1973) Angiographic criteria for successful tibial arterial reconstructions. Surgery 74(6):830-838
13. Jacob A, Stock K, Proske M et al (1996) Lower extremity angiography: improved image quality and outflow vessel detection with bilaterally antegrade selective digital subtraction angiography. A blinded prospective intraindividual comparison with aortic flush digital subtraction angiography. Invest Radiol 31(4):184-193
14. Dorweiler B, Neufang A, Kreitner K et al (2002) Magnetic resonance angiography unmasks reliable target vessels for pedal bypass grafting in patients with diabetes mellitus. J Vasc Surg 35(4):766-772
15. Kreitner K, Kalden P, Neufang A et al (2000) Diabetes and peripheral arterial occlusive disease: prospective comparison of contrast-enhanced three-dimensional MR angiography with conventional digital subtraction angiography. AJR 174:171-179
16. McDermott V, Meakem T, Carpenter J et al (1995) Magnetic resonance angiography of the distal lower extremity. Clin Radiol 50(11):741-746
17. Baum R, Rutter C, Sunshine J et al (1995) Multicenter trial to evaluate vascular magnetic resonance angiography of the lower extremity. American College of Radiology Rapid Technology Assessment Group. JAMA 20;274(11):875-880
18. Owen R, Carpenter J, Baum R et al (1992) Magnetic resonance imaging of angiographically occult runoff vessels in peripheral arterial occlusive disease. N Engl J Med 326(24):1577-1581
19. Harrington E, Harrington M, Schanzer H et al (1992) The dorsalis pedis bypass–moderate success in difficult situations. J Vasc Surg 15(2):409-414
20. Strauch B, Yu H (1993) Atlas of Microvascular Surgery. New York: Theime Medical Publishers
21. Cronberg C, Sjoberg S, Albrechtsson U et al (2003)

Peripheral arterial disease. Contrast-enhanced 3D MR angiography of the lower leg and foot compared with conventional angiography. Acta Radiol 44(1):59-66

22. Kaufman J, McCarter D, Geller S et al (1998) Two-dimensional time-of-flight MR angiography of the lower extremities: artifacts and pitfalls. Am J Roentgenol 171:129-135

23. Rofsky N, Adelman M (2000) MR angiography in the evaluation of atherosclerotic peripheral vascular disease. Radiology 214(2):325-338

24. Wang Y, Winchester P, Khilnani N et al (2001) Contrast-enhanced peripheral MR angiography from the abdominal aorta to the pedal arteries: combined dynamic two-dimensional and bolus-chase three-dimensional acquisitions. Invest Radiol 36:170-177

25. Winchester P, Lee H, Khilnani N et al (1998) Comparison of two-dimensional mr digital subtraction angiography of the lower extremity with x-ray angiography. J Vasc Interv Radiol 9:891-899

26. Maki J, Wilson G, Eubank W et al (2003) 3D Gd-enhanced peripheral MR angiography using multi-station SENSE (WakiTrak LS) – an update. In: Eleventh Scientific Meeting and Exhibition. Toronto, Canada: International Society of Magnetic Resonance in Medicine 257

27. Huber A, Scheidle J, Wintersperger B et al (2003) Moving-Table MR Angiography of the Peripheral Runoff Vessels: Comparison of Body Coil and Dedicated Phased Array Coil Systems. AJR 180:1365-1373

28. Maki J, Wilson G, Eubank W et al (2002) Utilizing SENSE to achieve lower station sub-millimeter isotropic resolution and minimal venous enhancement in peripheral MR angiography. J Magn Reson Imaging 15:484-491

29. Janka R, Fellner F, Fellner C et al (2000) Dedicated phased-array coil for peripheral MRA. Eur J Rad 10:1745-1749

30. Sodickson D, McKenzie C, Ohliger M et al (2002) Recent advances in image reconstruction, coil sensitivity calibration, and coil array design for SMASH and generalized parallel MRI. MAGMA 13(3):158-163

31. Weiger M, Pruessmann K, Kassner A et al (2000) Contrast-enhanced 3d MRA using SENSE. J Magn Reson Imaging 12:671-677

32. Brophy D, Patel S (1999) Optimal digital subtraction angiography of dorsalis pedis artery: effect of foot positioning on angiographic demonstration. J Vasc Interv Radiol 10(3):376-377

33. Hoogeveen R, Bakker C, Viergever M (1998) Limits to the accuracy of vessel diameter measurement in MR angiography. J Magn Reson Imaging 8:1228-1235

34. Wilson G, Haynor D, Maki J (2000) Resolution requirements for grading stenoses in 3D CE-MRA. Sixth scientific meeting of the International Society for Magnetic Resonance in Medicine. Denver, CO: 1787

35. Swan J, Carroll T, Kennell T et al (2002) Time-resolved three-dimensional contrast-enhanced MR angiography of the peripheral vessels. Radiology 225(1):43-52

36. Maki J, Wilson G, Eubank W et al (2003) Predicting venous enhancment in peripheral MRA using a two station timing bolus. In:Eleventh Scientific Meeting and Exhibition. Toronto, Canada: International Society of Magnetic Resonance in Medicine 91

37. Kadir S (1991) Atlas of normal and variant angiographic anatomy. Philadelphia: W. B. Saunders

38. Edwards E (1960) Anatomy of the small arteries of the foot and toes. Acta Anat 41:81-96

39. Roditi G, Robertson I, Cockburn M et al (2003) 1024 matrix coronal crural vessel imaging with SENSE, CLEAR, and CENTRA as an adjunct to standard moving table aorta and peripheral run-off MRA. In:Fifteenth scientific meeting of the Magnetic Resonance Angiography Club. Toronto, Canada

40. Carpenter J, Golden M, Barker C et al (1996) The fate of bypass grafts to angiographically occult runoff vessels detected by magnetic resonance angiography. J Vasc Surg 23(3):483-489

41. Hoch J, Tullis M, Kennell T et al (1996) Use of magnetic resonance angiography for the preoperative evaluation of patients with infrainguinal arterial occlusive disease. J Vasc Surg 23(5):792-800

42. Carpenter J, Baum R, Holland G et al (1994) Peripheral vascular surgery with magnetic resonance angiography as the sole preoperative imaging modality. J Vasc Surg 20(6):861-869

43. Nelemans P, Leiner T, de Vet H et al (2000) Peripheral arterial disease: meta-analysis of the diagnostic performance of MR Angiography. Radiology 217:105-114

44. Cambria R, Kaufman J, L'Italien G et al (1997) Magnetic resonance angiography in the management of lower extremity arterial occlusive disease: a prospective study. J Vasc Surg 25:380-389

45. Kreitner K, Kunz R, Kalden P et al (2001) Contrast-enhanced three-dimensional MR angiography of the thoracic aorta: experiences after 118 examinations with a standard dose contrast administration and different injection protocols. Eur Radiol 11:1355-1363

46. Oser R, Picus D, Hicks M et al (1995) Accuracy of DSA in the evaluation of patency of infrapopliteal vessels. J Vasc Interv Radiol 6:589-594

47. Hentsch A, Aschauer M, Balzer J et al (2004) Gadobutrol-enhanced moving-table magnetic resonance angiography in patients with peripheral vascular disease: a prospective, multi-centre blinded comparison with digital subtraction angiography. Eur Radiol 13(9):2103-2114

48. Leiner T, Ho K, Nelemans P et al (2000) Three-dimensional contrast-enhanced moving-bed infusion-tracking (MoBI-Track) peripheral mr angiography with flexible choice of imaging parameters for each field of view. J Magn Reson Imaging 11:368-377

49. Ho V, Choyke P, Foo T et al (1999) Automated bolus chase peripheral MR angiography: initial practical experiences and future directions of this work-in-progress. J Magn Reson Imaging 10:376-388

50. Ho K, Leiner T, DeHaan M et al (1998) Peripheral vascular tree stenoses: evaluation with moving-bed infusion-tracking MR angiography. Radiology 206:683-692

51. Velazquez O, Baum R, Carpenter J (1998) Magnetic resonance angiography of lower-extremity arterial disease. Surg Clin North Am. 78:519-537

52. Ascher E, Hingoran IA, Markevich N et al (2002) Lower extremity revascularization without preoper-

ative contrast arteriography: experience with duplex ultrasound arterial mapping in 485 cases. Ann Vasc Surg 16(1):108-114

53. Ofer A, Nitecki S, Linn S et al (2003) Multidetector CT angiography of peripheral vascular disease: a prospective comparison with intraarterial digital subtraction angiography. AJR 180(3):719-724

54. Heuschmid M, Krieger A, Beierlein W et al (2003) Assessment of peripheral arterial occlusive disease: comparison of multislice-CT angiography (MS-CTA) and intraarterial digital subtraction angiography (IA-DSA). Eur J Med Res 8(9):389-396

55. Rubin G, Schmidt A, Logan L et al (2001) Multi-detector row CT angiography of lower extremity arterial inflow and runoff: initial experience. Radiology 221(1):146-158

56. Janka R, Fellner F, Fellner C et al (2000) Dedicated phased-array coil for peripheral MRA. Eur Radiol 10(11): 1745-1749

57. De Vries M, van Engelshoven J, Leiner T (2002) Perihperal CE-MRA using thress station SENSE. In:XIV Annual International Workshop on MR Angiography. Essen, Germany 58

58. Herborn C, Ajaj W, Goyen M et al (2004) Peripheral vasculature: whole-body angiography with mid-femoral venous compression – initial experience. Radiology 230(s): 872-878

59. Bilecen D, Schulte A, Aschwanden M et al (2003) Infragenual compression for optimized CE-MRA of the crural arteries. In:Eleventh Scientific Meeting and Exhibition of the ISMRM. Toronto, Canada 85

60. Knopp M, von Tengg-Kobligk H, Floemer F et al (1999) Contrast agents for MRA: future directions. J Magn Reson Imaging 10:314-316

61. Herborn C, Lauenstein T, Ruehm S et al (2003) Intraindividual comparison of gadopentetate dimeglumine, gadobenate dimeglumine and gadobutro for pelvic 3D magnetic resonance angiography. Invest Radiol 38:27-33

62. Knopp M, Schoenberg S, Rehm C et al (2002) Assessment of Gadobenate Dimeglumine (Gd-BOPTA) for MR Angiography: Phase I Studies. Invest Radiol 37:706-715

63. Goyen M, Lauenstein T, Herborn C et al (2001) 0.5 M Gd chelate (Magnevist) versus 1.0 M Gd chelate (Gadovist): dose-independent effect on image quality of pelvic three-dimensional MR-angiography. J Magn Reson Imaging 14:602-607

64. Tombach B, Reimer P, Prumer B et al (1999) Does a higher concentration of gadolinium chelates improve first-pass cardiac signal changes? J Magn Reson Imaging 10:806-812

65. Perreault P, Edelman M, Baum R et al (2003) MR angiography with gadofosveset trisodium for peripheral vascular disease: phase II trial. Radiology 229(3):811-820

66. La Noce A, Stoelben S, Scheffler K et al (2002) B22956/1, a new intravascular contrast agent for MRI: first administration to humans–preliminary results. Acad Radiol 9 Suppl:S404-406

67. van Bemmel C, Wink O, Verdonck B et al (2003) Blood pool contrast-enhanced MRA: improved arterial visualization in the steady state. IEEE Trans Med Imaging 22(5):645-652

68. Lei T, Udupa J, Saha P et al (2001) Artery-vein separation via MRA- an image processing approach. IEEE Trans Med Imaging 20(8):689-703

69. Zhang H, Bush H, Kent K et al (2003) Soft tissue enhancement of diabetic feet on time-resolved peripheral MRA: preliminary study. In:Eleventh Scientific Meeting and Exhibition of the ISMRM. Toronto, Canada 90

VII.4

Whole Body 3D MR Angiography

Mathias Goyen

Clinical Indications/Background

Peripheral vascular disease (PVD) is a major health problem accounting for more than 100,000 surgical procedures annually in the United States alone [1]. PVD is caused by the systemic process of atherosclerosis, and is frequently associated with coronary, renal and carotid arterial disease. The management of a patient with PVD has to be planned in the context of the epidemiology of the disease and, in particular, the apparent risk factors or markers predicting spontaneous deterioration [2]. It is obvious that proper management of arterial disease requires a comprehensive assessment of the underlying vascular morphology. Localizing and gauging the severity of arterial lesions is crucial for therapeutic decision making. For this purpose, several imaging modalities, including conventional catheter angiography, duplex ultrasound, as well as CT- and MR-angiography (MRA) are in clinical use.

To date the display of the peripheral arterial system was accomplished with catheter-based X-ray angiography. High cost, invasiveness and associated risks [3-5] have motivated the development and evaluation of non-invasive peripheral vascular imaging techniques including ultrasound, computed tomographic (CT) angiography, and MR angiography (MRA). MR has advantages relative to CT angiography including the availability of a large field of view, use of non-nephrotoxic contrast material, and lack of ionizing radiation. Compared to ultrasound, MR is less operator-dependent and overcomes difficulties related to acoustic window limitations. Lack of ionizing radiation and safe contrast agents [6], in conjunction with high diagnostic accuracy have driven the rapid implementation of MRA as the modality of choice for assessing arterial disease in many centers throughout the world [7-10].

Since atherosclerotic disease effects the entire arterial system, extended coverage allowing the concomitant assessment of the arterial system from the supraaortic arteries to the distal runoff vessels appears desirable. Subsequent parenchymal enhancement and contrast dose limitations had initially curtailed contrast-enhanced 3D MRA to the display of the arterial territory contained within a single field-of-view extending over 40-48 cm.

The implementation of "bolus chase" techniques extended coverage to encompass the entire run-off vasculature, including the pelvic, femoral, popliteal and trifurcation arteries [11-14, see chapter VII.2. The implementation of faster gradient systems has laid the foundation for a further extension of the bolus chase technique: whole body coverage extending from the carotid arteries to the run-off vessels with 3D MRA has become possible [15].

Normal Anatomy

see respective chapters

Technique

The whole-body MRA-concept is based on the acquisition of five slightly overlapping 3D data sets acquired in immediate succession. The first data set covers the aortic arch, supraaortic branch arteries and the thoracic aorta, while the second data set covers the abdominal aorta with its major branches including the renal arteries. The third data set displays the pelvic arteries, and the last two data sets cover the arteries of the thighs and calves, respectively.

After planning the 3D acquistions using a True-FISP moving vessel scout and determining the contrast arrival time using the test-bolus technique, a commercially-available fast FLASH-3D sequence is employed (Magnetom Sonata˙, Siemens,

Table 1. Sequence parameters for whole-body MR angiography

TrueFISP moving scout	
TR	4.45 ms
TE	2.22 ms
FOV	400 mm
Flip angle	70°
Slice thickness	10 mm
No. of slices	6
Acquisition time	9 s
Spatial resolution	3.1_1.6_10 mm^3
Matrix	256
Test bolus	
TR	1, 000 ms
TE	1.58 ms
FOV	400 mm
Plane orientation	Coronal
Flip angle	8°
Slice thickness	10 mm
No. of slices	60
Acquisition time	60 s
Spatial resolution	3.0_1.6_10 mm^3
Matrix	256
Contrast injection	Test bolus, 1 ml Gd-BOPTA, flow, 1.3 ml/s+30 ml NaCl; flow, 1.3 ml/s; scan, proximal third descending aorta
Contrast-enhanced 3D FLASH	
TR	2.2 ms
TE	0.74 ms
FOV	390 mm
Plane orientation	Coronal
Flip angle	20°
Slice thickness	1.5
No. of slices	64
Acquisition time	12 s
Spatial resolution	1.8_1.5_1.5 mm^3
Matrix	256
Contrast injection	0.2 mmol/kg bw Gd-BOPTA, diluted with NaCl to 60 ml; biphasic injection protocol, 1.3 ml/s for the first half, 0.7 ml/s for the second half of the bolus+30 ml NaCl; flow, 1.3 ml/s

Erlangen/Germany: TR/TE 2.1 ms/ 0.7 ms, flip angle: 25°, 40 partitions interpolated by zero-filling to 64, slab thickness: 120 mm, slice thickness: 3.0 mm interpolated to 1.9 mm, FOV: 390 x 390 mm, matrix: 256 x 225 interpolated by zero-filling to 512 x 512, read-out bandwidth = 863 Hz/pixel, acquisition time: 12 s) (Table 1). To avoid any gaps, the 3D data sets are overlapped by 3 cm, resulting in a cranio-caudal coverage of 176 cm. Each 3D data set is collected over 12 seconds [16].

A weight-adjusted dosage of 0.2 mmol/kg bw gadobenate dimeglumine (Gd-BOPTA, Multi-Hance, Bracco Imaging, Milan/Italy) [17] diluted with 0.9% of normal saline to a total volume of 60 ml is used. Gd-BOPTA is automatically (MR Spec-

tris·, Medrad, Pittsburgh, PA) injected using a biphasic protocol: the first half is injected at a rate of 1.3 ml/s, while the second half is administered at a rate of 0.7 ml/s. The contrast is flushed with 30 ml of saline injected at 1.3 ml/s.

The performance of whole-body 3D MRA can be improved by using the AngioSURF (Angiographic System for Unlimited Rolling Field-of-views, MR-Innovation GmbH, Essen/Germany) system which integrates a torso-surface coil for signal reception thereby improving spatial resolution [16, 18]. Patients are placed feet first within the bore of the magnet and examined in the supine position on the AngioSURF platform which is placed on the existing table top. Up to six 400mm

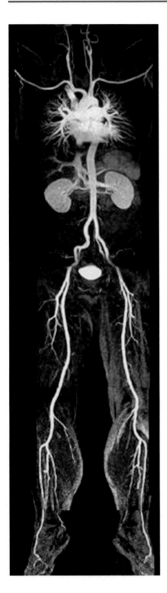

Fig. 1. AngioSURF–based 3D whole-body MR angiogram consisting of five 3D data sets collected over 72 seconds. The acquisition time for each 3D data set amounts to 12 seconds. During a 3 second acquisition break the table is manually repositioned to the center of the subsequent image volume. With 5 successive acquisitions craniocaudal coverage was extended over 180 cm, while the total data acquisition time amounted to 72 s. Multihance (Bracco Imaging, Milan/Italy) was administered at a dose of 0.2 mmol/kg BW at a rate of 1.3 ml/sec for the first half and 0.7 ml/sec for the second half of the contrast volume, followed by a 30 ml saline flush using an automated injector (MR Spectris, Medrad). The scan delay was determined with a 2ml test bolus at the level of the descending aorta. The quality of the whole body MR angiogram is sufficient to assess the arterial system from the supraaortic arteries to the run-off vessels

3D data sets can be acquired in immediate succession, with markers permitting adjustment of the desired field-of-view. Signal reception is accomplished using posteriorly located spine coils and an anteriorly located torso phased array coil, which remains stationary within the bore. While the two utilized elements of the spine coil are integrated in the patient table, the standard torso phased array coil is anchored in a height-adjustable holder, which remains fixed to the stationary patient table. Thus, data for all 5 stations are collected with the same stationary coil set positioned in the isocenter of the magnet.

Using the latest high performance scanners and gradients, the acquisition time for a complete 3D data set can be reduced significantly. By shortening the repetition time to 2.1 ms, a 3D data set can be collected in only 12 s. Thus, up to five 3D data sets can be collected within the short intraarterial contrast phase of slightly more than 60 seconds (Figs.

1, 2). To assure maximal arterial enhancement, Gd-BOPTA, a paramagnetic contrast agent with high intravascular relaxivity owing to some degree of albumin-binding [19] is employed. Improved signal within the arterial system due to usage of a phased-array torso surface coil directly translates into an increase in achievable spatial resolution, which amounts to 0.8x0.8x2 mm (post-interpolation voxel size) in the applied protocol. This enables better delineation of smaller vessels such as the tibial vessels.

In patients with PVD it is desirable to localize and gauge the severity of occlusive arterial lesions to assist in planning an intervention (Fig. 3). The TransAtlantic Inter-Society Consensus (TASC) on Management of Peripheral Arterial Disease recommends that – depending on local availability, experience, and cost - duplex scanning or magnetic resonance angiography can be used as a preliminary, noninvasive examination before angiography [20].

Accuracy of Technique Published in Literature / Critical Review of Clinical Applications

In a preliminary study, 5 healthy volunteers and 6 patients with angiographically documented peripheral vascular disease were examined using Gd-BOPTA at a dose of 0.3 mmol/kg bodyweight. Compared with conventional DSA, two independent blinded readers noted overall sensitivities of 91% (95% CI 0.76-0.98) and 94% (0.8-0.99), and specificities of 93% (0.85-0.97) and 90% (0.82-0.96), for the detection of substantial vascular disease (luminal narrowing >50%) [15]. Furthermore, inter-observer agreement for the assessment of whole-body MR angiograms was excellent (kappa=0.94; 95% CI 0.9-0.98), indicating that the approach was accurate and robust for morphologic vasculature screening.

More recent studies have further defined the value of Gd-BOPTA in whole body 3D CE-MRA (17, 18). In an initial study aimed at establishing the optimum dose to employ, Goyen et al (17) examined 10 healthy volunteers three times each with an ascending dose of Gd-BOPTA (0.1/0.2/0.3 mmol/kg bodyweight) using the AngioSURF rolling table platform system, an integrated torso surface coil, and a 3D FLASH sequence run at five stations from the carotid arteries to the trifurcation vessels. SNR and CNR values were calculated for 30 segments per patient and qualitative evaluation was performed using a 4-point visualization scale. Overall, significantly (p<0.05) higher SNR and CNR values were determined for the 0.2 and 0.3 mmol/kg dose groups compared to the 0.1

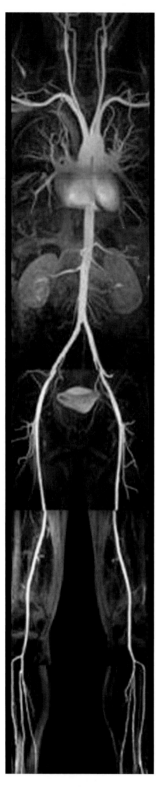

Fig. 2. AngioSURF-based whole-body 3D MR angiogram of a 42-year-old male patient with hypertension. The exam consists of five slightly overlapping 3D data sets collected over 72 s. The acquisition time for each 3D data set amounts to 12 s. During a 3s acquisition break, the table is manually repositioned to the center of the subsequent image volume. With five successive acquisitions, craniocaudal coverage was extended over 176 cm, while the total data acquisition time amounted to 72 s. Finding: high-grade stenosis of the right renal artery

mmol/kg dose group. Similarly, qualitative evaluation revealed the image quality to be significantly (p<0.05) superior for the 0.2 and 0.3 mmol/kg dose groups compared with the 0.1 mmol/kg dose group. Interestingly, neither qualitative nor quantitative assessment was able to demonstrate a statistically significant difference between the 0.2 and 0.3 mmol/kg dose groups (p>0.05), indicating that Gd-BOPTA at a dose of 0.2 mmol/kg bodyweight is sufficient for satisfactory diagnostic image quality.

Confirmation of the suitability of the 0.2 mmol/kg dose of Gd-BOPTA for whole-body CE-MRA was subsequently demonstrated in 3 volunteers and 10 patients with peripheral vascular disease using the same multi-station 3D imaging approach and rolling table platform system [18]. Similarly high SNR and CNR values were obtained for all subjects. More importantly, sensitivity and specificity values of 95.3% and 95.2%, respectively, were obtained for the detection of significant stenoses (luminal narrowing > 50%) when compared with conventional DSA as reference standard.

A more complete evaluation of both the imaging procedure and contrast agent dose has recently been performed in 102 consecutive patients with peripheral vascular disease [21]. Using an identical whole-body 3D CE-MRA imaging approach, Gd-BOPTA at a dose of 0.2 mmol/kg bodyweight, and similar image assessment criteria based on 30 vascular segments per patient from the carotid arteries to the tibial vessels, two experienced MR radiologists in consensus noted clinically relevant disease in 33 segments in 25 patients that was additional to the known disease in the peripheral vessels. Specifically, the additional disease comprised renal artery narrowing (n=15), carotid arterial stenosis (n=12), subclavian artery stenosis (n=2), and abdominal aortic aneurysms (n=4). The study confirmed the whole body 3D CE-MRA approach with 0.2 mmol/kg Gd-BOPTA to be quick and risk-free and to allow a comprehensive evaluation of the arterial system in patients with atherosclerosis.

The high degree of concomitant arterial disease in patients with peripheral vascular disease is not surprising. It merely underscores the systemic nature of atherosclerosis. Patients with intermittent claudication are at particularly high risk of atherosclerotic disease affecting other parts of the circulation. PVD, due as it is to atherosclerosis, is rarely an isolated disease process.

The extent of coexisting cardiovascular disease needs to be appreciated to ensure that the clinician will treat PVD in a true context. Studies on the prevalence of coronary artery disease (CAD) in patients with PVD show that history, clinical examination, and electrocardiography typically indicate the presence of CAD in 40% to 60% of such patients, although this may often be asymptomatic

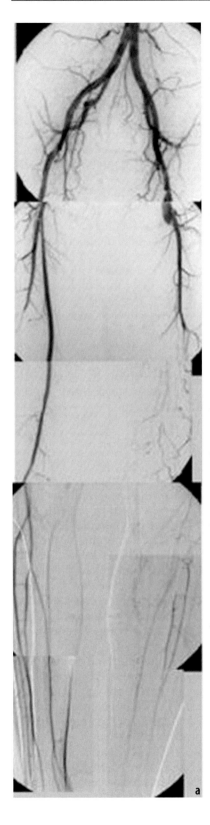

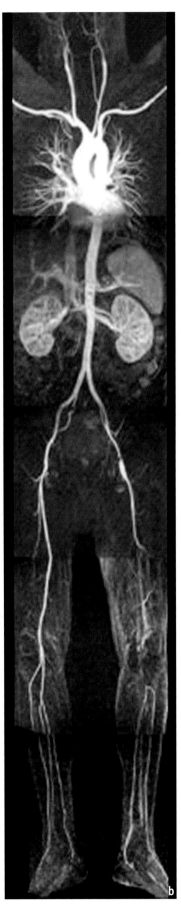

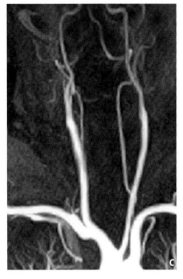

Fig. 3a-c. Invasive catheter angiogram (**a**) and whole-body MR angiogram (**b**) in a 54 year old male patient with PVD, history of bypass-graft left leg. The catheter angiogram shows a high-grade stenosis of the proximal anastomosis of the bypass-graft and an occlusion of the superficial femoral artery/popliteal artery on the left. The whole-body MR angiogram reveals these pathologic findings to the same advantage. (**c**) In addition, due to the extended coverage of the anatomy, a high-grade stenosis of the right internal carotid artery was detected which was clinically not susupected as it is masked by exercise restrictions in these patients [22]. The link between PVD and cerebrovascular disease (CVD) seems to be weaker than that with CAD. Using duplex sonography, carotid disease has been found in 26% to 50% of patients with PVD [23, 24]. Most of these patients will have a history of cerebral events or a carotid bruit and seem to be at increased risk of further events [25].

The fact that in this series twelve unsuspected carotid lesions in ten patients were identified highlights the often too symptom-focused means of patient questioning. Since all studied patients presented with symptoms suggestive of peripheral vascular disease, the patients' histories were focused on that region. Only very direct questioning revealed additional symptomatology suggesting carotid disease in three patients.

Approximately one fourth of PVD patients have hypertension, and in these patients consideration should be given to the possibility of renal artery narrowing.

In this cohort 13 patients (13%) showed renal artery disease with a luminal narrowing > 50%.

There is ongoing controversy about the value of screening all patients with PVD, symptomatic or not, for carotid disease and aortic aneurysms [24, 26]. There is no doubt that claudicant patients are more likely to have significant asymptomatic disease in these areas than the general population, but the treatment of asymptomatic carotid disease is still controversial, and there is the issue of yield versus cost of such screening tests.

It has to be mentioned that our approach – although referred to as a whole-body MRA-exam - does not cover the intracranial or coronary arteries, which still require a dedicated approach for diagnostic assessment.

However, noninvasiveness, three-dimensionality, extended coverage and high contrast conspicuity are the characteristics of whole body MR angiography that combine to allow a quick, risk-free, and comprehensive evaluation of the arterial system in patients with atherosclerosis.

Pitfalls and Limitations

Despite the encouraging results of initial evaluations, whole-body MR angiography faces some relevant limitations regarding spatial resolution for the depiction of tight stenoses and small vessels in the lower legs. This has resulted in some over- and undergrading of disease. Potential advantages associated with the acquisition of higher resolution data sets are offset by the development of venous overlap. Hence, delineation of small arteries, particularly those potentially needed for surgical grafting, remains challenging with whole-body MR angiography [15], as well as with most other

bolus-chase techniques [27].

Various strategies have been employed to achieve high-resolution peripheral MR angiography images without venous overlap. The mere increase in spatial resolution is not sufficient, as was recently illustrated [28]. The quality of the high-resolution images of the calf arteries was both quantitatively and qualitatively inferior in comparison with that of the standard protocol with an interpolated matrix. In addition, the longer acquisition times translated into considerable venous contamination of the high-resolution image set in comparison with the standard whole-body MR angiography protocol, thereby further reducing diagnostic confidence. The need for imaging at the two distal stations with high resolution is reflected by the localization of the infrapopliteal trifurcation in whole-body MR angiography; this important vascular region is acquired either at the penultimate or the last station, depending on the size of the patient. High resolution with submillimeter isotropic voxel size for the last station in multistation MR angiography has been described with parallel imaging techniques (eg, sensitivity encoding) [29] and thus might be extended to the last two stations in whole-body MR angiography.

Future Perspectives

Most recently, time-resolved imaging of contrast kinetics, or TRICKS, 3D MR angiography has been employed for peripheral vessels in patients with peripheral arterial occlusive disease [30]. This technique relies on repeated sampling of the central k space, which results in high temporal resolution and thereby prevents venous contamination [31]. Spatial resolution is maximized by sharing peripheral k-space data from temporally adjacent acquisitions. Initial clinical evaluations proved satisfactory, with high sensitivity and specificity regarding the reliable depiction of arterial disease in the lower extremities. Complex and voluminous reconstructions have limited the technique to only a few centers. Furthermore, only a single station can be imaged with this technique, thereby necessitating multiple contrast material injections for coverage of the entire runoff system.

In contrast to TRICKS 3D MR angiography, the high-resolution protocol with venous compression does not require voluminous data reconstructions and can be implemented into a multistation protocol. Its effect on image quality was similar: high resolution that permits better delineation of small calf arteries is achieved without venous contamination. The superiority of the high-resolution protocol with venous compression was evidenced by significantly higher SNR and CNR values of the arteries of the lower leg in comparison with those of both the standard and the high-resolution whole-body examinations. In addition, the visualization of small arteries was apparently improved at least in part because of the increased blood volume in the arterial bed. This finding was underlined by the improved differentiation between patent and occluded vessels when analysis was based on the high-resolution images with venous compression compared with the standard protocol. Furthermore, venous compression caused prolonged arterial and delayed venous filling and thus allowed for better arterial visualization.

Venous compression has so far been applied for MR angiography of the venous vessels [32] to prevent rapid washout following contrast material administration into a peripheral vein, which is similar to conventional fluoroscopic x-ray phlebography. Venous compression for arterial imaging has, to date, been employed for imaging of arteriovenous fistulas and has been described before for imaging of peripheral vascular disease (U.S. patent 5, 924, 987).

Recently, Bilecen et al described their first experience with a subsystolic continuous compression technique for optimized assessment of hand vascularization on contrast-enhanced MR angiography [33]. Herborn et al evaluated this technique (VENCO) for the peripheral vasculature [28]: five volunteers and 10 patients suspected of having peripheral vascular disease underwent multistation contrast material–enhanced three-dimensional whole-body magnetic resonance (MR) angiography. The first examination, based on standard protocol, lasted 72 seconds, while the following two examinations, performed with a high-spatial-resolution T1-weighted gradient-recalled-echo sequence for the last two stations (lower extremities) lasted 170 seconds. In the second high-resolution examination, midfemoral venous compression was used. Intraindividual comparison showed the high-resolution protocol with venous compression resulted in the best qualitative and quantitative image quality through higher signal-to-noise and contrast-to-noise ratios in the calf arteries. Despite prolonged acquisition times, there was no venous contamination. The data suggest that midfemoral venous compression should be incorporated in multistation protocols of the lower extremities to improve depiction of calf arteries without disturbing venous overlap. The technique is simple and appears to be highly effective.

Herborn et al. conclude that multistation whole-body MR angiography with high spatial resolution of the femoral and trifurcation arteries in conjunction with venous compression at the midfemoral level leads to a vastly improved display of the arterial vasculature of the lower extremities. The high resolution is achieved without any venous contamination. Venous compression whole-body MR angiography is simple to implement and is likely to enhance the performance of all other multistation MR angiography strategies for assessment of the peripheral arterial tree.

New MR Contrast Agents and Whole-Body MRA

Currently, only a few extracellular non-binding gadolinium (Gd) chelates have regulatory approval as agents for MR angiography [34]. Modified paramagnetic Gd-based agents with varying degrees of protein as well as superparamagnetic compounds are currently undergoing clinical evaluation [35]. Some new agents such as MultiHance which was mainly used in the above mentioned studies on whole-body MR-angiography have higher relaxivity and dual routes of excretion but still distribute into the extracellular spaces. Contrast compounds with higher concentration formulations such as Gadovist 1.0 M (Schering, Berlin/Germany) might be advantageous with regard to arterial enhancement [36] as compared to conventional 0.5 M extracellular contrast agents. Blood pool or intravascular contrast agents are large enough, or bind to large enough molecules when injected, that they do not leak out of the capillaries but stay within the intravascular compartment. However, in view of the rapid progress of MRA techniques based on the use of extracellular agents, the future of intravascular contrast agents for morphologic imaging of the arterial vascular tree outside the coronary arteries remains questionable. On the other hand, with regard to whole-body MRA, intravascular contrast agents might be advantageous in allowing a preliminary screening-like whole-body MRA exam, followed, without further contrast administration, by a steady-state mono-station high-resolution acquisition of culprit lesions identified by whole-body MRA.

References

1. Rutkow IM, Ernst CB (1986) An analysis of vascular surgical manpower requirements and vascular surgical rates in the United States. J Vasc Surg 3:74-83
2. Management of peripheral arterial disease (PAD) (2000) TransAtlantic Inter-Society Consensus (TASC). J Vasc Surg 31, part 2 (Supplement):S5
3. Hessel SJ, Adams DF, Abrams HL (1981) Complications of angiography. Radiology 138:273-281
4. AbuRahma AF, Robinson PA, Boland JP et al (1993) Complications of arteriography in a recent series of 707 cases: factors affecting outcome. Ann Vasc Surg 7:122-129
5. Shehadi WH (1982) Contrast media adverse reactions: occurrence, recurrence, and distribution patterns. Radiology 143:11-17

6. Shellock FG, Kanal E (1999) Safety of magnetic resonance imaging contrast agents. J Magn Reson Imaging 10:477-84

7. Prince MR (1994) Gadolinium-enhanced MR aortography. Radiology 191:155-164

8. Prince MR, Narasimham DL, Stanley JC et al (1995) Breath-hold gadolinium-enhanced MR angiography of the abdominal aorta and its major branches. Radiology 197:785-792

9. Meaney JF, Weg JG, Chenevert TL et al (1997) Diagnosis of pulmonary embolism with magnetic resonance angiography. N Engl J Med 336: 1422-1427

10. Goyen M, Debatin JF, Ruehm SG (2001) Peripheral MR-Angiography Top Magn Res Imaging 12:327-335

11. Meaney JF, Ridgway JP, Chakraverty S et al (1999) Stepping-table gadolinium-enhanced digital subtraction MR angiography of the aorta and lower extremity arteries: preliminary experience. Radiology 211:59-67

12. Ho KY, Leiner T, de Haan MW et al (1998) Peripheral vascular tree stenoses: evaluation with moving-bed infusion-tracking MR angiography. Radiology 206:683-692

13. Ruehm SG, Hany TF, Pfammatter T et al (2000) Pelvic and lower extremity arterial imaging: diagnostic performance of three-dimensional contrast-enhanced MR angiography. Am J Roentgenol 174:1127-1135

14. Goyen M, Ruehm SG, Barkhausen J et al (2001) Improved Multi-Station Peripheral MR Angiography with a Dedicated Vascular Coil J Magn Reson Imaging 13:475-480

15. Ruehm SG, Goyen M, Barkhausen J et al (2001) Rapid magnetic resonance angiography for detection of atherosclerosis. Lancet 357: 1086-1091

16. Ruehm SG, Goyen M, Quick HH et al (2000) Whole-body MRA on a rolling table platform (AngioSURF) RöFo 172:670-674

17. Goyen M, Herborn CU, Lauenstein TC et al (2002) High-Resolution Whole-Body 3D MR-Angiography using AngioSURF: Assessment of Optimal Contrast Dosage Invest Radiol 37:263-268

18. Goyen M, Quick HH, Debatin JF et al (2002) High Resolution Whole Body 3D MR Angiography (AngioSURF): Initial Clinical Experience Radiology

19. Cavagna FM, Maggioni F, Castelli PM et al (1997) Gadolinium chelates with weak binding to serum proteins. A new class of high-efficiency, general purpose contrast agents for magnetic resonance imaging. Invest Radiol 32:780-796

20. Management of peripheral arterial disease (PAD) (2000) TransAtlantic Inter-Society Consensus (TASC). J Vasc Surg 31, part 2 (Supplement):S69

21. Goyen M, Herborn CU, Kröger K et al (2003) Detection of atherosclerosis: systemic imaging for systemic disease with whole-body three-dimensional MR angiography – initial experience. Radiology 227:277-282.

22. Von Kemp K, van den Brande P, Peterson T et al (1997) Screening for concomitant diseases in peripheral vascular patients. Results of a systematic approach. Int Angiol 16:114-122

23. Klop RB, Eikelboom BC, Taks AC et al (1991) Screening of the internal carotid arteries in patients with peripheral vascular disease by colour-flow duplex scanning. Eur J Vasc Surg 5:41-45

24. Alexandrova NA, Gibson WC, Norris JW et al (1996) Carotid artery stenosis in peripheral vascular disease. J Vasc Surg 23:645-649

25. McDaniel MD, Cronenwett JL (1989) Basic data related to the natural history of intermittent claudication. Ann Vasc Surg 3:273-277

26. Marek J, Mills JL, Harvich J et al (1996) Utility of routine carotid duplex screening in patients who have claudication. J Vasc Surg 24:572-577 discussion 577-9

27. Kreitner KF, Kalden P, Neufang A et al (2000) Diabetes and peripheral arterial occlusive disease: prospective comparison of contrast-enhanced three-dimensional MR angiography with conventional digital subtraction angiography. AJR Am J Roentgenol 174:171-179

28. Herborn CU, Ajaj W, Goyen M et al (2004) Peripheral vasculature: whole-body MR angiography with midfemoral venous compression—initial experience. Radiology. 230: 872-878

29. Maki JH, Wilson GJ, Eubank WB et al (2002) Utilizing SENSE to achieve lower station sub-millimeter isotropic resolution and minimal venous enhancement in peripheral MR angiography. J Magn Reson Imaging 15:484-491

30. Swan JS, Carroll TJ, Kennell TW et al (2002) Time-resolved three-dimensional contrast-enhanced MR angiography of the peripheral vessels. Radiology 225:43-52

31. Korosec FR, Frayne R, Grist TM (1996) Time-resolved contrast-enhanced 3D MR angiography. Magn Reson Med 36:345-351

32. Ruehm SG, Zimny K, Debatin JF (2001) Direct contrast-enhanced 3D MR venography. Eur Radiol 11:102-112

33. Bilecen D, Aschwanden M, Heidecker HG et al (2004) Optimized assessment of hand vascularization on contrast-enhanced MR angiography with a subsystolic continuous compression technique. AJR Am J Roentgenol 182:180-182

34. Goyen M, Ruehm SG, Debatin JF (2000) MR-Angiography: The Role of Contrast Agents European Journal of Radiology 34: 247-56

35. Knopp MV, von Tengg-Kobligk H, Floemer F et al (1999) Contrast agents for MRA: future directions. J Magn Reson Imaging 10:314-316

36. Goyen M, Lauenstein TC, Herborn CU et al (2001) 0.5 M Gd-Chelate (Magnevist) vs. 1.0 M Gd-Chelate (Gadovist): Dose-independent Effect on Image Quality of Pelvic 3D MRA J Magn Reson Imaging 14:602-607

SECTION VIII

MR Angiography in Pediatrics

VIII

MRA in Pediatric Patients

Peter Fries, Roland Seidel and Günther Schneider

Introduction

Congenital vascular malformations represent an important group of pediatric diseases. The clinical importance of vascular anomalies ranges from uncomplicated and asymptomatic alterations such as hemangiomas of the skin which have only esthetic therapeutic consequences, up to life threatening pathologies such as anomalies of the great vessels or large angiomatoid tumors manifesting with hypoxia due to compression of the airways or because of inadequate oxygen saturation due to right-to-left shunting.

Most of the vascular malformations arise between the third and seventh weeks of embryonic development and may affect the arterial or venous blood vessels, capillaries, lymphatic vessels or venous sinuses. Typically most of the clinically relevant malformations are found in the thorax, however sometimes they also may be incidental findings in other areas (Fig. 1). Malformations may present as changes of the size or course of vessels or as alterations of the vessel wall anatomy. Some malformations involve only an isolated vessel or parts of a vessel, while others may affect a larger part of the vascular system [1].

Vascular malformations, due to the diversity of their clinical manifestations and resulting therapeutic consequences, require an adequate diagnostic tool. MR imaging with its high spatial resolution, free choice of image orientation and lack of ionising radiation is increasingly considered the imaging modality of choice, especially in newborn or small children. A recent study has shown that MRA of the pulmonary vessels in children is superior to echocardiography [2]. Specifically, MRA may clarify uncertain diagnoses in up to one third of the patient population, and reveal an additional diagnosis in another third.

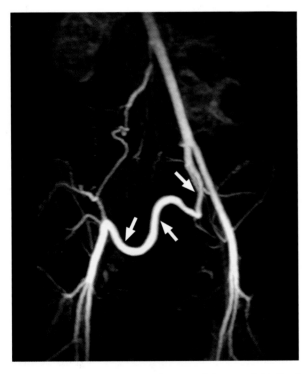

Fig. 1. MIP reconstruction of a 3D CE MRA dataset of the distal aorta and iliac arteries (Gd-BOPTA, 0.1 mmol/kg). Preoperative evaluation of a 14 year old female patient referred for surgery of the urinary bladder revealed an unclear vascular malformation of the pelvic vessels. The MIP image shows that the right common iliac artery derives blood from an atypical vessel originating from the left common iliac artery at the origin of the internal left iliac artery. This atypical vessel crosses the pelvis dorsal to the urinary bladder and supplies the right lower extremity (*arrows*)

Technique

Technical progress in MR imaging has enabled significant reductions of acquisition times to the point that acquisition of real-time images is now possible. Nevertheless, motion artefacts remain critical since patient movement can severely reduce image quality and subsequent diagnostic accuracy. To avoid motion artefacts in pediatric patients, sedation or even anesthesia with intubation and controlled ventilation is often required. MR imaging may be performed in spontaneous breathing patients if respiratory-gated sequences are utilized. A pressure sensor attached to a belt encircling the patient's upper abdomen can be used to record respiratory motion. Synchronization between the detected abdominal wall excursion and the MR acquisition has been shown to decrease motion artefacts considerably. However, the technique is limited by the indirectness of the mechanic coupling between the abdominal wall motion and the structures to be imaged in the chest. Nevertheless, the technique is suitable for the evaluation of intraabdominal pathologies.

With the introduction of navigator sequences a new method of respiratory monitoring has become available. For these navigator sequences a single slab measurement perpendicular to the diaphragm detects the motional excursion of the diaphragm and can be used as a trigger signal for the MR acquisition. This allows for compensation of respiratory motion. However, acquisition of high resolution cross-sectional images in the thorax has to be combined with ECG gating and thus measurement times may drastically increase.

As a consequence, controlled ventilation combined with breath-holding is often preferred for examinations of intrathoracic lesions in order to reduce motion artefacts. State of the art MR imaging equipment now permits many acquisitions to be completed in just a few seconds making anesthesiologically controlled breath-hold imaging possible in children.

The strong magnetic field inherent to MRI requires special equipment for patient monitoring such as special pulse oximetry devices or ECG paddles. In addition, a ventilation unit and medical perfusor devices have to be MR compatible or should be placed outside the magnetic field and connected by long infusion lines.

Patient positioning within the magnet may be head-first or feet-first since this has no influence on the quality of imaging. However, patient positioning should be consistent with the requirements for careful monitoring and possible ventilation.

For the functional evaluation of flow phenomena, phase related imaging with monitoring of the cardiac cycle is mandatory. To better detect the R-R interval, MR-compatible ECG electrodes should preferably be placed on the left lateral chest wall.

Depending on the patient's size or the size of the malformation to be examined, different kinds of coils may be used.

In small children the use of phased array body surface coils covering almost the whole body permits examination of the entire intracorporal vas-

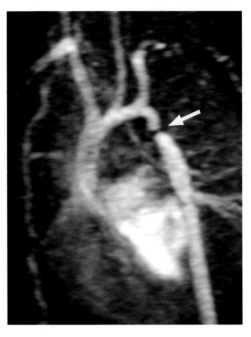

Fig. 2. MIP reconstruction of the arterial phase of a thoracic MRA in a premature baby (30th week of pregnancy) (Gd-BOPTA, 0.2 mmol/kg, total contrast agent volume 0.15 ml). Limitations of resolution are apparent due to the extremely small size of the anatomic structures (diameter of aorta approx. 1.5 – 2 mm). Nevertheless, diagnosis of a typical aortic coarctation (*arrow*) with a stenosis distal to the left subclavian artery was possible

cular architecture in one imaging study. In small babies, newborns or for more localized malformations, wrap around surface coils may be used, however even with these coils the borders of resolution may be reached in premature babies (Fig. 2). Alternatively extremity coils can be used for imaging of children. Head coils are generally not advisable since the geometry of the thorax of a baby does not fit the volume for which head coils are optimized.

Imaging Protocol and Strategy

Every examination begins with the acquisition of localizing images obtained in the axial, coronal and sagittal planes using SSFP sequences or GRE sequences with ECG gating. Alternatively, fast gradient-echo sequences without ECG-gating can be used. The aim is to obtain a detailed description of anatomic structures (e.g. heart or major vessels) in the region of interest in order to further characterize the underlying anomaly.

ECG-gated CINE images may be acquired for evaluation of the heart and the great vessels. These fast gradient echo images may demonstrate flow and functionality of the vessel anatomy and subsequent pathological processes. The anatomic course of a vessel and flow direction can be demonstrated

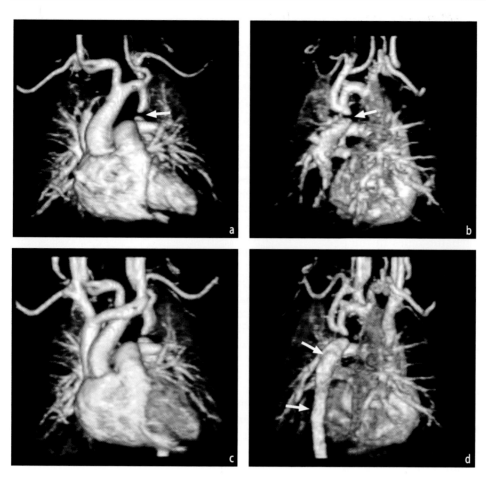

Fig. 3a-d. This case demonstrates a patient with coarctation distal to the left subclavian artery. Evaluation of the aortic arch and supraaortic branching vessels is clearly possible on early arterial phase imaging (**a**) anterior-posterior view; (**b**) posterior-anterior view (*arrows*). However, no assessment of the descending aorta distally to the stenosis is possible at this time. On images acquired directly after this first phase the thoracic arterial and venous vessels are apparent (**c**) anterior-posterior view. Note that at this time-point the descending aorta distal to the stenosis is also depicted and is available for further evaluation (**d**) (*arrows*). This case demonstrates that several acquisitions after contrast agent administration may provide additional information on arterial and venous vessel status as well as on the direction of blood flow (Gd-BOPTA, 0.1 mmol/kg)

immediately. In cases of vascular stenosis, for example in patients with aortic coarctation, a post-stenotic jet phenomenon can often be observed.

T1w spin-echo sequences can be used for the evaluation of wall structures. Due to their excellent anatomic resolution small endoluminal webs and baffles can be demonstrated. In cases of endovascular thrombus formation T1w fat suppressed images can be acquired to increase the signal intensity of the blood clot and thereby better emphasize the thrombotic material.

For investigation of vessels after endovascular stenting ECG-gated double- or triple-inversion recovery fast spin-echo sequences can be used to clearly elaborate the post-surgical vascular anatomy. Since these images are acquired in the diastolic phase during a solitary breath-hold, and demonstrate very low susceptibility artefacts in the presence of metallic implants, the image quality is only slightly reduced and vascular structures can be evaluated satisfactorily.

Notwithstanding the value of non-contrast sequences, it is contrast-enhanced 3D MR angiography (CE-MRA) in conjunction with the use of extracellular gadolinium contrast agents that plays the key role in the diagnosis of vascular malformations. CE-MRA permits differentiation between arterial, venous and lymphoid vessels, depicts the blood supply of tumoral lesions, and may highlight the nature of a pathological process. With the 3D acquisition technique an entire volume of interest can be covered with one slab, allowing precise characterisation of the vessel shape and course. Furthermore, the detection of collateral vessels, the extension of a stenosis or the 3D relationship to other anatomic landmarks such as the heart or other great vessels can be revealed with one acquisition. Multiplanar reconstruction as a postprocessing option can be helpful for a detailed evaluation of complicated vessel anatomy.

In order to evaluate the vascular architecture of the thorax or even the whole body in small children, contrast agent application during ongoing image acquisition may demonstrate the arterial and venous anatomy in one extended breath-hold (Fig. 3). The administration of a test bolus or automatic bolus triggering is rarely helpful in small children firstly because the amount of contrast agent required for a test bolus often approximates the total contrast agent dose required, and secondly because variable congenital shunting or post surgical variations sometimes render the order of enhancement of the pulmonary, and systemic arterial and venous structures unpredictable. With acquisition times of 6 to 8 seconds several perfusion phases of the volume of interest can be detected in one single breath-hold to better characterize arterial perfusion, venous return, arterio-venous shunting or pooling of the contrast agent in the case of tumor tissue. Additionally, VIBE (Volume Interpolated Breath-hold Examination) sequences may be acquired after contrast agent application in order to depict intramural pathologies and their correlation to surrounding anatomic structures.

Pathology

Whereas most vascular pathologies in the pediatric population are congenital in nature, a small percentage may be due to infection, systemic disease, trauma or iatrogenic causes. In terms of anatomic localisation, vascular pathologies may be sub-classified as thoracic lesions, as intraabdominal lesions, and as soft-tissue tumors of the head and neck, thoracic or abdominal wall, and limbs.

Congenital Anomalies of the Aorta

Anomalies of the aorta may range from asymptomatic changes such as atypical, aberrant supraaortic vessels to life-threatening malformations such as vascular rings with compression of the trachea, complex anomalies in association with cardiac malformations, or aneurysms with high-risk of rupture.

For many years conventional thoracic x-ray films, with and without a barium esophagogram was the primary diagnostic tool for evaluation of congenital anomalies of the aorta. Typically, conventional angiography also had to be performed in order to clarify the diagnosis. Nowadays, MRI and CE-MRA have replaced x-ray based imaging modalities for visualization of pathologies of the heart, aorta and great vessels [3, 4].

Congenital anomalies of the thoracic aorta may be sub-divided according to the course and diameter of the ascending aorta and aortic arch, the position of the supraaortic vessels and descending aorta, as well as the relationship of the thoracic aorta to the ductus and to the ligamentum arteriosum. Although these are the principal sub-divisions, adequate diagnosis also depends on careful and systematic examination of all subsequent parts of the aorta.

Aneurysm of the Aortic Sinus (Sinus of Valsalva)

The aortic sinuses are located at the aortic root, directly superior to the aortic valve. They comprise the right coronary sinus and the left coronary sinus, which correspond to the relevant coronary arteries, and the posterior, acoronary sinus. In cases of an abnormal or even congenitally missing media of the vessel wall in the aortic root, aneurysmatic dilation of a sinus of Valsalva may occur. Typically, these congenital aneurysms involve the right coronary sinus (90%). However, they may also be acquired in response to arteriosclerosis, post-inflammatory changes or trauma. The clinical manifestation ranges from asymptomatic to mediastinal hemorrhage and rupture into the chambers of the heart [5, 6].

Malformation of the Aortic Arch

Malformations of the aortic arch may be classified on the basis of position relative to the trachea, esophagus and the origin and course of the subclavian arteries. Many different classifications of malformations of the aortic arch have been described. However, most reasonable classifications derive from the hypothetical double aortic arch of *Edwards*, in which two aortic arches form a ring around the trachea and the oesophagus with separate origins of the subclavian and carotid arteries and a left and a right ductus arteriosus.

Double Aortic Arch

A double aortic arch develops if both embryologic arches persist and form a vascular ring around the trachea and the oesophagus. Usually these patients are asymptomatic and a double aortic arch is an isolated condition. If the vascular ring results in a stenosis of the trachea or the oesophagus typical symptoms may include stridor, dyspnea, recurrent pneumonia and dysphagia. Typically, in a double aortic arch the "four-artery sign" is found with each arch giving rise to a ventral carotid artery and a dorsal subclavian artery (Fig. 4).

Right Aortic Arch

In cases of a right aortic arch, the aorta is located right-sided in relation to the trachea and esophagus and passes the mediastinum posteriorly and laterally near the right lung. It may be found in up to 0.1% of adults [7]. Three different kinds of right aortic arch may be identified:
- a right aortic arch with an aberrant left subclavian artery
- a right aortic arch with mirror image branching, and
- a right aortic arch with isolated left subclavian artery, [8, 9].

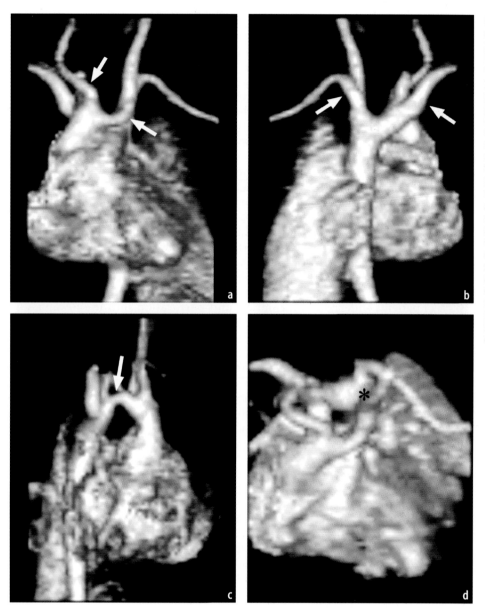

Fig. 4a-d. Surface rendered reconstruction of a 3D CE MRA dataset (Gd-BOPTA, 0.1 mmol/kg) in a 9 week old girl with incomplete double aortic arch. **a** Anterior-posterior view; **b** posterior-anterior view. Note that a total of four supraaortic vessels, two common carotid arteries anterior (*arrows* in **a**) and two subclavian arteries posterior (*arrows* in **b**) derive from the aortic arch. Additionally, note the typical Y-configuration of the subclavian vessels and the descending aorta. On a lateral view (**c**) a moderate stenosis of the right aortic arch can be seen (*arrow*). On a cranial-caudal view (**d**) the vascular ring with a hypoplasia of the anterior left part (*asterisk*) is also clearly depicted

Right aortic arch with aberrant left subclavian artery.

This occurs with an incidence of 0.06 to 0.1% in adult patients and is the most common right aortic arch malformation [10]. This anomaly may occur in association with other severe malformations of the heart such as tetralogy of Fallot. Corresponding to the course of the ligamentum arteriosum or the ductus arteriosus, formation of a vascular ring results in compression of the trachea or the esophagus leading to characteristic clinical symptoms. A right aortic arch with aberrant left subclavian artery is the second most common cause of a vascular ring formation after a double aortic arch [11].

Based on the hypothetical double aortic arch of *Edwards*, an embryologically right aortic arch with aberrant left subclavian artery develops due to an interruption of the left aortic arch between the left common carotid artery, which passes anterior to the trachea, and the left subclavian artery, which is located posterior to the esophagus. Typically, it is the localisation of the ligamentum arteriosum that determines whether a vascular ring is formed (left-sided between the left pulmonary artery and the left subclavian artery) or not formed (right-sided or left-sided between the left pulmonary artery and the left subclavian artery).

Right aortic arch with mirror image branching.

In this malformation, the supraaortal vessels are located anterior to the trachea and no retroesophageal vessel is found. Formation of a vascular ring does not occur and therefore airway compression is not a typical sign of right aortic arch with mirror image branching. Typically, the left common carotid artery and left subclavian artery derive from a left-sided bracheocephalic trunk while the right common carotid artery and right subclavian artery have separate origins.

Right aortic arch with mirror image branching is the result of a defect of the left descending aorta distal to the left subclavian artery. A high correlation exists between this malformation and other congenital malformations of the cardiovascular system such as tetralogy of Fallot, ventricular septal defect and truncus arteriosus. Moreover, right aortic arch with mirror image branching is frequently diagnosed in combination with congenital heart disease [7, 10].

Right aortic arch with isolated left subclavian artery.

The third most common right aortic arch anomaly is found in approximately 2% of patients with right aortic arch and occurs in association with tetralogy of Fallot. In this malformation an interruption of the embryogenic left arch takes place between the left common carotid artery and the left subclavian artery and additionally between the left ductus and the descending aorta. These interruptions result in a connection between the left subclavian artery and the left pulmonary artery which leads to a congenital subclavian steal syndrome.

Typical findings are a left common carotid artery arising as the first branch from the right aortic arch and a left subclavian artery that attaches to the left pulmonary artery through a patent ductus arteriosus. No vascular ring or retroesophageal components are found.

Left Aortic Arch

In embryological development, a right and a left aortic arch together with a potential persistent ductus arteriosus is found on each side. These two arches may fuse dorsally to the trachea and the esophagus and form the future descending aorta. Normal anatomy may develop in response to an interruption of the right aortic arch distally to the origin of the right subclavian artery. Fusion of the right common carotid artery and the right subclavian artery forms the brachiocephalic vessel.

Left aortic arch with aberrant right subclavian artery.

A left aortic arch with aberrant right subclavian artery represents a mirror image of a right aortic arch with aberrant left subclavian artery. It is the most common malformation of the left aortic arch occurring with prevalence of 0.4% to 2%, and is usually asymptomatic [12]. Left aortic arch with

aberrant right subclavian artery is based on an interruption of the right aortic arch between the right common carotid artery and the right subclavian artery. Occasionally, the origin of the right subclavian artery may show an ectasia (the so-called diverticulum of Kommerell), which represents a persistent part of most distal aspect of the right aortic arch [7, 10].

Left aortic arch with aberrant right subclavian artery may be an isolated finding or may occur in conjunction with other congenital cardiovascular malformations. As the aberrant right subclavian artery passes the mediastinum dorsally to the trachea and the esophagus no vascular ring is formed. In elderly patients, the aberrant right subclavian artery may show ectatic changes and tortuousity, thereby causing compression of the trachea and esophagus, which may manifest with dysphagia and dyspnea [3, 4]. In some cases aneurysm formation and perforation into the oesophagus has been described.

Aortic Coarctation

Aortic coarctation is the most common congenital abnormality of the thoracic aorta, occurring with a frequency in newborns of 4/10000. It can be found in 7% of patients with congenital heart disease [12, 13]. Coarctation of the aorta develops secondarily to a deformity of the aortic media in which a fibrous ridge protrudes into the vascular lumen. The anomaly most frequently occurs distal to the left subclavian artery or near the branching of the ductus arteriosus (Fig. 5). Different forms of stenotic vascular segments can be found: the lesion may be focal, as in a juxtaductal coarctation; diffuse, as in a hypoplastic aortic isthmus; or complete, as in an aortic arch interruption. Depending on the grade of the stenosis, collateral circulation may develop via intercostal arteries, internal mammary arteries, lateral thoracic arteries, the anterior spinal artery, scapular arteries or transverse cervical arteries.

MR imaging has similar sensitivity to conventional angiography and higher sensitivity than echocardiography for the evaluation of stenotic segments and collateral vessels and for therapeutic monitoring (Fig. 6) [14]. Axial and left anterior oblique spin-echo sequences can determine the localisation and extension of the lesion. The vessel diameter can be measured on axial images perpendicular to the ascending and descending aorta. Expression of the severity of stenosis is possible as a percentage ratio between the minimal diameter of the isthmus and the mean diameter of the ascending and descending aorta subtracted from 100 [15]. A relevant stenotic segment can be presumed if a measured segment has a diameter of less than 50%.

CINE imaging with left anterior oblique orien-

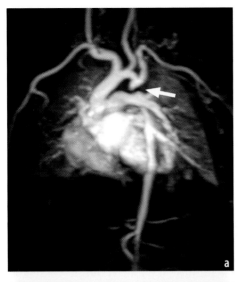

Fig. 5a-c. This case demonstrates a 2 week old male newborn with aortic coarctation. **a** After intravenous contrast agent application (Gd-BOPTA 0.1 mmol/kg bodyweight) the systemic arterial system from the supraaortic vessels down to the abdominal vessels are clearly depicted on the MIP reconstruction. Note the subtotal stenosis of the aortic isthmus distal to the branching of the left subclavian artery (*arrow*) depicting as complete interruption of contrast enhancement within the vessel. The subsequent increased blood pressure and blood flow leads to a kinking of the supraaortic vessels. **b** demonstrates the corresponding surface rendered image reconstruction in anterior-posterior and posterior-anterior (**c**) view

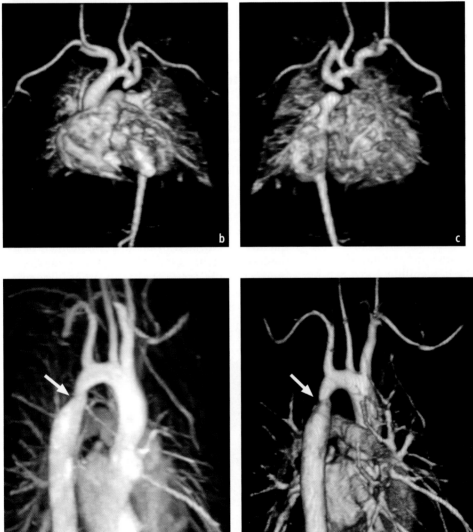

Fig. 6a, b. MIP reconstruction of a 3D CE MRA dataset of the thoracic aorta (Gd-BOPTA, 0.1 mmol/kg) in a patient undergoing surgical intervention for aortic coarctation 6 years prior to the current imaging study. Although blood flow is significantly improved and the pressure gradient is relatively shallow, a late recurrence of reduced vessel diameter is depicted (*arrow*). **b** represents the corresponding surface reconstruction

tation can demonstrate flow phenomena such as poststenotic jet phenomenon. Measurement of peak flow velocity is possible with the use of phase contrast images in through plane orientation and with this information the pressure gradient over the stenosis can be estimated on the basis of the Bernoulli equation.

Collateral vascularisation is best demonstrated on 3D CE MRA since the whole spectrum of possible collateral vascular pathways is demonstrable with one acquisition.

Aortic Pseudocoarctation

Aortic pseudocoarctation is an uncommon congenital abnormality of the thoracic aorta. Characterized by an elongation of the first descending part of the aortic arch, an abnormal kinking at the level of the ligamentum arteriosum can be observed (Fig. 7). It occurs when the third and seventh aortic dorsal segments fail to fuse properly to form the aortic arch. A degree of stenosis may be present due to the aortic kinking, although pressure gradients are typically not detected [16].

MRI is an effective tool in the workup of this abnormality. On spin-echo images the high anatomic position of the aortic arch and kinking of the proximal descending aorta can be identified clearly. Velocity encoded imaging is helpful for the exclusion of relevant pressure gradients. Due to turbulent flow phenomena caused by the tortuous course of the vessel a region of flow void may be detected in aortic pseudocoarctation, however this should not be confused with aortic stenosis or coarctation. On 3D MR angiography the complete anatomic course of the descending aorta can be depicted and the absence of collateral vessels can be demonstrated [17].

Venous Malformations

Congenital Venolobar Syndrome

This term comprises a heterogeneity of uncommon abnormalities that may occur singly or in combinations involving anomalous connections of the lung parenchyma, the pulmonary and systemic vasculature, and, rarely, the gastrointestinal tract. Most of the patients present as asymptomatic. In cases of concurrent cardiac anomalies or severe forms of pulmonary atresia or hypoplasia clinical symptoms may occur at an early age. Surgical therapy may be required in selected cases of intractable infections, hemoptysis, and congestive heart failure or pulmonary hypertension due to excessive shunting. Precise anatomic identification of abnormal pulmonary and systemic vessels as well as tracheobronchial anomalies is mandatory for preoperative evaluation of affected patients [18, 19].

Sequestration

In cases of bronchopulmonary sequestration, parts of the pulmonary parenchyma may be found without or with an atypical connection to the tracheobronchial tree. Pulmonary sequestration may be classified as either extralobar or intralobar sequestration.

Extralobar sequestration is usually located in the posterior costodiaphragmal recessus and is typically more left sided than right sided. Less frequently it is located in the upper abdomen or the mediastinum. In about 50% of cases, extralobar sequestration is associated with other congenital anomalies. Extralobar sequestration is usually surrounded by a proper layer of pleura. The arterial

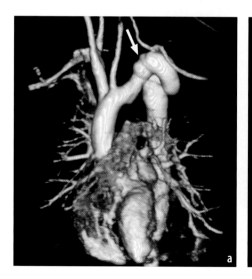
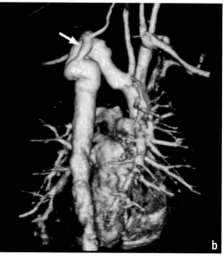

Fig. 7a, b. A 5 year old boy who presented with an unclear pulsating mass in the left supraclavicular fossa of the lower left neck. On the surface rendered image of the thoracic vessels (Gd-BOPTA, 0.1 mmol/kg) a notable tortuous course of the aortic arch distal to the left common carotid artery is apparent (**a**, *arrow*). The corresponding dorsal oblique view demonstrates that the left subclavian artery originates from a tortuous part of the aortic arch (**b**, *arrow*). These findings are indicative of a pseudocoarctation of the aortic arch

blood supply usually derives from the thoracic or abdominal aorta through small branches (Fig. 8) while venous blood drains into the azygous or hemiazygous vein [20].

Intralobar sequestration is usually surrounded by normal pulmonary parenchyma and is located within the normal pleural space. These lesions may be found incidentally in children with no further congenital anomalies. Arterial blood may derive from the pulmonary arteries or aortic branches while venous drainage is usually into the pulmonary veins [21].

Most pulmonary sequestrations are found incidentally on x-ray chest films and therefore require further diagnostic imaging. These anomalies are usually hyperintense on T2w MR imaging while on CE-MRA the anatomic localisation and arterial and venous blood vessel architecture may be suggestive of pulmonary sequestration.

Partial Anomalous Pulmonary Venous Return

In cases of partial anomalous venous return one or more, but not all of the pulmonary veins drain into a systemic vein, resulting in a left-to-right shunt (Fig. 9). Partial anomalous venous return is usually an isolated finding located on the right side. Most patients are either mildly symptomatic or asymptomatic.

Hypogenetic Lung Syndrome / Scimitar Syndrome

In scimitar syndrome one lung is hypoplastic and drained by an anomalous pulmonary vein. The feeding pulmonary artery might be hypoplastic or atretic with systemic collaterals. Abnormal bronchial branching or bronchial hypoplasia in coexistance with abnormal pulmonary segmentation might occur. It is located predominantly on the right and is associated with congenital heart disease in approximately 25% of the patients. Most commonly the atrial septum is involved [22].

If the scimitar vessel drains into the junction of the inferior vena cava with the right atrium a left-to-right shunt is the result [23].

When symptomatic, scimitar syndrome usually occurs in the setting of congestive heart failure. However, the anomaly is often an asymptomatic finding on chest radiographs obtained for other reasons. The typical radiographic sign is an anomalous pulmonary venous trunk coursing vertically along the right atrium toward the right cardiophrenic angle, imitating the appearance of a scimitar or a sword (Fig. 8). Multiplanar MR imaging can visualize the anatomic structures, a hypoplastic lung parenchyma and the abnormal course of the draining vein. For better detection of vascular structures and determination of the venous insertion site CE-MRA is superior to cross sectional imaging.

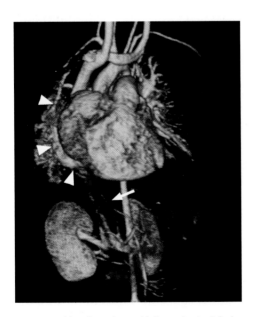

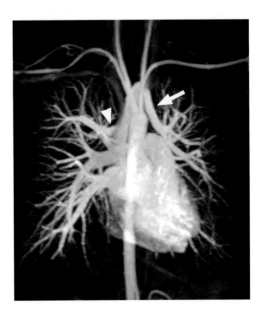

Fig. 8. A 4 year old male patient with hypoplastic right lung and pulmonary sequestration located in the lower lobe of the right lung. A surface reconstruction of a 3D CE MRA dataset in anterior-posterior view reveals an atypical artery which is responsible for the blood supply of the sequester which derives from the abdominal aorta (*arrow*). In addition a malformation of the right pulmonary veins is found which corresponds to a scimitar vessel (*arrowheads*)

Fig. 9. An 8-year-old girl with partial anomalous pulmonary venous return of both upper pulmonary veins. On the MIP reconstruction of the pulmonary CE MRA study (Gd-BOPTA, 0.1 mmol/kg) the upper left pulmonary vein shows a connection to the anonymous vein (*arrow*) with the connection defined as a so-called vertical vein and which is a remnant of the left superior caval vein. The corresponding right upper pulmonary vein also shows an anomalous connection to the superior caval vein (*arrowhead*)

Pulmonary Arteries

Interruption of the pulmonary arteries is possible both on the left and on the right side, with a higher prevalence of interruptions on the right. In case of an interruption of a pulmonary artery the distal pulmonary arteries in both lungs are usually intact being supplied by systemic collateral arteries. Interruption of the left pulmonary artery is less common and is usually associated with congenital heart disease such as tetralogy of Fallot or a ventricular septal defect. In the absence of other congenital anomalies there is almost always a right aortic arch [24].

The affected lung and hilum are usually decreased in size and the pulmonary vessels are either absent or of smaller caliber, causing a radiolucent and asymmetric aspect on chest radiographs. Peripheral arterial perfusion is supplied by systemic mediastinal and transpleural vessels, which can be observed as serrated pleural thickening or subpleural bands on CT or MR imaging. MRA provides a good overview of the location of the interruption of the pulmonary vessels as well as the collateral vascularization.

Pulmonary Stenosis / Atresia

Pulmonary artery stenosis is seen without ventricular septal defect in about 8% of patients with congenital heart disease. In most cases the finding is asymptomatic, although it may be accompanied by cyanotic congenital heart disease. Due to turbulent blood flow, ectasia of the pre- and/or poststenotic part of the vessel may occur.

In cases of pulmonary atresia the continuity between the right ventricle and the pulmonary trunk is interrupted. The right ventricular outflow tract shows hypoplasia and may end blindly. In addition, the main pulmonary artery appears hypoplastic or even atretic and the left and right pulmonary arteries are usually underdeveloped. In most cases, this anomaly is associated with a large ventricular septum defect and formation of collaterals such as dilated intercostal and bronchial arteries as well as a persistent ductus arteriosus Botalli (Fig. 10) [25].

Typically Spontaneous Aortopulmonary Arterial Connections

Accurate imaging of this anomaly is crucial for the planning of reconstructive surgery and MRI is the method of choice to demonstrate all malformations within one examination. Essential for the feasibility of surgical repair of this malformation is to demonstrate the presence of a central confluence of the pulmonary artery even in cases of an absent main pulmonary artery. In addition, depiction of collateral vessels (MAPCA; Major Aorto Pulmonary Collateral Arteries) is important as ligation of these vessels has to be included as part of the surgical repair (Fig. 11) [26].

Vasculitis

Vasculitis involving arterial structures is rare in children. However, inflammatory changes of arterial vessels can be detected in the context of Wegener's granulomatosis, Churg-Strauss syndrome (Fig. 12) and systemic connective tissue diseases such as lupus erythematodes (LE) or dermatomyositis [27]. Wegener's granulomatosis is a necrotizing vasculitis with granuloma formation that involves the respiratory tract and the kidneys [28].

The most common radiographic finding in children involves diffuse interstitial and alveolar opacities. CT detects centrilobular, perivascular faint, or groundglass opacities. MR imaging can demonstrate vascular irregularities on CE-MRA and focal wall enhancement or enhancement of the surrounding tissue in cases of inflammatory infiltrations (Fig. 13). In addition to specific laboratory findings, biopsy is usually required for definitive diagnosis.

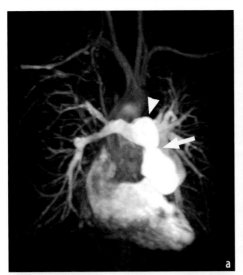

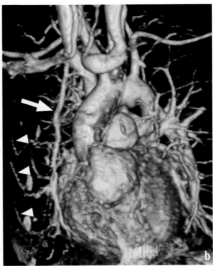

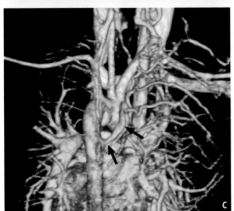

Fig. 10a-d. A 12 year old female patient with obstruction of the right ventricular outflow tract (RVOT). The MIP reconstruction of the arterial phase pulmonary MRA (Gd-BOPTA, 0.1 mmol/kg) (**a**) reveals a stenosis of the RVOT (*arrow*) and a subsequent dilatation of the pulmonary trunk (*arrowhead*). The corresponding surface reconstruction of a second acquisition in anterior-posterior view (**b**) demonstrates ectasia of the internal mammarian artery as one of numerous collateral vessels (*arrow*). Collateral blood flow takes place through intercostal vessels (*arrowheads*) with connection to a major aorto-pulmonary collateral artery (MAPCA), which is depicted on the VRT reconstruction in the posterior-anterior view (**c**, *arrows*). The connection between the aorta and the pulmonary artery is confirmed on axial multiplanar reconstructions (**d**, *arrows*)

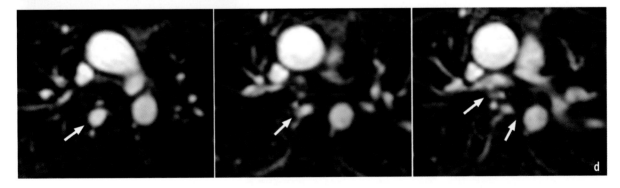

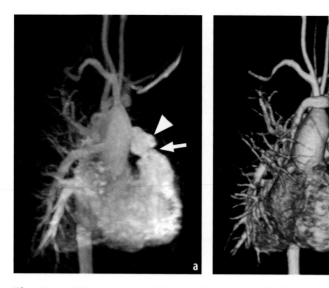
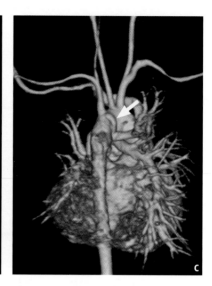

Fig. 11a-c. MIP reconstruction (**a**) and surface rendering (**b, c**) of a 3D CE MRA dataset of a patient with pulmonary stenosis (*arrows* in **a, b**) and subsequent post-stenostic dilatation of the pulmonary trunk (*arrowheads* in **a, b**). Formation of a MAPCA (*arrow*) between the aortic arch and the left superior pulmonary artery is demonstrated on the surface rendered image in posterior-anterior view

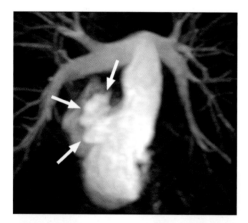

Fig. 12. A 14 year old patient with Churg-Strauss syndrome. On screening echocardiography a pathologic dilatation of the right ventricular outflow tract was found. MIP reconstruction of a pulmonary MRA demonstrates an aneurysm (*arrows*) of the RVOT

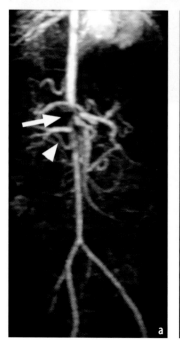
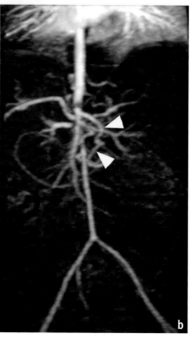

Fig. 13a, b. MIP reconstruction of an abdominal MRA (Gd-BOPTA, 0.1 mmol/kg) in a 2 month old male baby. **a** The abdominal aorta shows a subtotal occlusion due to aortitis (*arrow* in **a**) in the area of the celiac trunk. Distal to the occlusion the diameter of the aorta is significantly reduced. Note the subsequent formation of various collaterals (*arrowheads* in **a, b**) which establish blood supply distal to the stenosis through connections between the celiac trunk and the superior and inferior mesenteric artery

Takayasu Arteritis

Takaysu arteritis is a chronic inflammatory arteritis of unknown origin resulting in thrombosis, stenosis, dilatation and aneurysm formation of the aorta, aortic branch vessels, and pulmonary arteries. Mural calcification and thickening of the aortic wall can also be observed [29]. Symptoms of the disease include an onset beginning in the second decade of life up to the seventh decade, with a mean within the third decade. Early symptoms include dyspnoea and haemoptysis, progressing vascular dissection, cerebrovascular accident and aortic insufficiency with resulting heart failure [30].

T1w MR imaging demonstrates structural wall inhomogeneities and focal thrombi. With SSFP sequences aspects of valvular function can be investigated, permitting detection of possible aortic valve insufficiency. 3D CE MRA can demonstrate the extent of the disease, the grade of arterial stenosis and the formation of aneurysms. On contrast enhanced cross sectional images the inflammatory activity of the disease may be assessed. Intramural neovascularity, high signal of the thickened vascular wall and periaortic tissues reflect activity of the disease. Mural enhancement is also seen in chronic active disease. In this context MR imaging is a good diagnostic tool for therapeutic control [31].

Marfan's Syndrome

Marfan's syndrome is a connective tissue disorder with an autosomal dominant inheritance of variable penetrance. Two of four major criteria involving the cardiovascular, ocular and skeletal systems and family history have to be present for diagnosis. Cardiovascular complications include aortic root dilatation, aortic dissection and aortic valve insufficiency [32].

Non-invasive evaluation of the aorta with MR imaging is very effective for delineation of the aortic configuration and thus detection of aneurysmal dilatation, dissection, and aortic insufficiency. In addition, detection of aneurysms of the pulmonary artery, abdominal aorta or aortic branch vessels, also encountered in Marfan's syndrome, is possible. Pre- and postoperative evaluation of vascular structures can be performed reliably using spin-echo sequences, cine imaging and MR angiography [33].

Arterial Tortuosity Syndrome

Arterial tortuosity syndrome (ATS) is a rare hereditary disorder with variable clinical presentation involving tortuosity and elongation of the ma-

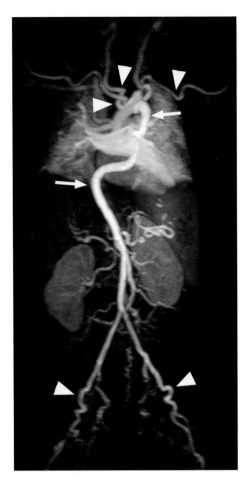

Fig. 14. MIP reconstruction of a 3D CE MRA dataset (Gd-BOPTA, 0.1 mmol/kg, total contrast agent volume 0.3 ml) in a male newborn with arterial tortuosity syndrome. Imaging was performed with a wrap around shoulder coil covering the whole body of the baby. Note the kinking of the thoracic and abdominal aorta (*arrows*) as well as of the supraaortic and iliac vessels (*arrowheads*)

jor arteries. Aneurysm, pulmonary artery stenosis, pulmonary hypertension, skin and joint laxity can be associated and are suggestive of a connective tissue disorder. The transmission of ATS follows an autosomal recessive pattern [34].

Genetic analyses of inbred families have revealed a gene localization on chromosome 20q13, which is different to the locations for other connective tissue disorders such as Marfan's, Beal's or Williams' syndromes. As yet, the causative gene has not been completely identified [35].

The tortuous course of the major arterial vessels as well as associated vascular abnormalities can be excellently demonstrated on 3D CE-MRA (Fig. 14). Additionally, stenotic or ectatic vascular changes can be detected. In pediatric patients, for whom conventional angiography is very challenging and combined with a high risk for vascular damage especially in cases with increased vessel tortuosity, CE-MRA should be the preferred technique for diagnostic evaluation.

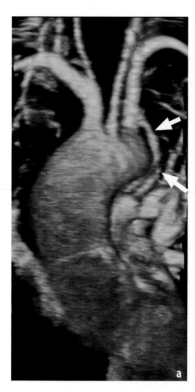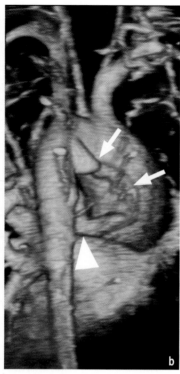

Fig. 15 a, b. Surface rendering of a 3D CE MRA dataset (Gd-BOPTA, 0.1 mmol/kg) of the thoracic vessels. Due to atresia of the RVOT a Blalock-Taussig anastomosis connecting the left subclavian artery with the left pulmonary artery (*arrow*) was created. On the corresponding posterior-anterior view an additional MAPCA is depicted (*arrows*). Distally, the MAPCA connects to the pulmonary trunk (*arrowhead*)

Postoperative Evaluation of Vascular Structures

Evaluation of the postoperative vascular status can be a diagnostic challenge because of confusing anatomy with aberrant circulatory characteristics. Strategies for thoracic surgery comprise a large variety of anastomotic or conduit techniques involving the connection of major vascular or cardiac structures for the restitution of adequate physiologic hemodynamic status. A typical example is represented by the Blalock-Taussig shunt which connects the right or left subclavian artery with the main pulmonary artery branch of the ipsilateral side in order to bypass pulmonary atresia or stenosis (Fig. 15). In addition, a combined patent ductus arteriosus can usually be found. Another example of surgical strategies which can be performed in cases of double outlet right ventricle, is a Glenn-shunt which connects the right superior vena cava with the corresponding pulmonary artery branches (Fig. 16). Under these circumstances a modified Fontan conduit connecting the inferior vena cava to the left or right pulmonary artery is often combined. Evaluation of a postsurgical vascular status of this type with catheter angiography would require an invasive preparation of the left

internal jugular vein, puncture of an iliac vein and arterial catheterisation. In cases in which the left superior vena cava persists, even both jugular veins may have to be punctured.

MR imaging is a valuable diagnostic tool for non-invasive assessment of the postsurgical outcome. In particular, CE 3D MR angiography is very helpful for a complete anatomic description of the area of interest. Due to the requirement for accurate detection of arterial and venous perfusion, multiphase acquisitions involving up to six perfusion phases, are mandatory. Best results are obtained under breath-hold conditions after intubation. For the diagnostic evaluation, thick slab MIP reformations or 3D surface rendered reconstructions may provide an overview of the anatomic situation. Vessel anastomosis or single vascular areas should be assessed by means of multiplanar reformations with reconstruction of thin slabs of variable thickness covering the individual structure of interest. With a focussed diagnostic approach, reliable detection of vessel stenosis in an area of anastomosis can be achieved even when the vessel diameters are extremely small [36].

Common therapeutic approaches in cases of aortic coarctation include interventional treatment with dilatation of the stenosis (Fig. 17), sur-

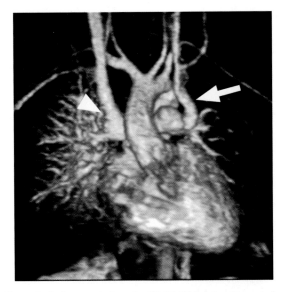

Fig. 16. Surface rendering of a 3D CE MRA dataset in anterior-posterior view in a patient with pulmonary atresia (Gd-BOPTA, 0.1 mmol/kg). This study demonstrates the postoperative situation following bilateral Glenn anastomosis. A persistent left upper vena cava was connected to the left pulmonary artery (*arrow*) and the normal right upper vena cava was connected to the right pulmonary artery (*arrowhead*)

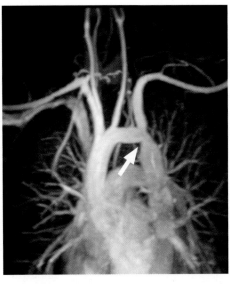

Fig. 17. Patient with coarctation following percutaneous transarterial angioplasty. On MR angiography a remaining low grade stenosis distal to the branching left subclavian artery can be seen (*arrow*). However, no dissection or rupture of the vessel wall due to angioplasty was found. The case shows that MRA is an excellent imaging modality for follow-up of post-operative or post-therapeutic studies of aortic coarctation

gical resection of the involved segment combined with end-to-end anastomosis (Fig. 18) and patch angioplasty. When a concomitant hypoplastic aortic arch is present, flow turbulence can lead to aneurysm formation with the possibility of fatal complications. Finally, the combination of coarctation and aortic valve malformation has to be considered in follow up studies of patients with aortic stenosis (Fig. 19).

MR angiography is extremely reliable in detecting aneurysm formation in the postsurgical follow up of patients and diagnosis based on MR fre-

quently results in therapeutic approaches such as surgical intervention with graft implantation [37]. In addition MR angiography is a valuable diagnostic instrument for the detection of pulmonary artery stenosis, pulmonary shunting or pulmonary vein stenosis after thoraco-surgical treatment [38].

For complete postoperative evaluation MR angiography should always be combined with unenhanced multiplanar T1w and T2w imaging techniques to detect or exclude perivascular complications such as hematoma or seroma as a possible cause for vascular obstruction [39].

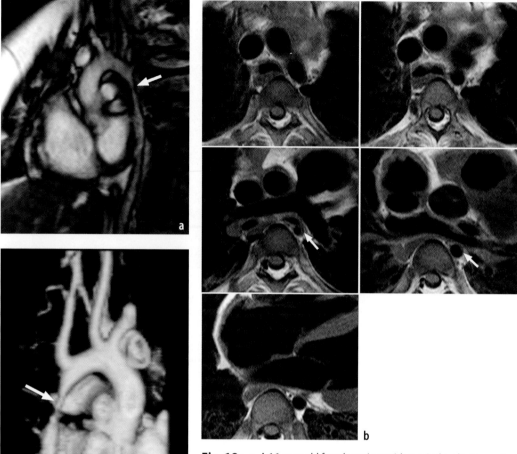

Fig. 18a-c. A 16-year-old female patient with surgical and interventional therapy of aortic coarctation. **a** shows a CINE trueFISP sequence orientated along the axis of the descending aorta. Recurrent stenosis (*arrow*) indicated by a jet phenomenon as a sign of accelerated blood flow can be seen distal to the left subclavian artery. On T1w sequences orientated perpendicular to the axis of the aorta a thickening of the wall of the descending aorta is demonstrated (*arrows* in **b**). Surface rendering of a 3D CE MRA dataset of the same patient (**c**) reveals a significant stenosis distal to the left subclavian artery (*arrow*)

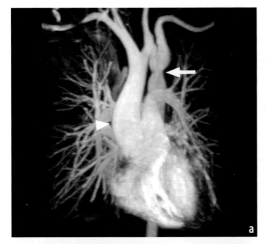

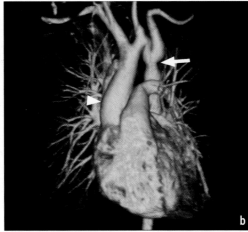

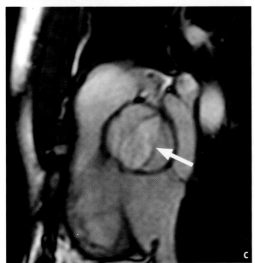

Fig. 19a-c. MIP reconstruction (**a**) of a thoracic CE MRA study (Gd-BOPTA, 0.1 mmol/kg) in a patient with surgical reconstruction of aortic coarctation. This follow-up study revealed a slight residual stenosis distal to the branching of the left subclavian artery (*arrow* in **a**, **b**). However a newly developed ectasia of the aortic root was also depicted on both the MIP (**a**) and the surface rendered image (*arrowheads*). Further examination using CINE trueFISP sequences perpendicular to the aortic valve (**c**) revealed a biscupid aortic valve (*arrow*). This may occur in approximately 30% of patients with aortic coarctation and may result in aneurysm formation of the ascending aorta due to flow turbulence

Conclusion

Detection of vascular malformations in newborns or small children is still a challenge. Due to the varying manifestations and the different clinical and therapeutic consequences, interdisciplinary cooperation between paediatricians, paediatric cardiologists, paediatric surgeons, thoracic surgeons and radiologist is indispensable.

In order to make or confirm a diagnosis, adequate visualisation of the pathology or patho-anatomic circumstances has to be performed. While sonography, echocardiography and plain film radiography are economic and widely disposable screening tools, MR imaging is undoubtedly superior in facilitating a definitive diagnosis. CE-MRA is a safe, non-invasive and accurate imaging modality for anatomic evaluation of vascular abnormalities. In particular, MR angiography may obviate the need for conventional x-ray angiography in evaluating vascular malformations in the paediatric patient population.

References

1. Pascual-Castroviejo I, Pascual-Pascual SI (2002) Congenital vascular malformations in childhood. Semin Pediatr Neurol; Dec 9(4):254-73
2. Valsangiacomo ER, Levasseur S, McCrindle BW et al (2003) Contrast enhanced MR angiography of pulmonary venous abnormalities in children. Pediatr Radiol; Feb 33(2):92-8
3. Van Dyke CW, White RD (1994) Congenital abnormalities of the thoracic aorta presenting in the adult. J Thorac Imaging 9:230-245
4. Gomes AS, Lois JF, George B et al (1987) Congenital abnormalities of the aortic arch: MR imaging. Radiology 165:691-695
5. Coscina WF, Kressel HY, Gefter W et al (1986) MR imaging of the doubleaortic arch. J Comput Assist Tomgr 10:673-675
6. Ho VB, Kinney JB, Sahn DJ (1995) Ruptured sinus of Valsalva aneurysm. cine phase-contrast MR characterization . J Comut Assist Tomgr 19:652-656
7. Kersting-Sommerhoff BA, Sechtem UP, Fisher MR et al (1987) MR imaging of congenital anomalies of the aortic arch. AJR 149:9-13
8. Glanz S, Gordon DH (1981) Right aortic arch with

left descent. J Comput Assist Tomogr 5:256-258

9. Friese KK, Dulce MC, Higgins CB (1992) Airway obstruction by right aortic arch with right-sided patent ductus arteriosum: demonstration by MRI. J Comput Assist Tomogr 16:888-892

10. Van Dyke CW, White RD (1994) Congenital abnormalities of the thoracic aorta presenting in the adult. J Thorac Imaging 9:230-245

11. Kleimman PK, Spevak MR, Nimkin K (1994) Left-sided esophageal indentation in right aortic arch with aberrant left subclavian artery. Radiology 191:565-567

12. Schulthess GK von, Higashino SM, Higgins SS et al (1986) Coarctation of the aorta. Radiology 158:469-474

13. Stefens JC, Bourne MW, Sarkuma H, et al (1994) Quantification of collateral blood flow in coarctation of the aorta by velocity encoded cine magnetic resonance imaging. Circulation 90:937-943

14. Soler R, Rodríguez E, Requejo L et al (1998) Magnetic resonance imaging of congenital abnormalities of the thoracic aorta. Eur Radiol 8:540-546

15. Rees S, Sommerville J, Ward C et al (1987) Corctation of the aorta: MR imaging in late postoperative assessment. Radiology 173:499-502

16. Munial AK, Rose WS, Wiliams G (1994) Magnetic resonance imaging of pseudocoarctation of the aorta: a case report. J Thoracic imaging 9:88-91

17. Soler R, Pombo A, Bargiela A et al (1996) MRI of pseudocoarctation of the aorta: morphological and cine MRI findings. Comp Med imaging Graphics 19:431-436

18. Felson B (1973) Chest roentgenology. Philadelphia, Pa:Saunders 87-92

19. Woodring JH, Howard TA, Kanga JF (1994) Congenital venolabar syndrome revisited. Radiographicss 14:349-369

20. Rosado-de-Christenson ML, Frazier AA, Stocker JT (1993) Extralobular sequestration: radiologic-pathologic correlation. Radiographics 13:425-441

21. Frazier AA, Rosado-de-Christenson ML, Stocker JT et al (1997) Intralobar sequestration: radiologic-pathologic correlation. Radiographics 17:715-745

22. Sener RN, Tugran C, Savas R et al (1993) CT findings in scimitar syndrome. AJR Am J Roentgenol 160:1361

23. Panicec DM, Heizmann ER, Randall PA et al (1987) The continuum of pulmonary developemental anomalies. Radiographics 7:747-772

24. Ellis K (1991) Developmental abnormalites in the systemic blood supply of the lungs. AJR Am J Roentgenol 156:669-679

25. Didier D, Ratib O, Beghetti M, Oberhaensli I et al (1999) Morphologic and functional evaluation of congenital heart disease by magnetic resonance imaging. J Magn Reson Imaging 10:639-655

26. Kersting-Sommerhoff BA, Sechtem UP, Higgins CB (1988) Evaluation of blood supply by nuclear magnetic resonance imaging in patients with pulmonary atresia. J Am Coll Cardial 11:166-171

27. Conolly B, Manson D, Eberhard A et al (1996) CT appearance of pulmonary vasculitis in children. AJR Am J Roentgenol 167:901-904

28. Wadsworth DT, Siegel MJ, Day DL (1994) Wegener´s granulomatosis in children: chest radiographic manifestations. AJR Am J Roentgenol 163:901-904

29. Park JH, Chung JW, IM JG et al (1995) Takayasu arteritis: evaluation of mural changes in the aorta and pulmonary artery with CT angiography. Radiology 196:89-93

30. Yamada I, Numano F, Suzuki S (1993) Takayasu arterits: evaluation with MR imaging. Radiology 188:89-94

31. Choe YH, Kim DK, Koh EM et al (1999) Takayasu arteritis: diagnosis with MR imaging and MR angiography in acute and chronic avctive stages. J Magn Reson Imaging 10:751-757

32. Kawamoto S, Bluemke DA, Traill TA et al (1997) Thoracoabdominal aorta in Marfan syndromme: MR imaging findings of progression on vasculopathy after surgical repair. Radiology 203:727-732

33. Soulen RL, Fishman EK, Pyeritz RE et al (1987) Marfan syndrome: evaluation with MR imaging versus CT. Radiology 165:697-701

34. Franceschini P, Guala A, Licata A et al (2000) Arterial tortuosity syndrome. Am J Med Genet 91:141-143

35. Gardella R, Zoppi N, Assanelli D et al (2004) Exclusion of candidate genes in a family with arterial tortuosity syndrome. Am J Med Genet 126A(3):221-228

36. Takayuki M, Mtoyuki K, Shigeru K et al (2000) Gadolinium-enhanced MR angiography in the evaluation of congenital cardiovascular disease pre- and postoperative states in infants and children. J Magn Reson Imaging 12:1034-1042

37. Bogaert J, Dymarkowski S, Budts W et al (2001) Graft dilation after redo surgery for aneurysm formation following patch angioplasty for aortic coarctation. Eur J Cardiothorac Surg 20(2):430-431

38. Duerinckx A, Wexler L, Banerjee A et al (1994) Postoperative evaluation of pulmonary arteries in congenital heart surgery by magnetic resonance imaging: comparison with echocardiography. Am Heart J 128(Pt 1):1139-1146

39. Van Rijn R, Berger R, Lequin M et al (2001) Development of a perigraft seroma around modified Blalock-Taussig shunts: Imaging evaluation. AJR 178:629-633

SECTION IX

MR Venography

IX

MR Venography

Stefan G. Ruehm

Introduction

The ability of MR imaging to depict flow, in combination with the inherent soft tissue contrast, has led to the rapid clinical implementation of this modality for vascular imaging. Slower flow and more homogeneous flow profiles make MR venography technically less demanding than MR arteriography. Since venous pathology usually tends to be more extensive, high resolution MR imaging is not required for routine MR venography to the same extent as it is needed for imaging of the arterial system. Conventional time-of-flight (TOF) and phase contrast (PC) MR techniques, which do not require the use of a paramagnetic contrast agent, have therefore evolved as reliable and clinically accepted methods for assessment of the venous system. However, these techniques do have limitations in that they are susceptible to pulsatility, in-plane saturation effects, and spin dephasing when laminar flow is disturbed. Furthermore, lengthy acquisition times coupled with the technique's inability to reliably display small deep veins in the calf or superficial and perforating veins running horizontal to the imaging plane have restricted the routine clinical application of conventional MR techniques [1]. To overcome these limitations, the use of contrast-enhanced three-dimensional (3D) contrast-enhanced MR venography has been suggested and is now used with increasing frequency in many institutions.

Techniques for MR Venography

Both TOF and PC MR venography sequences have been employed for morphological evaluation of the vascular system. Although they have limited applicability for assessment of the arterial system, they remain valuable for assessment of the portal and systemic venous systems. Since these techniques are rather time consuming and of limited use in the presence of inordinately slow flow or tortuous venous anatomy, the use of contrast-enhanced 3D MR venography has been proposed to overcome these limitations.

Time-of-Flight MR Venography

Time-of-Flight (TOF) MR angiography is based on a GRE sequence with rapid succession of alpha pulses and short repetition times (TR). Thus the signal of stationary tissue is suppressed, whereas flowing spins in the vessel are consistently refreshed. Two-dimensional (2D) or three-dimensional (3D) TOF images with bright intravascular signal can be obtained (Fig. 1) [2-4]. For vessels coursing within the acquired section ("in-plane flow"), the inflow effect becomes less effective. Intravascular signal may be reduced to the level of surrounding stationary spins, prohibiting differentiation of flowing blood from stationary tissues. Potential difficulties in TOF MR venography may therefore arise in situations where longer vessel sections lie within the imaged section.

Since vessels appear bright on TOF MR venography independently of flow direction, differentiation of arteries from veins can be difficult. Flow in a particular direction can, however be saturated by using spatial flow presaturation bands (Fig. 2). Spins being washed into the section from the presaturated area do not carry any magnetization, resulting in a lack of inflow enhancement [5]. These saturation bands can thus be used to obtain selective TOF arteriograms or venograms.

Commonly, two types of 2D TOF sequences are used for MR venography. The first type (spoiled sequences) relies on the inflow of blood alone to create vascular signal. FLASH (fast low angle shot) [6] and spoiled GRASS (gradient-recalled acquisition in a steady state) sequences belong to this cat-

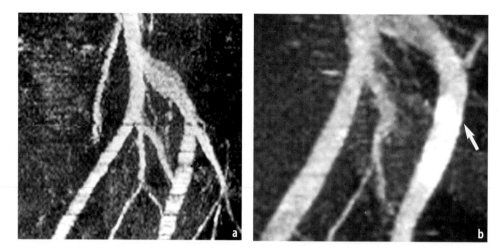

Fig. 1a, b. Maximum Intensity Projection (MIP) display of pelvic venous anatomy based on a 2D MR venography protocol with single slice acquisition in the transverse plain. **a** Regular display of venous anatomy. **b** Missing visualization of left internal iliac vein (*arrow*) due to thrombosis

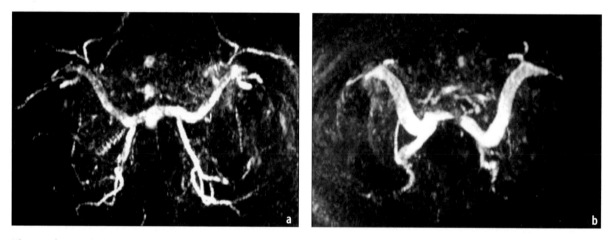

Fig. 2a, b. MIP display (inferior view) of TOF MR angiography of pelvic vasculature with selective visualization of flow from (**a**) superior to inferior (arteries) and (**b**) inferior to superior (veins) using presaturation bands

egory. With the second type of sequence some T2*-weighting is associated resulting in additional brightness of the blood vessels. However, stationary tissues containing fluid, such as bowel or bladder, may also be bright. FISP (fast imaging sequence with partial refocusing) sequences are included in this category, as are GRASS sequences as well. When imaging is performed to study deep vein thrombosis (DVT) spoiled sequences are usually employed.

Blood brightness can be increased by using longer repetition times (TR). Increasing the TR results in an increased number of relaxed spins entering the imaging plane. This is accomplished, however, at the cost of a longer acquisition time. The echo time (TE) should be short although the exact value is not defined and is of minor importance. A TE of 8 msec (on a 1.5 T magnet) has been proposed so that the signal from water and fat are out of phase to enable the signal from fat to be reduced.

Selection of the appropriate flip angle is important. Too large a flip angle may lead to saturation of the venous signal, whereas too small a flip angle results in noisy images. The best flip angle depends on whether the image slice is oriented perpendicular or parallel to the axis of the vessel. For longitudinal flow an angle of 20° to 25° is regarded as appropriate, whereas an angle of 45° should be chosen for imaging in the transverse plane.

Image slices need not be contiguous if only a survey of the venous system is desired. However, thin contiguous or overlapping slices are required if Maximum Intensity Projection (MIP) images need to be calculated.

Phase-Contrast MR Venography

Phase-contrast (PC) MR venography is based on the observation that spins moving through a magnetic field gradient acquire a different phase (phase shift) as compared with static spins. For PC imaging two interleaved views are acquired over successive TRs. There is only one difference between the two views: the second view has an added bipolar gradient along one direction [7]. This bipolar gradient only affects moving spins which acquire a different phase based on their specific flow characteristics. The difference between the phase data of the two successively acquired images is thus limited to phase shifts from moving spins. A true velocity map is therefore acquired. The measured phase difference in individual pixels with flow is directly related to the flow velocity along the direction of the first moment change, which is referred to as the "velocity-encoded direction", and which may be along the x-, y-, or z-axis. By convention, flow is bright if it flows from right to left (x-plane), anterior to posterior (y-plane) and superior to inferior (z-plane). Flow in the opposite direction is depicted as black. The technique is unique in the sense that it is a direct velocity map, in which the voxel intensity values are proportional to the actual flow velocity in a particular flow direction. The flow sensitivity can be adjusted. The "velocity encoding value" (VENC) helps to determine the largest measurable velocity. The appropriate VENC value should be chosen to exceed the maximum expected velocity by about 25%. For some time PC imaging was the preferred MR technique for assessing the portal venous system [8] since it permitted direct quantitative characterization of flow dynamics over time [9].

3D Contrast-Enhanced MR Venography Techniques

Contrast-enhanced MR venography can be performed using an indirect or direct approach. For the indirect approach, contrast agent is usually administered via an antecubital vein and imaging is performed during the equilibrium contrast phase [10, 11]. Typically a large dose is required since the contrast agent undergoes considerable dilution before it reaches the venous vascular territory under investigation. Images should be obtained in the early equilibrium phase to avoid significant redistribution of the contrast agent in the extracellular fluid compartment.

Typically, image subtraction needs to be performed to improve the contrast-to-noise ratio (CNR) of vessels versus background in order to improve the quality of the 3D displays. Image sub-traction requires the acquisition of pre- and post-contrast data. Image subtraction works less well in the chest and abdomen due to potential spatial misregistration artifacts caused by respiratory motion. The advantage of the indirect approach is that there is no requirement for direct cannulation of the vein in the affected extremity.

For the direct approach diluted paramagnetic contrast agent is continuously injected upstream on the side of the affected extremity. This approach permits a full display of the deep and superficial venous system in a manner similar to that achieved with conventional venography. Compared to the indirect approach the direct injection technique results in superior CNR values although considerably less contrast agent is required. To avoid T2-shortening effects the dilution factor should be in the range of 1:10-20. The 3D data set should be collected during contrast administration. Repeated acquisitions can be performed, e.g. with and without placement of a tourniquet or with the extremity in different positions to evaluate for functional obstruction of veins [12, 13], e.g. in patients with suspected thoracic outlet syndrome.

The use of a surface coil to increase signal-to-noise ratio (SNR) and resolution is advantageous. For data collection, a 3D data set with very short TR and TE values and a flip angle of 30-40° should be used. Imaging should start following the injection of the first 50-60 ml of diluted contrast agent. To allow for continuous contrast agent infusion, a tubing set is helpful which permits the simultaneous attachment of two 60 ml syringes. Contrast agent injection should continue during data collection with sequential k-space filling. This enables central k-lines to be acquired in the middle of the data acquisition and helps avoid artifacts arising from changing gadolinium concentration. In addition, this approach allows more time for filling of venous collaterals in the presence of a venous occlusion.

Direct Thrombus Imaging

In contrast to most imaging techniques, which delineate thrombus as flow void or contrast filling defect, magnetic resonance direct thrombus imaging visualizes thrombus against a suppressed background (Fig. 3). During the process of thrombus formation, a predictable reduction in the T1 value of the clot occurs reflecting the presence of methemoglobin. High signal intensity occurs initially at the periphery of the clot which, over time, extends toward the center. In addition to the signal generated by the thrombus itself, further contrast of a clot against blood can be created by nulling the unclotted blood signal using an inversion recovery pulse. Background signal on the T1-weighted image can be further suppressed through selective radio-fre-

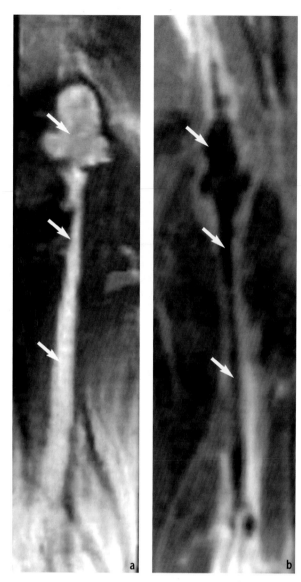

Fig. 3a, b. Oblique reformatted display of thrombus extending from the calf vein into the politeal vein displayed by (**a**) direct thrombus imaging (no contrast administration) and (**b**) indirect contrast-enhanced MR venography. Whereas the thrombus (*arrows*) shows bright signal intensity with the direct thrombus imaging approach, on the contrast enhanced image the thrombus is visualized as filling defect

quency excitation of water molecules to reduce the fat signal. The technique has been shown to be useful for the detection of acute DVT [14].

Pitfalls and Limitations

Interpretation of MR venography for the detection of thrombus is usually based on the depiction of a dark intraluminal defect. On MIP images such a central filling defect can be masked by the bright signal of blood surrounding the thrombus. On TOF MR venography, reduced intravascular intensity may be mistaken for thrombus on MIP dis-

plays because the vein enters the slice obliquely. Similarly, compression of a vein by an adjacent structure may be mistaken for thrombus on both non-contrast-enhanced and contrast-enhanced techniques alike. It is therefore mandatory to scrutinize the source images rather than to simply rely on MIP displays alone.

Some patients show exaggerated respiratory variations in venous flow. If flow sensitive TOF MR venography is used the vein will appear dark if the central part of the acquisition is obtained while the venous flow is substantially reduced during exhalation. Under these circumstances data acquisition should be performed during breath-holding. The left common iliac vein is compressed as it passes behind the aorta or iliac artery. On TOF MR venography in particular this can be misinterpreted as a stricture or a filling defect on the MIP display.

With the direct MR venography technique insufficient dilution of the contrast agent will induce T2 and T2* shortening effects resulting in complete signal drop of the venous lumen. To avoid this artifact, a standard 0.5 molar extracellular contrast agent should be diluted at least by a factor of 10.

In the presence of venous occlusion, the period of contrast agent injection might not be enough to allow complete filling of collateral veins and reconstitution of the leading venous vessel distally to the occlusion. To overcome this potential pitfall, several data sets should be collected during and immediately after infusion of the contrast agent. If the image quality is still inadequate a longer infusion period in combination with a larger contrast agent volume should be used.

Venous anatomy may be less predictable than arterial anatomy, especially if collateral veins need to be displayed in the presence of post-thrombotic changes. To ensure that all veins are included thicker 3D volumes frequently need to be prescribed. Analysis of a pre-contrast data set can help to ensure the complete display of all veins in the 3D volume.

With the indirect MR venography approach timing of the 3D acquisition needs to be planned so that the acquisition of the center of k-space coincides with the venous phase of the contrast agent bolus. Adequate image quality is usually obtained when a large contrast agent dose (0.3 mmol/kg) is used. When image subtraction is employed potential misregistration artifacts due to respiratory motion need to be considered.

Superior Vena Cava (SVC) and Upper Extremity

The superior vena cava is (SVC) formed proximally by the confluence of the right and left brachiocephalic veins in the superior mediastinum at the level of the right first costal cartilage. From there, the SVC runs for about 5-7cm inferiorly in a slightly anterior-medial orientation. It ends at the superior vena caval orifice in continuity with the right atrium at the level of the third right costal cartilage in the middle mediastinum. Superior to this point it becomes ensheathed by pericardium. Posteriorly, at the level of the second costal cartilage, the azygous vein runs anteriorly over the root of the right lung to merge with the posterior aspect of the SVC.

The brachiocephalic veins and the SVC represent the major veins in the superior mediastinum. They drain venous blood from the subclavian veins and internal jugular veins, thus providing venous blood return from both the territories of the upper extremities and the head and neck.

The right brachiocephalic vein is shorter than the left brachiocephalic vein. Usually near the convergence of the internal jugular vein and the subclavian vein the right brachiocephalic vein receives lymphatic supply from the right lymphatic duct, right jugular lymph trunk and subclavian lymph trunk. At the confluence of left subclavian vein and left internal jugular vein the left brachiocephalic additionally receives the inferior thyroid veins, the thoracic duct, the thymic veins and the superior intercostal vein.

The axillary vein is a continuation of the basilic vein from the arms. It extends along the chest to the first rib, where it becomes the subclavian vein. The cephalic vein belongs to the superficial venous system of the upper extremity. It merges with the axillary vein just before it becomes the subclavian vein.

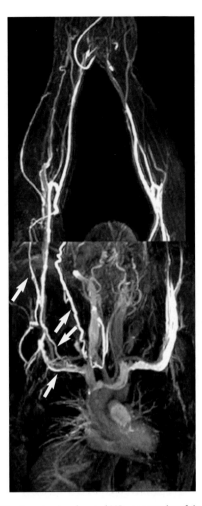

Fig. 4. Direct contrast-enhanced MR venography of the upper extremity and central thoracic veins. Diluted (1:15) contrast agent was injected into a vein on the dorsum of the hand bilaterally. The data set shows normal filling of the left sided veins. On the right side an occlusion of the axillary/subclavian vein is well depicted. Note the prominent collateral veins on right side (*arrows*)

Imaging Techniques

Because of the variable orientation of the chest and upper extremity veins conventional 2D TOF MR venography usually requires data acquisition in variable planes with the scan plane oriented perpendicular to the venous vessels in order to obtain adequate image quality. This results in rather long examination times. Contrast-enhanced MR venography is a particularly well suited technique for this anatomic region and can be especially advantageous in patients with impaired renal function, who have a dialysis shunt, fistula or long time central catheter placement. For bilateral evaluation of the axillary, subclavian and brachiocephalic veins and for assessment of the superior vena cava, simultaneous injection into the right and left upper extremities can be performed (Fig. 4). Usually two operators are needed for this approach, each with two 60 ml syringes containing diluted contrast agent. The bilateral injection needs to be coordinated so that both operators complete the injection of the first syringe at approximately the

same time. Acquisition of the imaging data should be commenced as soon as half of the contrast volume of the second syringe has been injected.

Alternatively, the indirect approach (Fig. 5) can be chosen, with a single injection in an antecubital vein in combination with the acquisition of the 3D data set in the equilibrium contrast phase. The indirect approach is especially useful in patients for whom bilateral venous access is problematic or when information on both arterial and venous vessels is needed, e.g. when the anastomosis of a dialysis fistula needs to be displayed.

Clinical Applications

Indications for MR imaging of the central thoracic veins include the investigation of superior vena cava syndrome, assessment of mediastinal abnor-

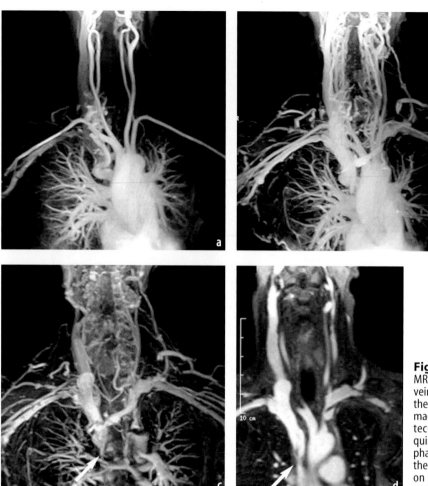

Fig. 5a-d. Indirect contrast-enhanced MR venography of the central thoracic veins. Imaging was performed following the administration of 0.3 mmol/kg paramagnetic contrast agent in the right antecubital vein. 3D data sets were acquired (**a**) in the arterial and (**b**) venous phase. A high grade stenosis (*arrows*) of the superior vena cava is best depicted on the (**c**) subtracted data set and (**d**) coronal reformatted image

malities with potential vascular involvement, and evaluation of anatomical variants such as a left-sided superior vena cava or arteriovenous (AV) malformations. MR venography can also be employed to monitor therapeutic success in cases of DVT.

Superior vena cava syndrome is characterized by cyanosis and swelling of the head, neck and arm in combination with the distension of veins on the neck and trunk. The most common cause accounting for approximately 90% of cases is mediastinal neoplastic disease, usually primary or secondary lung tumors, and lymphoma. The most common benign causes are mediastinal fibrosis and thrombosis secondary to central venous catheters or transvenous pacing wires. Obstruction of any of the major veins which drain into the SVC may occur as part of thoracic outlet syndrome.

Persistent left SVC syndrome [15] occurs in about 0.3% of the population. It is found with higher frequency (ca. 4.3%) in patients with congenital cardiac disease. Left SVC syndrome may occur in isolation but is more frequently found in association with a right SVC. The left SVC commonly drains into the coronary sinus or less frequently into the left atrium.

Inferior Vena Cava (IVC) and Lower Extremity

Anatomy

The inferior vena cava (IVC) is a retroperitoneal structure which arises dorsally to the right common iliac artery from the junction of the right and left common iliac veins. It ascends posterior to the right gonadal artery, the transverse colon, mesenteric root, pancreas and duodenum to reach the sulcus venae cavae on the posterior surface of the liver. It then penetrates the diaphragm to enter the right atrium. The common iliac veins, lumbar veins, right gonadal vein, renal veins, right adrenal vein, phrenic vein and hepatic veins drain into the IVC.

Congenital anomalies of the IVC occur in less

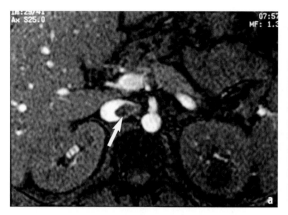
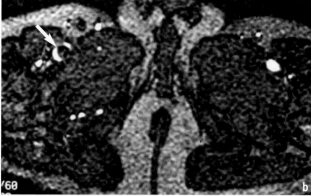

Fig. 6a, b. Two-dimensional (2D) TOF MR venography at (**a**) the level of the inferior vena cava and (**b**) femoral vein. Thrombus (*arrows*) in the inferior vena cava and right femoral vein appearing with dark signal intensity is well depicted

than 1% of cases although the incidence is higher in patients with congenital heart disease. A left-sided IVC is the commonest of these anomalies. In these patients the left-sided IVC terminates in the left renal vein, which then usually drains into a normally located distal segment of the IVC. A double IVC is a less frequent finding. The left vena cava again usually terminates in the left renal vein but may occasionally drain into the lumbar and hemiazygos venous system, the coronary sinus or the left atrium. The suprarenal segment of a normal or abnormal IVC may occasionally drain into the azygos and hemiazygos vein instead of passing through the liver. In the presence of agenesis or hypoplasia of the IVC, blood from the pelvis and lower extremities drains mainly into the lumbar, hemiazygos and azygos veins, which act as collateral vessels.

The venous drainage of the lower limbs can be anatomically categorized into two separate systems - the superficial and deep systems. The deep veins usually follow the course of the main arteries. In the lower extremity, the deep venous system includes the superficial and deep femoral veins, the popliteal vein, and the anterior tibial, posterior tibial, and peroneal veins. The veins are commonly paired at the tibial level, and may, as normal variants, be duplicated at the popliteal and femoral levels as well. The deep femoral vein, which usually lies in the upper two-thirds of the calf, may connect with its lower part and with the superficial femoral or popliteal veins.

The greater saphenous vein is the longest superficial vein. It runs from the dorsal arch of the foot medial to the tibia up the medial thigh to the femoral vein. The lesser saphenous vein runs from the lateral arch of the foot postero-laterally in the calf to join the popliteal vein. Beyond being used as graft vessels for arterial bypass procedures, the superficial venous system is an important collateral pathway in the event of DVT.

Imaging techniques

Following the development of gradient echo techniques, TOF MR venography quickly evolved as a clinically reliable method for detecting DVT of the pelvic and lower extremity veins (Fig. 6) [16-18]. Although TOF venography can detect venous thrombosis in the femoral and trifurcation veins [19], lengthy acquisition times have limited its use mainly to the pelvis. Due to in-plane flow saturation preventing reliable depiction of perforating veins which run in the horizontal plane, and the technique's lack of sensitivity to slow or retrograde flow, TOF MR venography has not been employed for assessing varicose veins or post-thrombotic changes. Contrast-enhanced 3D MR venography overcomes the limitations inherent to TOF venography. Specifically, direct MR venography with unilateral or bilateral injection of diluted paramagnetic contrast agent allows the display of all vessels, regardless of the underlying flow characteristics and the orientation of the vessel (Fig. 7, 8). Thus in-plane saturation is eliminated and imaging along the vessel axis is possible. Perforating and superficial veins containing slow or even retrograde flowing blood are fully depicted. The underlying 3D data sets provide high spatial resolution, which permits delineation of very small vessels.

In the pelvic veins, dilution from draining venous tributaries can cause a reduction of the very bright signal. Thus for display of the pelvic veins and IVC by means of the direct MR venography technique, it is of advantage to use a slightly lower dilution of the contrast agent, e.g. a dilution of 1:10. Whereas the indirect "equilibrium" MR venography approach is commonly sufficient for the diagnostic display of pelvic veins and IVC (Fig. 9), the direct imaging approach usually results in superior CNR which translates into better image quality and a more detailed depiction of the more peripheral venous anatomy.

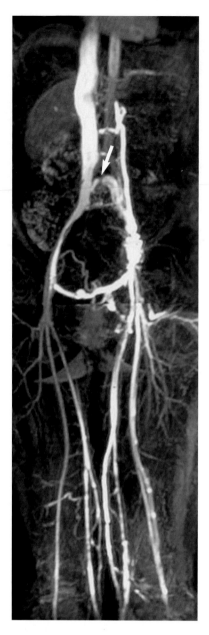

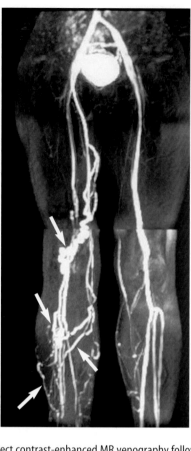

Fig. 8. Direct contrast-enhanced MR venography following bilateral injection of diluted contrast agent into a dorsal pedal vein showing marked postthrombotic changes on the right side with collateralization (*arrows*) via superficial veins. The left leg shows normal deep venous anatomy

Fig. 7. Direct contrast-enhanced MR venography of the veins of the upper thigh, and pelvis as well as of the inferior vena cava. A filling defect in the left proximal iliac vein (*arrow*) is present in the region where the right common iliac artery crosses anteriorly. Pelvic suprapubic and retroperitoneal collaterals are visualized. Normal drainage of the right pelvic veins into the inferior vena cava is visualized

Clinical Applications

Indications for MR venography of the IVC include assessment of extrinsic or intrinsic caval obstruction, evaluation of congenital anatomic variations and pre-operative or pre-interventional display of venous anatomy.

Thrombosis of the pelvic veins or IVC leads to the development of multiple collateral vessels. In patients with unilateral iliac thrombosis blood may drain to the contralateral side utilizing a wide variety of collaterals including the sacral, rectal, vesical, uterine or prostatic plexus. Complete thrombosis of the IVC leads to drainage of blood into the abdominal epigastric veins and via the thoracic epigastric veins into the SVC. In addition,

Subject Index